Plunkett's
Procedures for the
Medical
Administrative
Assistant

Fourth Edition

D1303492

Plunkett's

Procedures for the
Medical
Administrative
Assistant

Fourth Edition

Elsbeth McCall

Sir Sandford Fleming College
Peterborough Regional Health Centre

Lorna Plunkett

formerly of Sir Sandford Fleming College

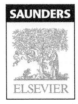

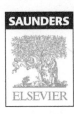

NOTICE

The content and procedures in this book are based on information currently available. They were reviewed by instructors and practising professionals in various regions of Canada. However, employer policies and procedures may vary from the information and procedures in this book. In addition, research and new information may require changes in standards and practices.

Standards and guidelines from your regional Medical Secretaries Association may change as new information becomes available. Federal, provincial, or territorial organizations and agencies also may issue new standards and guidelines. Government legislation also may change.

You are responsible for following the policies and procedures of your employer and the most current standards, practices, and guidelines as they relate to the safety of your work.

Library and Archives Canada Cataloguing in Publication

Plunkett, Lorna, 1939-
    Plunkett's procedures for the medical administrative assistant / Lorna Plunkett, Elsbeth McCall.—4th ed.
    Previous ed. published under title: Procedures for the medical administrative assistant. Includes index.
    ISBN-13 978-0-7796-9911-7   ISBN-10 0-7796-9911-4
    1. Medical assistants—Canada.   2. Medical secretaries—Canada.
    3. Office practice.   I. McCall, Elsbeth   II. Title.   III. Title: Procedures for the medical administrative assistant.
    R728.8.P58 2006
    651'.961   C2005-904275-3

ISBN-13 978-0-7796-9911-7
ISBN-10 0-7796-9911-4

Publisher: Ann Millar
Managing Developmental Editor: Martina van de Velde
Projects Manager: Liz Radojkovic
Managing Production Editor: Lise Dupont
Publishing Services Manager: Melissa Lastarria
Project Manager: Gail Michaels
Designer: Amy Buxton
Copy Editor: Michelle Harrington
Typesetting and Assembly: SNP Best-set Typesetter Ltd., Hong Kong
Printing and Binding: Courier Westford
Cover Printer: Phoenix

Elsevier Canada
420 Main Street East, Suite 636, Milton, ON Canada L9T 5G3
416-644-7053

Last digit is the print number: 10 9 8

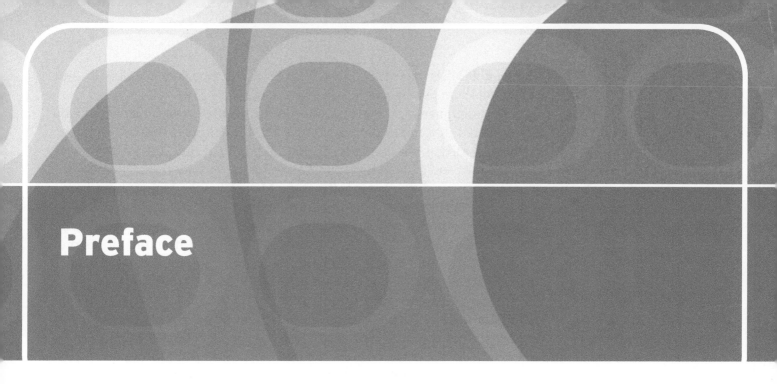

Preface

The healthcare field is such a dynamic environment that instructional publications must be constantly revised to keep up to date with change. It does not seem that long ago when I worked with Lorna on the third edition, and now the fourth edition is complete.

You are embarking on a very exciting career as a medical administrative assistant, one that will present everyday challenges, as well as many opportunities for change and advancement. *Plunkett's Procedures for the Medical Administrative Assistant* will provide you with the learning outcomes you require to be a successful contributor to health care and to a healthcare team.

The medical office is a diverse environment that requires skills and knowledge, not only in office procedures but also in communications, human behaviour, stress management, various computer programs, medical transcription, terminology, and anatomy. The focus of this text is on office procedures in a medical office, complementary care office, and hospital environment. All other topics require more in-depth instruction than could be integrated into the chapters of this text.

The text covers the most essential procedures that a medical administrative assistant is required to know. Topics include booking appointments and suggested patient flow; records management; accounting; healthcare billing; hospital records, reports and requisitioning; meeting organization; ordering procedures; and medical legal issues. In addition, we have included appropriate formats for letters, memos, and forms. On the accompanying CD-ROM, we have provided timed writings and interactive exercises to assist in the learning process.

In addition, there are four useful appendices: Appendix A offers a quick reference to common abbreviations used in the healthcare field. Appendix B lists laboratory tests and their turnaround times. Appendix C provides names of the most commonly prescribed drugs, including brand and generic names.

Appendix D lists names of sources like medical dictionaries, handbooks, and other books on health care to which you can refer.

The assignments in the text attempt to simulate tasks that would be encountered in a medical environment. Dr. J.E. Plunkett will be the physician who assigns the majority of your tasks. In reality, Dr. Plunkett was Lorna's husband's Uncle Elmer. In 1931, after graduating from Queen's University and spending nine months at the Mayo Clinic in Minneapolis, he set up his medical practice at 278 O'Conner Street in Ottawa. He was a dedicated surgeon and physician until his untimely demise in 1952. The inscript on the letterhead used for the assignments was taken from one of his prescription pad pages on which his wife, Marion, had written a recipe. All other names and all medical information used in the book are fictitious.

We have also provided information on 15 fictitious patients. You will notice throughout the book that some exercises and examples deal with these patients. This was intended to provide a patient database to be used as needed.

With respect to the Peterborough Regional Health Centre forms that appear throughout the text, as well as the forms that were supplied by other health institutions, please note that they are designed to represent information in use at the time of publication and that they may no longer be up-to-date. To ensure currency of information, the forms are not recommended for use without a thorough review by the agency adopting them.

CONFIDENTIALITY

Healthcare professionals have access to confidential material, and the medical administrative assistant is no exception.

You will hear, read, and observe things that are extremely confidential. It is of utmost importance that you respect the nature of the information and ensure that it is not passed on to others.

Throughout the text, the importance of confidentiality will be continually reinforced.

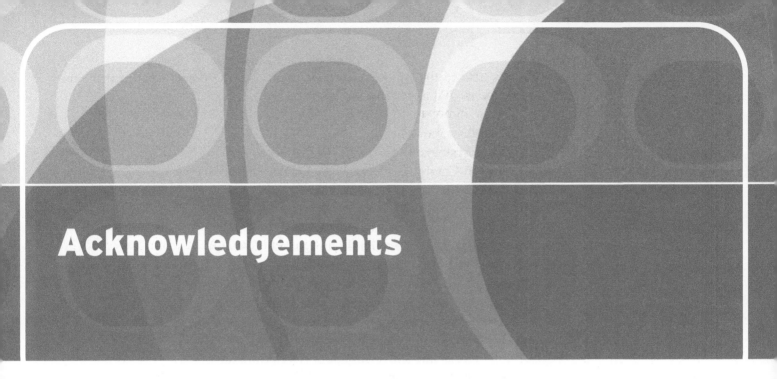

Acknowledgements

There are many individuals to thank for their assistance on this fourth edition, but I especially want to thank Lorna Plunkett for having the confidence and trust in me to step back and ask me to update her textbook. I truly appreciate the incredible work and dedication that she has put into this text.

I want to thank the following people for letting me tap into their knowledge and expertise in order to make this text the best I could for the students and instructors who will be using it:

Kerri-Lynn Baker
Ashley McCall
Robert Moncrief
Pradeep Naik
Donald Harterre, MD
Maureen Condon
Dale Noble
Colleen Howson
Allan Barolet, MD
John Ross, MD

The following instructors provided feedback for this edition:

Gillian Ball, Heartbeat Training Institute, British Columbia
Fernanda Farinho, National Academy of Health and Business, Ontario
Patricia A. Faulkner, Holland College, Prince Edward Island
Irene Lacoursiere, Vancouver Community College, British Columbia
Ann Robinson, ARC Advantage, Ontario
Janet Schreier, Douglas College, British Columbia
Christiane Tarrey, Trillium College, Ontario

Thanks also to the following organizations for the permission to print the many forms that appear in the text:

The Bank of Nova Scotia
Bibbero Systems, Inc.
Canadian Centre for Occupational Health and Safety
Canadian Medical Association
Dean et fils, Inc.
Manitoba Health Services Commission
Régie de l'assurance maladie du Québec (RAMQ)
Nova Scotia Department of Health
Ontario Medical Association
Ontario Ministry of Health and Long-Term Care
Peterborough Regional Health Centre (formerly Peterborough Civic
    Hospital and St. Joseph's Hospital)
Public Works and Government Services Canada
Workplace Safety and Insurance Board

Ann Millar and Martina van de Velde from Elsevier Canada have been my lifeline throughout, and I thank them for their patience and professionalism.

Last, but certainly not least, my thanks go to my family for putting up with me: my husband, Ron, and my children, Michael, Ashley, Craig, and Christopher.

Elsbeth McCall

Contents

APPENDICES

Plunkett's

Procedures for the

Medical

Administrative
Assistant

Fourth Edition

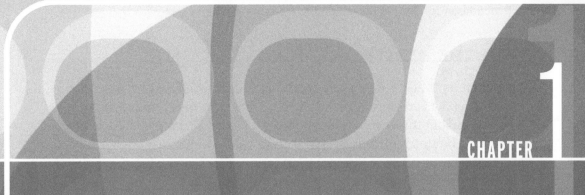

CHAPTER 1

Your Future as a Medical Administrative Assistant

CHAPTER OUTLINE

Becoming Part of the Healthcare Team
Career Qualifications
Customer Service

Stress Management
Career Opportunities
Topics for Discussion

LEARNING OBJECTIVES

After reading this chapter, you should understand

- Personal qualities required for employment in a medical environment
- Skill requirements of the medical administrative assistant
- Professional appearance for a medical administrative assistant

- The importance of customer service
- The importance of stress management
- Potential areas of employment

KEY TERMS

Confidentiality: The dictionary defines confidential as "entrusted with secrets." In the medical field this term applies to patient identification as well as patient information, diagnosis, prognosis, and medical records access (manual and computer).

Medical administrative assistant: A healthcare professional with additional training in scheduling, office records management, medical billing, and general office procedures who performs administrative and/or clinical duties in a medical office environment.

Medical machine transcriptionist: An individual who creates a written or typed copy of a dictated medical note. Above standard accurate keyboarding skills and an excellent understanding of anatomy and terminology are required for this position.

BECOMING PART OF THE HEALTHCARE TEAM

A position as a healthcare professional is exciting and rewarding. You are embarking on a career path that will allow you, as a **medical administrative assistant**, to join this stimulating specialty. Historically, medicine has been a mysterious but intriguing subject; the news media frequently affords it headline status; innovations in the control of serious illnesses are happening every day. As a medical administrative assistant your education is not finished when you complete your course. As the medical field advances very quickly you will be required to upgrade your skills and education to maintain your efficiency. It is important to remember that the medical environment is a team environment (see Figure 1.1). In your office the team can include the housekeeping staff, building maintenance staff, the courier service, the front line worker (which includes the nurse and medical administrative assistant), and the physician. In a hospital setting, the team is not only the staff working directly with you on your floor or department but also the rest of the hospital, including the volunteers.

FIGURE **1.1   Regardless of the field chosen, the medical administrative assistant works with a whole team of professionals.**

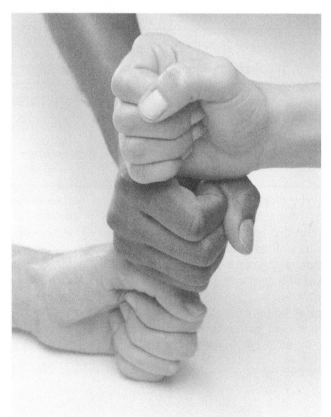

SOURCE: Eggers, D.A. & Conway, A.M. (2000). *Mosby's Front Office Skills for the Medical Assistant* (p. 9: Figure 1.3). St. Louis: Mosby.

CAREER QUALIFICATIONS

The job turnover rate in your chosen career is surprisingly low. This would indicate that medical administrative assistants derive a great deal of satisfaction from their positions. It also indicates that those seeking employment in this field must have superior personal qualifications and skills.

Personal Qualities

If you think about why you have chosen this profession, you will recognize that you possess the following qualities:

1.1 Personal Qualities of a Medical Administrative Assistant
Pleasing personality
Genuine interest in people
Ability to assume responsibility
Ability to remain calm under pressure
Respect for the privacy of others
Empathy, compassion, and serenity
Honesty and reliability
Professional attitude
Dedication and loyalty
Sense of humour
Tact
Patience
Understanding and helpfulness
Efficiency

Skill Requirements

The medical office environment can be extremely busy and cause many stressful moments for the medical administrative assistant. At all times, you need to present a calm, professional appearance. Having the ability to prioritize your workload and multi-task are essential. You must also master additional job-related skills:

1.2 Job-Related Skills of a Medical Administrative Assistant

Effective communication skills
Good organizational ability
Fast and accurate keyboarding skills *computer skills*
Sound understanding of medical terminology and anatomy
Excellent medical machine transcription skills
Knowledge of basic computer programs and software billing systems
Ability to multi-task
Ability to work efficiently on an individual basis as well as part of a team

Personal Appearance

Professional attitude and skills are complemented by a professional personal appearance, which includes the following:

1.3

Neat hairstyle
Tasteful make-up
Comfortable attire appropriate for the office
Comfortable footwear suitable for a working environment
No fragrance, as many individuals have allergies

CUSTOMER SERVICE

Never underestimate the importance of first impressions! You are the voice of your doctor's practice. You are the first person to greet the patients when they visit the doctor. Many people judge the physician's practice by their first impression.

Gum chewing, cigarette smoking, and eating while on duty and dealing with the public are unacceptable. Tattoos and piercings may be acceptable in certain environments, but not in most medical offices or departments. Tattoos should be covered and no more than two earrings per earlobe should be worn. Long nails are inappropriate and can be unsafe when working with patients. If nail polish is worn, it should be clear or muted polish.

It is important to be friendly and greet patients with a pleasant voice and expression (see Figure 1.2). Remember that people who visit the doctor's office are usually under stress. It is your responsibility to put them at ease in order to alleviate some of their fears and concerns. Be sure to acknowledge

FIGURE **1.2**   **A good attitude goes a long way in patient and staff relationships.**

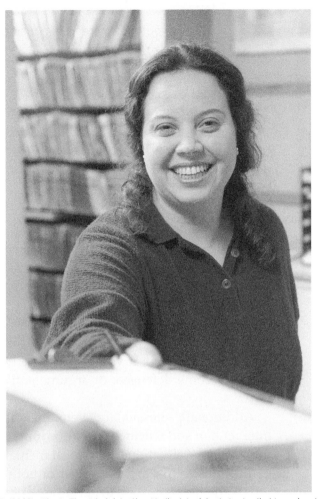

SOURCE: Young, A.P. (2003). *Kinn's The Administrative Medical Assistant: An Applied Learning Approach* (5th ed., p. 56: Figure 4.4). St. Louis: Elsevier/Saunders.

them as quickly as possible. If the physician is behind schedule, inform the patients when they arrive that there is a delay.

The subject of **confidentiality** will be stressed continually throughout this text. When patients approach your work area, it is important that you are discreet in conversing with them. Do not discuss their illness or reason for seeing the doctor in a voice that may be heard by others in the waiting area. If your conversations with patients may be overheard by others, move to an area where you can talk privately. If you have a questionnaire that needs to be filled out, have the patients do it themselves and be available for assistance if it is needed.

> **1.4** Confidentiality
>
> Throughout your career as a medical administrative assistant, you will encounter many "secrets." You will hear, read, and observe things that are extremely confidential. It is your responsibility to make sure that these "secrets" are not passed on to others. A breach of confidentiality can result in termination of employment.

STRESS MANAGEMENT

The healthcare environment is very busy and demanding, often creating stressful situations for the administrative assistant. It is important that you consider situations that cause undue stress and take action to correct them, for example, by being well organized.

If you encounter a difficult patient, remain calm and in control. Let angry patients talk out their frustrations, and try to be reassuring. Their anger is not usually directed at you and is usually caused by anxiety. Remain calm, do not become defensive or argumentative, and maintain eye contact with them.

Additional professional development in Non-Violent Crisis Prevention & Intervention and Suicide Prevention, or both, may be helpful for dealing with these kinds of situations. Your local mental health association may be helpful in directing your search for either or both of these courses.

It is equally important to get enough physical exercise, rest, and relaxation, and to eat nutritious meals—all essential ingredients for a reduced stress level.

CAREER OPPORTUNITIES

Hospitals or Clinics

Employment opportunities exist at all stages of health care, from the admission of the patient to the discharge, or in the management of documents in the medical records department. The clinics and hospitals of today have advanced technically to include many new and state-of-the-art departments that require high-end professionals. One example of these new departments would be a complete cardiac service that includes catheterization, angioplasty, echocardiograms, and pacemaker checks. Another example would be renal (kidney) dialysis units. Many departments include in-patient as well as out-patient treatment, and have added wellness and health teaching to their programs. Upon completion of your training, many job opportunities will be available to you in the healthcare field. Chapter 14 will discuss your job search in more detail, as well as preparation procedures.

1.5 Examples of Job Opportunities for Medical Administrative Assistants

Medical machine transcriptionist
Medical administrative assistant in X-ray, laboratory, physiotherapy, and admissions departments
Ward secretary in emergency departments and nursing units
Operating room booking secretary
Office administrator in a health services organization or community health centre
Office administrator in Nurse Practitioner clinics

Government Facilities

Many opportunities also exist within the public sector. A career in this environment will provide challenge and opportunity for advancement. Areas where you will be eligible for employment include the following:

1.6

Health units
Provincial laboratories
Food and drug administration offices
Nursing homes
Institutions for the physically/mentally disadvantaged
Provincial and federal healthcare plan offices
Medical, nursing, and research departments of universities and colleges

Private Practices

Opportunities are also abound in the private sector. Positions in this area allow employees to learn all facets of office administration. The following is a listing of the types of private practice that exist:

1.7

Offices of physicians engaged in general practice or
   specialty services
Practitioners' offices (optometrists, chiropractors, massage
   therapists, naturopaths, podiatrists)
Dentists' offices
Veterinarian hospitals and offices
Home care organizations
Medical supply companies
Medical foundations
Insurance companies
Pharmaceutical companies
Occupational health offices in large corporations

All of the preceding positions play a vital role in delivering quality health care.

ASSIGNMENT **1.1**

Set up a personal file (portfolio) to begin collecting evidence of your achievements, challenges, academic documents, and other relevant data. This will allow you to maintain a record of documents to be used within this program and throughout your career, for example, letters of reference, performance evaluations, work-related "thank you" letters, diplomas/certificates, educational transcripts, copies of successfully completed projects/assignments.

ASSIGNMENT **1.2**

Write a short essay (one to two pages) stating why you have chosen a career as a medical administrative assistant. Outline the personal qualities you possess that will enable you to be an effective healthcare professional. Be prepared to defend your ideas.

ASSIGNMENT **1.3**

 Take a few moments to complete the rating sheet from the CD, as shown in Figure 1.3. Be as objective and honest as you can. Keep the sheet in your portfolio to be used in Assignment 14.2.

ASSIGNMENT **1.4**

 Do you currently possess all of the skills and personal qualities required for a healthcare environment? Perhaps you have some of the skills and some of the personal qualities, but not at the level necessary to secure the position you are seeking.

FIGURE **1.3**   **Rating Sheet**

**RATING SHEET
A FIRST IMPRESSION**

Place a check mark (✔) in the space that best describes your personal attributes.

Facial Expression

☐ Happy Smile   ☐ Serious Outlook   ☐ Blank Expression

Voice

☐ Loud Tone   ☐ Soft Spoken   ☐ Well Modulated

Communication Ability

☐ Control Conversation ☐ Shy and Withdrawn   ☐ Outgoing and Friendly

Language Skills

☐ Adequate   ☐ Excellent   ☐ Poor

Hair Style

☐ Acceptable for Business ☐ Unacceptable   ☐ Just Acceptable

Make-up (for female employees)

☐ Accentuated   ☐ Light   ☐ Heavy

Nails

☐ Manicured   ☐ Suitable   ☐ Rough

Clothes

☐ High Fashion   ☐ Comfortable   ☐ Sloppy

Hygiene

☐ Excellent   ☐ Good   ☐ Needs Improvement

OVERALL FIRST IMPRESSION

☐ Excellent   ☐ Acceptable   ☐ Poor

In order to assess your current skills and personal qualities as they relate to a position as a medical administrative assistant, complete the skills and personal qualities inventory sheet found in the CD.

Be as objective as possible as you assess your skills and qualities; retain your inventory sheet in your portfolio for use in Assignment 14.2.

TOPICS FOR DISCUSSION

1. Relate an experience you have had

    a. When a first impression was positive. Why?
    b. When a first impression was negative. Why?
    c. When your first impression was inaccurate. Why?

2. List 10 areas within a hospital where a medical administrative assistant would be required.

3. Some physicians prefer that their receptionists wear a uniform. Discuss pros and cons of wearing or not wearing uniforms.

4. Discuss how confidentiality could be breached and how such a breach can be avoided.

5. Why is it important to know the members of the team you are working with?

CHAPTER 2

Reception, Booking Appointments, and Clinical Responsibilities

CHAPTER OUTLINE

Reception
Booking Appointments

Clinical Responsibilities
Topics for Discussion

LEARNING OBJECTIVES

After reading this chapter, you should be able to

- Explain the responsibilities of the medical administrative assistant regarding patient reception
- Demonstrate the methods for scheduling patient appointments
- Demonstrate the methods for scheduling diagnostic appointments

- Demonstrate the procedure for booking surgery
- Explain the clinical responsibilities of the medical administrative assistant

KEY TERMS

Benign: Not recurrent or progressive; non-malignant. Not cancerous (*Taber's Cyclopedic Medical Dictionary*, 20th Edition).

Encounter: When a patient sees the physician for one symptom or problem, for example, a sore throat, this is considered one encounter. If the same patient wants another symptom or problem (e.g., a mole) looked at by the doctor within the same appointment time, this would be a second encounter. Many doctors will see a patient for one encounter per visit. If the patient needs to see the doctor for a second encounter, he or she will need to book another appointment.

Most responsible physician (MRP): The MRP is the physician who assumes primary care for a patient admitted to the hospital. The MRP may change during the patient's hospital stay, depending on the patient's medical needs. For example, a patient may be admitted for a cholecystectomy (surgical removal of the gallbladder). The patient recovers from the surgery only to develop a secondary condition (not related to the surgery) before being discharged. The MRP responsibility may then be transferred to another physician who treats the patient for the secondary condition.

Stream scheduling: With stream scheduling, patients are booked at fixed times depending on the nature of their appointment. This system makes it easier to ensure a steady flow or stream of patients during the day.

Venipuncture: To puncture a vein, typically to obtain a specimen of blood (*Taber's Cyclopedic Medical Dictionary*, 20th Edition).

Version code: A version code consists of one or two letters the Ministry of Health assigns to an Ontario health card which needs to be replaced by the patient. Following are some reasons that a card may need to be replaced: a stolen card, a lost card, an expired card, a name change, a card that has been damaged. The original card number does not change, but without the current version code, the health card is invalid.

Wave scheduling: Wave scheduling is based on the average time spent with each patient within a half hour or an hour. If a physician spends 10 minutes with each patient, then three patients can be seen within a half hour. Three patients would be given the same time at the beginning of the hour, for example 10:00. Another three patients would be given the same time on the half hour, for example 10:30.

Now let's take a look at some of the responsibilities you will have when you go to work, specifically, receptionist duties. You will see that these are quite different from those in a non-medical environment. We will also discuss pertinent points concerning the doctor's appointment schedule. In your role as a medical administrative assistant you will also have clinical responsibilities to perform.

2.1 RESPONSIBILITIES

Office reception
Booking appointments
Collecting patient information for data entry
Arranging diagnostic tests
Arranging referrals to specialists/practitioners
Booking out-patient procedures and surgery, or both
Maintaining charts in the appropriate format
Filing patient information
Billing provincial healthcare plans and Workers Safety
 Insurance claims
Billing patients for services not covered by their healthcare
 plans
Billing third-party insurances
Calling in prescriptions to pharmacies
Ordering and maintaining supplies
Maintaining examination rooms
Sterilizing instruments
Assisting the physician when required
Medical transcription

RECEPTION

Waiting Area

The waiting room should be a peaceful, comfortable area for patients to await their appointment (see Figure 2.1). Appealing decor, comfortable chairs, interesting magazines (current issues), enjoyable music, and children's books and toys are items that should be considered. Of course, cleanliness and tidiness are the two most important features. During the day, the waiting area will need to be tidied periodically. As many patients will be handling the magazines, books, and doorknobs, it is good practice to have an antibacterial hand wash at the reception desk when patients arrive. Have all patients, their children, and any non-patient visitors wash their hands on arrival before they are seated in the waiting room. Some offices have toys for young children. These should only be toys that can be washed or sprayed with disinfectant during and at the end of the day (depending on usage); therefore soft plush toys are not suitable. Books for small children that can be washed with disinfectant are encouraged.

FIGURE **2.1** **The waiting area should be peaceful and comfortable for your patients.**

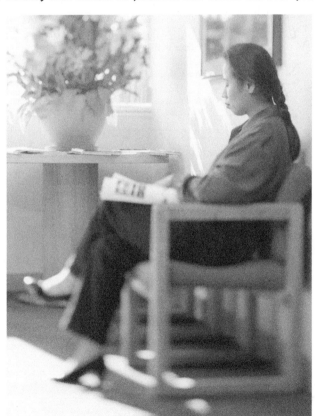

SOURCE: Eggers, D.A. & Conway, A.M. (2000). *Mosby's Front Office Skills for the Medical Assistant* (p. 181: Figure 7.9). St. Louis: Mosby.

Patient Information

You are responsible for establishing and maintaining a current and accurate file of information for all new and old patients. To obtain the required information from a new patient, you may ask the patient to complete a patient information form, as shown in Figure 2.2. If questions are to be answered orally, move to a private place to protect confidentiality. If a private place is not available, have patients fill out the information on their own. Provide them with a clipboard and pen and be available if they are in need of assistance. Ask them to print so you are able to read their information. This is the information you will depend on for accurate medical billing. You must make sure that *all* information is current, including the mailing address and telephone number. You should regularly ask if there are any changes in the patient information.

FIGURE **2.2**　**Patient Information Form**

PATIENT INFORMATION

(Please Print Clearly)　　　　　　　　　　Date _____

NAME _____ AGE _____ SEX _____

ADDRESS _____

CITY _____ PROV. _____ CODE _____

_____　☐ Mar.　☐ Sing.　☐ Wid.　☐ Div.
　　Date of Birth

PHONE: Home _____ Work _____

EMPLOYED BY _____

CITY _____ PROV. _____

OCCUPATION _____

SPOUSE'S NAME _____

EMPLOYED BY _____

CITY _____ PROV. _____

PHONE _____ OCCUPATION _____

REFERRED BY _____

_____

HEALTH CARD NO. _____ VERSION CODE _____

ALLERGIES _____

SERIOUS ILLNESS _____

EMERGENCY CONTACT _____ _____ _____
　　　　　　　　　　　　　　　　Name　　　　　Relation　　　Phone

Role play—Assume the role of a medical administrative assistant as you complete a patient information form for one of your classmates. Remember to maintain a friendly and relaxed manner. A blank form to complete the assignment can be found on the accompanying CD.

Your instructor may choose to evaluate your performance of this assignment. Insert the results of your evaluation in your portfolio.

Greeting Patients

A warm, friendly smile and immediate attention are two things to remember when greeting patients. If you are transcribing a letter, preparing a chart, or writing a prescription note, these activities can wait; the most important duty you have is to attend to patients. If you are busy with a patient and someone else comes into the office, look directly at the new arrival and acknowledge his or her presence ("I will be with you in just a moment"). If you are on the telephone, look at the person, smile or raise your hand to show you are aware someone has entered the office. Do not simply ignore the person. Attend to the person as soon as you are finished. Do not start on something else first.

Whenever possible, greet the patient by name. Initially, it is best to use the formal greeting (Mr., Mrs., Ms.) when receiving patients. Some patients will request that you refer to them by their first name after you have become acquainted. This practice is acceptable, but only after you have been instructed to take that liberty. The patient information form or the patient information in the computer will assist you in establishing the status of the patient, for example, single, married, separated, divorced, or widow(er). Checking this information for a patient with whom you are not familiar can help avoid some uncomfortable situations.

The majority of patients visiting the doctor are under stress. It is important for the medical administrative assistant to be considerate and caring.

Health Card Verification

All provinces in Canada provide eligible residents with a health card (see Chapter 6). Patients must present their health card when accessing services covered by the provincial healthcare system. When a patient arrives for an appointment, you must ask for the health card and verify that the card is current and belongs to the patient. In Ontario, health cards may have a version code. It is important to *ask* if the patient's card has been replaced for any reason. Some health cards have an expiry date. The majority of patients do not pay attention to this detail; therefore you can remind them if the expiry date is coming up when you check their card.

If there is a question about the validity of a health number, there is a toll-free number you can access on a touch-tone phone, 24-hours a day, 7 days a week. You will need to key in your personal identification number (PIN) and the health card number (plus version code in Ontario). An automated voice response will inform you if the insurance number is valid. This process takes time and ties up your phone line, so you would not use this for every patient. If the patient does not have their health card with them, you can have them complete a Health Number Release Form (see Figure 2.3). This will enable your office to access the correct health insurance number and to update your patient information and process your claim accurately when billing. In the physician's office, swiping the card or typing the number into the computer will bring up the patient's information. The medical administrative assistant can then confirm that the health card belongs to that patient. If there is a question about the authenticity of the health card, it is your responsibility to report this information to the provincial ministry. If a patient possesses two health cards, it is your responsibility to confiscate the outdated card. The patient must voluntarily submit this card to you.

Verification procedures may vary between offices, as well as provinces, ranging from manual to computerized systems. In most Ontario hospital settings a direct link is made to the Ministry of Health once the health card is swiped or when the number is typed into the computer. The system can then validate the number immediately. It is flagged if the number is invalid.

BOOKING APPOINTMENTS

The scheduling system is an important component in the smooth operation of the doctor's office. A successful system depends on good decision making by the medical administrative assistant. Systems vary and can consist of a manually processed appointment book, a computerized system, or a combination of the two. Not only does the system maintain a record of each day's functions in the office, but also it is an official record that can be used for billing purposes or as a legal document in case of legal action. When arranging your daily schedule, you must also be aware of the physician's schedule outside of the office. This would include meetings, hospital rounds, luncheon dates, speaking engagements, surgery schedule, whether the physician is on call, etc. It is the administrative assistant's responsibility to record such information, as well as a full schedule of operations and/or patient visits. The doctor frequently refers to a daily diary to keep on schedule. Many doctors will use portable digital assistants (PDAs) to view and update their schedules when away from the office. It is, therefore, imperative that you, the administrative assistant, be exact when making entries in the appointment schedule. Accuracy and legibility are essential.

FIGURE 2.3   Health Number Release Form

(Ontario logo) Ontario   Ministry of Health and Long-Term Care   Ministère de la Santé et des Soins de longue durée   Ministry Use Only/Réservé au ministère
Health Number/Numéro de carte Santé

Health Number Release   **Divulgation du numéro de carte Santé**

This form may be submitted to the Ministry of Health and Long-Term Care when the Health Number of a patient is not available.
La présente formule peut être envoyée au ministère de la Santé et des Soins de longue durée lorsque le numéro de carte Santé d'un patient ou d'une patiente n'est pas disponible.

Confidential when completed/Renseignements confidentiels

1   Patient/Patiente

A. General Information/Renseignements généraux

Last name/Nom de famille   First name/Prénom

Middle name/Deuxième prénom   Sex/Sexe   Birth date/Date de naissance
M   F   year/année   month/mois   day/jour

If an alternate last name is known, please provide/Si vous avez un deuxième nom de famille, inscrivez ici

B. Health Number Disclosure/Divulgation du numéro de carte Santé

The Ministry of Health and Long-Term Care will give your Health Number to the health care provider/facility.

I agree to allow the Ministry of Health and Long-Term Care to release my Health Number to the health care provider/facility listed below.

Le ministère de la Santé et des Soins de longue durée donnera votre numéro de carte Santé au fournisseur/à la fournisseuse ou à l'établissement de soins de santé.

J'autorise le ministère de la Santé et des Soins de longue durée à divulguer mon numéro de carte Santé au fournisseur ou à l'établissement de soins de santé dont le nom figure ci-dessous.

Signature of patient or guardian   Date   Home phone number   Business phone number
Signature du patient ou du tuteur   Téléphone (domicile)   Téléphone (bureau)
(   )   -   (   )   -

A parent or guardian may sign for a child under 16 years of age. A person holding power of attorney may sign for the represented individual.
Le père, la mère ou le tuteur, la tutrice peuvent signer pour un enfant de moins de 16 ans. Une personne titulaire d'une procuration peut signer pour la personne qu'elle représente.

2   Provider/Facility Fournisseur/Fournisseuse/Établissement

Date of service/Date de prestation du service
year/année   month/mois   day/jour

Provider no./N° du fournisseur   Provider's phone number N° de téléphone du fournisseur   Facility no./N° de l'établissement   Facility phone number N° de téléphone de l'établissement
(   )   -   (   )   -

The Health Number of the patient will be returned to the provider/facility listed here.

Le numéro de carte Santé du patient/de la patiente sera transmis au fournisseur/à la fournisseuse/à l'établissement de soins de santé dont le nom figure ci-dessous.

Provider name and address/Nom et adresse du fournisseur   Facility name and address/Nom et adresse de l'établissement

SOURCE: © Queen's Printer for Ontario, 2000. Reproduced with permission.

Figure 2.4 is an example of a manual system appointment book. There are several variations, but most have each hour broken down into specific time segments, depending on the doctor's practice and preference. If the office has two or more physicians or practitioners, a colour-coded appointment schedule is also available. Some books are designed to display six days on two pages, while others display a day at a time. A computerized system will also have variations in format. Figure 2.5 shows one example of a computerized scheduling system.

Many specialists book half-hour and one-hour appointments. General practitioners have ten- or fifteen-minute segments in their appointment schedule. Complementary Therapy clinics will also book half-hour and hour-long appointments, depending on the type of treatment required. Some chiropractic offices will book patients every 5 to 10 minutes.

Walk-in clinics and some private practices do not schedule appointments. Patients are seen on a first-come, first-served basis. This, of course, could lead to long waiting periods for some patients, as the most urgent cases would be seen first. In this type of practice, the office does not run at a steady pace. There is also no time to prepare for a patient's needs ahead of their visits.

Types of Scheduling

The most common type of scheduling is when patients are given a specific time for their appointments. This enables the medical administrative assistant to organize the day so that the patients arrive in a steady flow. This type of scheduling is also known as *stream* scheduling.

Wave scheduling is another method for booking appointments (see Figure 2.6). This method can help alleviate problems created by late arrivals. Assume that you use a schedule that books a patient every ten minutes, allowing three patients to be seen each half hour and at the time scheduled. If you changed to wave scheduling, three patients would be scheduled at the beginning of each half-hour interval and seen in order of arrival. Your initial schedule would be

1000	Mrs. Green
1010	Mr. Shultz
1020	Ms. Smith

Your revised schedule would be

1000	Mrs. Green
	Mr. Shultz
	Ms. Smith

If one patient were late for the appointment, it would not affect the other two, and the longest waiting interval would be twenty minutes.

Modified wave scheduling would have two patients booked at 1000 and one patient booked at 1020.

FIGURE **2.4** **Appointment Schedule: Manual System**

APPOINTMENT SCHEDULE

DOCTOR _Plunkett_

Day_____ Month_____ Year_____

TIME	PATIENT	PHONE	REASON FOR APPOINTMENT
0800	Erik Shultz	427-9977	Counselling
0815			
0830			
0845			Surgery Assist — Dr. Jones
0900			O.R. 6 St. Joseph's Hosp.
0915			Hemodyalisis & graft
0930			
0945			
1000			
1015			
1030			
1045			
1100			
1115			
1130			
1145			
1200			
1215			
1230			Kinsmen Luncheon
1245			
1300			
1315	Eliz. Green	427-3774	Annual Health Exam
1330	Y2 hr.		
1345			
1400			
1415			
1430			
1445			
1500	Coffee/Messages		
1515			
1530			
1545			
1600			
1615			
1630	Tim Peters	743-2525	Boil Lanced
1645			
1700	Dinner Engagement		

REMARKS: _Note: Kibber Kelli Skinner - did not Rebook._

FIGURE **2.5**   Appointment Schedule: Computer System

February 13, 2008
Wednesday

February 2008							March 2008						
S	M	T	W	T	F	S	S	M	T	W	T	F	S
					1	2							1
3	4	5	6	7	8	9	2	3	4	5	6	7	8
10	11	12	13	14	15	16	9	10	11	12	13	14	15
17	18	19	20	21	22	23	16	17	18	19	20	21	22
24	25	26	27	28	29		23	24	25	26	27	28	29
							30	31					

7 am

8 00 Erik Shultz (Counselling)

Surgery Assist - Dr Jones or @ St. Joe's Hosp (Hemodyalysis and Graft)

9 00

10 00

11 00 ☼ EXTRA

12 pm 12:30 KINSMEN LUNCHEON

1 00 Eliz Green (ANNUAL HEALTH EXAM)

2 00

3 00 Coffee/Messages

4 00

Tim Peters (BOIL LANCED)

5 00 Dinner Engagement

6 00

TaskPad
☐ ☑ TaskPad

Notes

FIGURE **2.6**   **Appointment Schedule: Wave Scheduling**

		APPOINTMENT SCHEDULE	
DOCTOR	*Plunkett*		Day_____ Month_____ Year_____

TIME	PATIENT	PHONE	REASON FOR APPOINTMENT
0930			
1000	*Eliz. Green*	*427-3774*	
	Erik Shultz	*427-9977*	
	Heather Smith	*576-3225*	
1030			
1100			
1130			
1200			
1230			
1300			
1330			

REMARKS: _____

Double booking is not recommended, except for appointments such as allergy shots, blood pressure checks, or flu shots. These appointments should take less than five minutes per patient.

We will not attempt to dictate a specific method for booking appointments. Each office varies and your doctor/employer will give you instructions about personal preferences for booking appointments. We will, however, make some suggestions.

When a patient requests an appointment, ask the reason for the visit in order to assess the time allotment required; for example, a minor sore throat or cold may need a ten-minute appointment, whereas counselling or a complete physical could require a half-hour appointment.

Always allow for travel time, from hospital to office for example, when required. It is wise to leave a fifteen-minute open appointment each morning and afternoon if possible. This allows for catch-up time if the doctor is behind schedule. If the doctor is on schedule, the time could be used to discuss telephone messages or even for a quick coffee break. However, every doctor may not want you to follow this procedure. Discuss with your employer what his or her booking preference is before implementing such a practice in the appointment schedule. When arranging your appointment schedule, it is important to anticipate that Mondays and Fridays tend to be very busy days.

An earache, chest pain, and high temperature are emergencies that are considered urgent and *must* be seen. On the other hand, a common cold may be seen the next day. When your daily schedule is completely filled and a patient insists on seeing the doctor, tell the patient you will check with the doctor and call back with instructions. Refusing a critically ill patient could result in legal action against the doctor. *Never* make such a decision on your own. Remember—your responsibility is to book appointments, not to make a diagnosis.

Never put off an emergency patient. If the doctor should become involved in an emergency and cancellations prove necessary, always make arrangements to have urgent patients seen by another physician. If another physician is not available to see your patients, it is then necessary to send them to a walk-in clinic or the nearest emergency department. This is also a physician preference that will need to be discussed with your employer. Routine appointments can be booked for a later date. If time allows, contact the patient before he or she leaves for the office.

A record of the patient's telephone number (home, work, or cellular phone number) on the appointment schedule is recommended in case it is necessary to change an appointment—this practice provides you with easy access to your patients.

ASSIGNMENT 2.2

Assume you are the administrative assistant and a patient has arrived for an appointment. Dr. Plunkett has been called to the hospital to deliver a baby—he expects to return in approximately one hour. You were unable to contact the patient. Think about how you would handle the situation, and then write a scenario.

Additional Recommendations Concerning the Appointment Book

1. If your office is using an appointment book, record the date at the top of the page in pen but record all appointments in pencil. If changes are required, it is advisable to draw a line through the original entry and record the new information just above or below the crossed-out entry.

FIGURE **2.7** **Appointment Reminder Card**

> **APPOINTMENT REMINDER**
>
> An appointment is scheduled with
>
> DR. J.E. PLUNKETT
>
> Date_____
>
> Time_____

Never erase an entered appointment. This may be more difficult in a computer schedule, due to lack of space. You may need to add another column.

2. Consider giving patients who book appointments preprinted appointment reminder cards (see Figure 2.7) to give to patients who book appointments in the office. Any special instructions to the patient can be recorded on the back of the card, for instance "Bring Medication." This eliminates misunderstandings and errors (see Figure 2.8). If time allows, missed appointments can be virtually eliminated by telephoning the

FIGURE **2.8** **Patients should be given a reminder card when an appointment is arranged for them.**

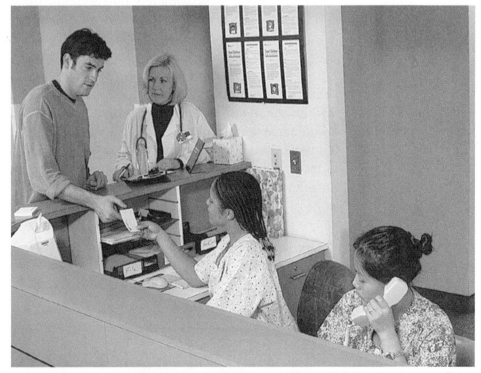

SOURCE: Young, A.P. (2003). *Kinn's The Administrative Medical Assistant: An Applied Learning Approach* (5th ed., p. 164: opener). St. Louis: Elsevier/Saunders.

patient the day before his or her scheduled visit. This practice is usually done by specialists, dentists, physiotherapy clinics, and Complementary Therapy clinics. It is not usually done in a family practice. If a patient is scheduled to return for an appointment in the future, arrange the appointment time before the patient leaves the office.

3. Make appointments for homemakers, preschoolers, and retirees early in the day. This leaves time open for school-age children after 4 p.m. and for working patients after 5 p.m.

4. If a patient cancels an appointment and does not request a rebooking, follow these steps:
   - Make a notation and advise the doctor.
   - If the missed appointment will jeopardize the patient's well-being, telephone the patient and suggest making another appointment.
   - Mark a line through the cancelled appointment and make a notation in the remarks area at the bottom of the appointment schedule, in the patient's chart, or both.
   - If you are employed in a specialist's office and a patient cancels or misses an appointment, advise the referring/family physician.

5. Do not book several long appointments together (unless your doctor/employer does all annual health exams on a specific day).

6. When the doctor is called away from the office for an emergency and a patient arrives for an appointment,
   - Apologize for the inconvenience.
   - Explain the doctor's absence (without going into too much detail).
   - Tell the patient approximately how long the doctor will be detained.
   - If the doctor is not going to be away too long,
     i. Suggest the patient might like to wait, and offer a magazine.
     ii. Suggest the patient might have some errands to run and would like to come back later.
     iii. Suggest rebooking for a future date.
   - Offer the use of a telephone to contact children left at home, or to call a taxi, and so on.

7. If a patient may be infectious to other patients, try to book him or her as the first appointment of the morning or as the first appointment of the afternoon. Take the patient into an examination room upon arrival so he or she will not be seated in the waiting room with other patients.

2.2	Some Abbreviations Used in Scheduling
F/U or FUp	Follow Up
Pap	Pap Smear
WB	Well Baby
BP	Blood Pressure
N/S	No Show
Inj	Injection
NP	New Patient

Arranging for Diagnostic Testing and Appointments with Specialists

At the end of the doctor's consultation with the patient, you may be required to complete requisition forms for specific tests. (A more thorough outline of completion of requisition forms will be covered in Chapter 11.) It may be necessary to arrange appointments for such tests—for example, ultrasound or blood work. It may also be necessary to arrange an appointment with a specialist.

Some points to consider when making arrangements for special tests follow:

1. Some patients who are very ill can tolerate only so much in one day. Be sure you don't overtax someone with too many tests at one time.
2. Ask about any required special preparations for the test. Ensure that instructions are clearly communicated to and understood by the patient. It is good practice to provide instructions both verbally and in written form.
3. If more than one test is required, determine whether the patient can be booked consecutively or the appointments must be booked on separate days.
4. If a series of weekly appointments need to be booked, try to arrange them for the same day and time each week. This will make it easier for the patient to remember.
5. Inform the patient of the approximate amount of time required to complete the test.
6. Try to be aware of your patients' comfort level with pending tests. Allay their fears, or encourage them to ask questions.
7. Discuss time availability with the patient before arranging for the testing.
8. Inform the receptionist at the testing location of any special needs of the patient.

2.3

Diagnostic tests require a requisition. If the facility does not receive the requisition, the appointment may be cancelled. Give the patient a copy of the requisition (give the original if you are not mailing it) and put a copy of the requisition in the patient chart.

When arranging a referral to a specialist you will also be required to do the following:

1. Provide the patient's sociological information (name, address, date of birth, telephone number, and health card number).
2. Supply the reason for the referral.
3. Fax or send a referral letter and relevant diagnostic test results.

Patients without Appointments

If a patient arrives and wishes to see the doctor without having first made an appointment, you would point out that the doctor sees patients by appointment only and that, in the future, arrangements should be made before coming to the office. If you are able arrange to have the doctor see the patient without inconveniencing anyone, you would then explain that there will be a waiting period (state time, for example, approximately one hour) before the patient can be seen by the doctor.

Of course, you may be faced with an emergency situation whereby a patient arrives at the office and needs to be seen immediately. In such an instance, you would usher the patient into the first available examining room, pull the patient's chart, and inform the doctor.

No Shows

Inevitably you will have patients who do not arrive for their scheduled appointments. When this occurs, you will need to call the patient and rebook if necessary. If you need to leave a message, be as confidential as possible. One way of leaving your message may be, "Please have Mr. Baxter call this number when he arrives" versus "This is Dr. Plunkett's office. Please have Mr. Baxter call this number when he arrives." Some health facilities and doctor's offices will choose to have "Private Name, Private Number" as opposed to the office number or facility name shown on a telephone's call display.

Be sure to document in your appointment schedule, as well as the chart, that the patient did not arrive for the appointment and the date of the new appointment, if applicable. Inform the physician, who can then adjust his or her daily schedule.

House Calls

The delivery of health care has changed radically over the years. If we compare health care in the early 1900s with healthcare delivery today, we see that early in the last century the doctor came to the patient's home, while today the patient usually sees the doctor in the office or in a hospital. There are occasions, however, when it may be necessary for the doctor to visit the patient at home. If you are responsible for making arrangements for a house call, you must get explicit instructions regarding the location of the house or apartment, as well as the name, telephone number, and complaint. You must also advise the patient about the approximate time of the doctor's arrival. If a doctor is making a house call, it will usually be after office hours, or before or after hospital rounds. It is important to have the patient's chart available, as the physician must take the patient's chart with him or her at the time of the house call. Make a note of the house call in your appointment schedule. (Note: Remember—house calls are expensive and time consuming. Always urge patients to come to the office if at all possible.)

New Patients/Patient Education

It is good practice to have a new patient arrive earlier than his or her appointment time so any required paperwork can be completed.

When a new patient arrives in your office, you should supply a brochure or outline of your office policies, including the following information:

- Office phone number
- Hours of operation
- Any additional costs not covered by the provincial healthcare plan
- What to do in the case of an emergency outside of office hours
- Office policy with regards to visits (i.e., if the physician will only see one **encounter** per visit)

Scheduling Surgery

In most areas, hospital operating rooms are booked to capacity many weeks in advance. Procedure requirements for booking surgery will differ according to hospital and area, but the following information will be required by any operating room scheduling officer or admitting department:

1. The patient's sociological information (name, address, phone or cellular phone number, as well as the medical care plan number)
2. Whether the surgery is elective or urgent
3. Type of surgery that will be performed
4. The admitting diagnosis
5. Surgeon performing surgery [**most responsible physician (MRP)**]
6. The name of the patient's family physician

In order to manage more efficiently, many hospitals utilize an Expected Date of Discharge program. If such a program is in place, the surgery registration card would include the patient's expected length of stay.

Some hospitals may accept this information by telephone; others may require the completion of a Surgical Admission Booking Card (see Figure 2.9). Many surgical offices will have a surgical booking sheet that will accommodate up to five patients on one sheet per surgical date (see Figure 2.10). This sheet is usually faxed to the operating room booking secretary. It outlines the necessary information needed to book the doctor's surgeries, including the length of surgery and type of anaesthetic to be used.

Many hospitals now have a pre-surgical information package to be completed prior to surgery. The package is supplied by the surgeon's secretary. Components of the required information may vary among institutions, but usually include the following forms:

2.4

FORM	COMPLETED BY
Letter of instruction to patient	Surgeon
Pre-anaesthetic questionnaire	Patient
Pre-registration questionnaire	Patient
History and physical examination form	Surgeon/Family physician
Consent form	Surgeon must ensure completion by patient
Order sheet (including pre-op testing requirements)	Surgeon

It is important to inform your patient that if he or she experiences fever, diarrhea, sore throat, or any other flu-like symptoms, he or she must contact your office immediately. If your office is closed, the patient must contact the hospital admitting department. There is a chance that surgery will need to be postponed if any of these symptoms occur.

Many hospitals will run a pre-op clinic in which the patient meets with the anaesthetist and relevant instructions for the surgery are given. This provides the patient with education and information as well as an opportunity to ask any questions.

FIGURE **2.9   Surgical Admission Booking Card**

SURGICAL ADMISSION BOOKING CARD

☐ PETERBOROUGH CIVIC HOSPITAL
☐ ST. JOSEPH'S HOSPITAL & HEALTH CENTRE

ADMISSION DATE: _____
                        MM   DD   YY

SURGEON: _____

PROCEDURE DATE: _____
                          MM   DD   YY

SURNAME: _____

GIVEN NAMES: _____

DATE OF BIRTH: _____
                      MM   DD   YY

PHONE NUMBER: _____

HEALTH CARD #: _____

ADMISSION DIAGNOSIS: _____

PROCEDURE: _____

COMORBID CONDITIONS: _____

IF NOT A.M. ADMIT, PLEASE GIVE REASON: _____

☐ DISCHARGE PLANNING REQUIRED
☐ HOMECARE REQUIRED

FOR HOSPITAL USE:
CMG #: _____

FORM #JF1585

FIGURE **2.10** **Surgical Booking Sheet**

O.R. Bookings

Surgeon Dr. _____   Date _____

1 Start time	Last name		First name .... Alias			
Code [ ] Procedure			Total time	Birthdate DD MM YY	Age	M ☐ F ☐
SOP ☐ AM ☐ IP ☐	( ) Phone .... ( )	GA ☐ Loc ☐ Spinal ☐ NNA ☐ Neuro ☐ StBy ☐	ICU ☐ CCU ☐ CC ☐	Anaes consult ☐	Assistant	

2 Start time	Last name		First name .... Alias			
Code [ ] Procedure			Total time	Birthdate DD MM YY	Age	M ☐ F ☐
SOP ☐ AM ☐ IP ☐	( ) Phone .... ( )	GA ☐ Loc ☐ Spinal ☐ NNA ☐ Neuro ☐ StBy ☐	ICU ☐ CCU ☐ CC ☐	Anaes consult ☐	Assistant	

3 Start time	Last name		First name .... Alias			
Code [ ] Procedure			Total time	Birthdate DD MM YY	Age	M ☐ F ☐
SOP ☐ AM ☐ IP ☐	( ) Phone .... ( )	GA ☐ Loc ☐ Spinal ☐ NNA ☐ Neuro ☐ StBy ☐	ICU ☐ CCU ☐ CC ☐	Anaes consult ☐	Assistant	

4 Start time	Last name		First name .... Alias			
Code [ ] Procedure			Total time	Birthdate DD MM YY	Age	M ☐ F ☐
SOP ☐ AM ☐ IP ☐	( ) Phone .... ( )	GA ☐ Loc ☐ Spinal ☐ NNA ☐ Neuro ☐ StBy ☐	ICU ☐ CCU ☐ CC ☐	Anaes consult ☐	Assistant	

5 Start time	Last name		First name .... Alias			
Code [ ] Procedure			Total time	Birthdate DD MM YY	Age	M ☐ F ☐
SOP ☐ AM ☐ IP ☐	( ) Phone .... ( )	GA ☐ Loc ☐ Spinal ☐ NNA ☐ Neuro ☐ StBy ☐	ICU ☐ CCU ☐ CC ☐	Anaes consult ☐	Assistant	

Emergency surgery usually results after a patient has been examined in the emergency department at the hospital. The arrangements for emergency surgery would then be made within the hospital by the emergency department ward secretary and the operating room scheduling officer.

Booking for Two or More Physicians/Practitioners

Many offices have multiple physicians or practitioners working out of a shared area. It is very important to be aware of equipment, facilities, and staff that need to be available for appointments. For example, at 1300 Robert Baxter is having a **benign** mole removed by Dr. Plunkett. This would be done in the Minor Treatment Room. This room is also used for **venipuncture**, baby weights, and blood pressures. Dr. Park shares office space with Dr. Plunkett and you book the appointments for both physicians. Amelia Jackson is being seen by Dr. Park on the same day as Robert Baxter and needs a blood test taken. You will need to make sure that the minor treatment room will be available for Amelia's appointment.

In a dentist's office, the medical administrative assistant may need to coordinate a patient's appointment around the hygienist, assistant, and the dentist. This would also apply in a Complementary Therapy clinic, where rooms are being shared by the therapists and assistants.

Drug and Supply Salespersons and Non-Patient Visitors

Drug and supply salespersons often have new and innovative medicines and supplies in which the doctor is interested. They are usually aware of doctors' preferences for booking time to see them, and they arrange their appointment times well in advance of their visit. Always ask for the drug representative's or salesperson's business card. It is good practice to clip it to the daily schedule. Not only does this serve as a quick visual reminder, but you will also have the contact number or e-mail address available if the appointment needs to be changed.

The appearance of someone without an appointment on a very busy day may present you with a problem. Most doctors/employers will have a preference for scheduling appointments for non-patient visitors and you will, therefore, have clear-cut guidelines on how to deal with them. If, however, there are no set rules, an efficient medical administrative assistant will tactfully, but firmly, advise all non-patient callers that the doctor will see them only by appointment. Remember, the patients are the doctor's first priority and their appointment times should not be interrupted by those who have failed to make an appointment.

Daily Schedule

Many doctors prefer to have their administrative assistants produce a daily appointment schedule to have on their desks. In this way they know which patients are scheduled to be seen that day. The schedule might be formatted as follows:

DR. PLUNKETT
APPOINTMENTS FOR JANUARY 23, 20___

Morning
0900-1130   Assist Dr. Jones in surgery—Gary Green—bypass
1200-1300   Speaking engagement—Kinsmen Lunch Bunch—
                 Holiday Inn, Green Room

Afternoon
1300-1315   Hazel Davis, O.B. checkup

If you are using a manual appointment book, you will need to photocopy the page (if your book shows one day at a time) or you will need to format the schedule into the computer and generate a hard copy. If your office uses a computer for scheduling, you can print off a copy. Some physicians can view their daily schedule from their office computer. If your physician is able to do this, make sure that the computer monitor is at an angle that cannot by viewed by someone who may be sitting in the physician's office.

24-Hour Clock

You will notice in the previous appointment example that times are written in a style that is different from the norm. In the medical environment, many areas use a 24-hour schedule to identify time.

Rather than dividing the day into two sections (morning and afternoon), the schedule begins at one minute after midnight and proceeds cumulatively through to midnight. At one minute after midnight, the time is written 0001 and referred to as 0-0-0-1 (pronouncing O rather than saying zero). One o'clock in the morning is written 0100 and spoken as "O one hundred hours" rather than 1 a.m. Twelve o'clock noon is written 1200 and spoken as "twelve hundred hours." After noon hour, the time does not begin at one again but continues to be cumulative. Therefore, 1 p.m. would be written as 1300 and spoken as "thirteen hundred hours," 5 p.m. would be written as 1700 and spoken as "seventeen hundred hours," and so on (see Figure 2.11).

FIGURE **2.11** **Example of a 24-Hour Clock**

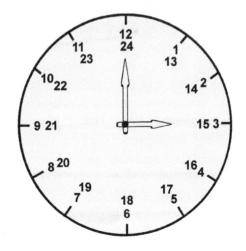

FIGURE **2.12 Common Instruments and Supplies Used in a General Practitioner's Office**

Blood Pressure Cuff	Bandages	Lancets
Syringes	Telfa	Peak Flow Meter
Needles	Ear Syringe	Slides (glass)
Alcohol	Otoscope	Fixative (cytology)
Sutures	Vaginal Speculum	Forceps
Needle Driver	Tongue Depressors	Curette
Scissors	Cotton Swabs	Height and Weight Chart
Mosquito Forceps	Reflex Hammer	Weight Scales
Skin Hooks	Eye Chart	Biological Supplies
Scalpel (and blade)	Gown	Ophthalmoscope
Cotton	Examining Table Paper	Silver Nitrate Sticks
Gauze	Stethoscope	Sample Bottles
Tensors	Hemoglobinometer	

CLINICAL RESPONSIBILITIES

Examining Rooms

The examining rooms should be prepared for the patients; instruments to be used should be readily available for the doctor; sufficient paper should be available to ensure a clean examination table at all times; light bulbs in examining lamps must be working; and all medical supplies required for the patient should be placed in an easily accessible area (see Figure 2.12). Of course, all areas of the medical office must be kept clean and medical instruments must be sterile.

All prescription pads *must* be kept only where the physician(s) or the medical administrative assistant can access them. They should never be left in view of non-medical personnel or patients. Never leave them in the examination rooms.

Now that you are ready, the patients can be allocated to the examination rooms. The patient's file should be readily available to the doctor, but not to the patient. If there is a holder outside the examination room door, the file is placed inside it. If such a holder is not available, the file can be placed somewhere on your desk so the physician knows who is to be seen next.

After each patient, you should change the paper on the examination table if necessary and ensure that all is in order in the examining room.

Consider your responsibilities in preparing the patient for the doctor. Does the patient need to disrobe? If so, most doctors provide a gown or sheet. Is a urine sample required? (See Box 2-5 for specimen collection instructions.) Particulars may be required if the patient is having a Pap smear. Many physicians will ask you to assist them when they need to perform any type of vaginal exam. Often the patient is more comfortable when you are in the room. This is not a legal requirement but it does protect the patient and the doctor if there are any accusations of inappropriate touching.

Some offices do not employ a licensed nurse; therefore, you may required to weigh and measure the patient. In addition, you may be require to perform such tasks as taking blood pressures and temperatures, checking pulses and respirations, and so on. These statistics are entered on the history sheet in the patient's file. The physician will instruct you if these responsibilities are required of you.

According to the Canadian Medical Protective Association, invasive procedures such as giving injections, taking blood (venipuncture), and other similar clinical procedures are beyond the terms of reference of a medical administrative assistant. These functions should be performed only by a trained nurse or by the doctor.

2.5 COLLECTION OF URINE SPECIMENS

Medical office personnel often collect urine specimens for a variety of tests that are performed at a hospital or outside lab.

Some are collected at the office, but some are to be collected by the patient at home so it is important that you are familiar with proper instructions. In either case, proper labelling is essential. Place the label on the container, not the lid, and use indelible markers.

Many specimens are kept under refrigeration as bacteria will grow as early as within one hour if the specimen is kept at room temperature.

ROUTINE URINALYSIS SPECIMEN

The preferred specimen for routine urinalysis is the first morning sample. Urine concentration varies considerably throughout the day from very dilute to very concentrated. As it is not practical to collect the first morning specimen at the medical office, the patient would collect this sample at home, and bring it into the office or drop it off at the designated lab (with a requisition).

24-HOUR URINE SPECIMEN

This specimen needs to be a full 24 hours. The patient would void on arising but this sample is not collected. The patient only needs to note the time of voiding. The test now begins with an empty bladder. The patient collects all urine voided in a small cup and pours it into the large 24-hour container (which can be picked up at a lab). The container is returned to the lab by the patient.

MIDSTREAM SPECIMEN

The patient collects the specimen *after* approximately one-third of the specimen is passed into the toilet. This acts to "flush" the lower urinary structures of normal contaminants—it is not saved. The patient then collects the second one-third portion (approx. 20 mL), and after collection, the patient completes urination into the toilet

In order to evaluate the patient's understanding of the proper procedures for a urine specimen collection, have him or her repeat the steps of the procedure to you.

ASSIGNMENT 2.3

Dr. Plunkett's office is very busy today. Due to an emergency, he is running behind schedule. An aggressive sales representative insists on seeing Dr. Plunkett that day because he is from out of town. He assures you he will only take five minutes of the doctor's time.

From past experience, you know that five minutes is not realistic. Dr. Plunkett has told you not to accept additional appointments today. The sales representative is very insistent.

Jot down some suggestions on how you would handle the situation.

ASSIGNMENT 2.4

For this assignment, refer to Figure 2.5 to complete an appointment schedule. Use the same style of form (i.e., manual system) from the CD provided.

a. The following appointments have been scheduled and entered in your book. Copy them from Figure 2.5.

Dr. Plunkett and his wife have a dinner engagement at 1700.

The president of the Downtown Kinsmen Club has asked Dr. Plunkett to speak to the Kinsmen Lunch Bunch at 1200. (Dr. Plunkett agreed.)

Dr. Jones, a vascular surgeon, is performing a bypass and graft for hemodialysis (synthetic) on Gary Green and has asked Dr. Plunkett to assist. Surgery will take approximately $2\frac{1}{2}$ hours beginning at 0900 in O.R. 6 at St. Joseph's Hospital. (Note: When a physician is asked to assist in surgery, the surgeon's office administrator will call the physician's office administrator and advise the time, date, place, type of surgery, patient's name, and approximate length of time for surgery).

Erik Shultz is "at the end of his rope" with his wife's drinking and needs to talk to the doctor immediately. (Note: Erik works from 0900 to 1900 and finds it difficult to arrange time off work. You feel there is some urgency in this situation. Since Dr. Plunkett usually comes into the office early in the morning, you book Erik in before Dr. Plunkett's scheduled surgery time. You discuss this with the doctor and he agrees.)

Elizabeth Green has requested an appointment for her annual health exam.

Tim Peters has a large boil on his forearm.

b. Complete the appointment schedule by entering the following appointments, allowing appropriate time periods. If you feel that some appointments do not need to be seen on this schedule, document when you would book them and your reasons for doing so.

Thomas Bell (427-5327) and Heather Smith (576-3225) have requested appointments for complete physicals.

Jean Belliveau and Mary Jane Brown have requested a premarital consultation and physicals. Mary Jane is a regular patient (427-3333) and her fiancé has requested that Dr. Plunkett consider him as a patient.

Hazel Davis (427-7006) is coming in for her monthly O.B. checkup.

There is a flu epidemic and the following patients are coming in with temperatures, sore throats, and congestion: Peter John Scott (427-2245), Mel

Thompson (427-5432), Amelia Jackson (748-3192), Bob Baxter (652-3179), and Lisa Basciano (742-2717).

Lois Elliott (748-3355) is coming in to have a dressing changed.

At 1 p.m. you receive a call from Mrs. Harris, whose 4-month-old baby, William, has been crying and upset all morning. He is screaming in obvious pain and Mrs. Harris is very upset. What will you do?

ASSIGNMENT **2.5**

Complete the daily schedule from your solution for Assignment 2.4.

You can use your creativity to set up a daily schedule. You may want to tabulate the time, patient's name, and reason for visit. Perhaps you would double space for readability.

ASSIGNMENT **2.6**

 Choose an appropriate scheduling system and prepare an appointment schedule (see blank form on the accompanying CD) for the following patients. Use today's date. The doctor will see patients from 9 a.m. to 6 p.m. with lunch from 12 to 1:30.

Rosie Smythe (236-7712) has a boil on her arm.

Sara Downs (471-3327) is becoming drug dependent and requests some counselling.

Gary Groves (236-8717) has been experiencing severe dizziness when he stands up and lies down.

Annabell Ford (236-3131) has an excruciating pain in her left thigh.

George Arthur (471-3728) has large sores in his mouth.

Ryan Elder (471-3515) has oozing sores on both ankles. He thinks it might be poison ivy.

Deanna Duggan (236-4131) has had intermittent chest pains over the past few days. The pain radiates into her neck and right shoulder blade.

Brad Nichols (471-3112) is experiencing tightness in his chest and his heartbeat races periodically.

James Noris (236-3449) has a bunion on his left toe; it is causing severe discomfort.

Walter Page (471-9952) is very uncomfortable because of constipation.

Janie Packer (471-8987) has several warts on her fingers.

Chuck Leahy (236-3577) has just been fired from his job and is very depressed.

Bunni Rill (471-8338) has had a cold; she now has a fever and is having trouble getting her breath.

Kendra Hall (236-1122) is experiencing severe pain in her lower back that radiates into her left leg.

Mohamed Nasir (471-8772) is booked to have stitches removed from a laceration on his right hand.

Sue Jessup (471-5567) has a broken wrist—her cast is getting loose. She is booked for a new cast.

Cheryl Page (236-3396) has had diarrhea for almost two weeks.

Diane Stevens (236-4747) is having hot flashes and experiences occasional periods of depression.

Jack Porter (236-3991) has a cloudy film over his left eye.

John Bard (471-9988) needs to have his blood pressure checked.

Harry Duffell (236-9991) has had pains in his stomach, some blood in his stool.

Ted Lang (236-6667) needs an allergy shot.

Harold Topper (236-1112) has severe laryngitis.

ASSIGNMENT 2.7

Your instructor will provide you with information to complete an appointment schedule for Dr. Plunkett. This assignment will be submitted for assessment.

TOPICS FOR DISCUSSION

1. What amenities add to the atmosphere of the waiting room? Discuss pros and cons of clocks and televisions in the waiting room.

2. Discuss with your classmates the types of special needs or any other considerations you may have to address when booking diagnostic tests or other referrals.

3. If a patient arrives in your office before you have had a chance to call them to rebook a cancelled appointment, how would you handle the situation?

4. Rate the following medical situations in terms of how urgently an office appointment is needed by circling a number on the scale provided; 1 is most urgent, 5 is least urgent.

	Most				Least
Annual checkup	1	2	3	4	(5)
Infected toenail × 1 week	1	2	(3)	4	5
Worried about moles (read about melanoma)	1	2	3	4	(5)
Painful urination × 3 days	1	(2)	3	4	5
Missed period—pregnancy test?	1	2	(3)	4	5
Baby coughing at night	1	2	(3)	4	5
Sore on leg won't heal	1	(2)	3	4	5
Camp medical (must be within 30 days)	1	2	3	4	(5)

5. As discussed in Chapter 1, it is necessary to prioritize your work in order to maintain an organized and efficient office. You are working alone in a physician's office. Number the following scenarios in the order you would deal with them, and discuss the reasons for your chosen order.

   a. The mail has just arrived.
   b. There are completed charts to be filed.
   c. There is correspondence (including diagnostic reports) to be filed.
   d. The doctor is looking for test results on a patient he is currently seeing.
   e. The phone is ringing.

f. The next two patients have arrived.

g. Mrs. Jackson is leaving and requires an urgent referral for a diagnostic test.

h. The examination room needs to be made ready for the next patient.

i. Mr. Baxter would like you to call him a taxi.

Patient Records Management

LEARNING OBJECTIVES

After reading this chapter, you will be able to outline

- The current status of technological advancements with respect to patient files
- The procedure for preparing patient file folders (charts)
- Rules for alphabetical filing

- General correspondence filing, subject and tickler filing, preparing correspondence for filing, charge-out systems, and updating files
- The purpose of colour-coding files
- Points to follow for efficient filing procedures

KEY TERMS

Charge-out card: The charge-out card is made of heavy cardboard and is inserted where a file has been removed. The patient's name, the date the file was removed, who removed it, and the present location are documented on the file

Cross-reference: Cross-referencing is used when charts are filed numerically. A system is required that will match the name of the patient or individual with the number that has been assigned. Cross-referencing can also be used when two names sound the same but are spelled differently, for example, "Thompson" and "Thomson." A cross-reference page would be filed with these charts. This page would be coloured (for easy identification) and lightweight (to conserve space).

Out-folder: The out-folder is similar to the charge-out card in that it is also inserted where a file has been removed. Information that is to be filed in the missing chart is placed in the folder and can be easily filed when the chart is returned to the filing system.

Purging: The removal of inactive files from active files. These files would include patients who have moved out of town, transferred to another physician, or are deceased. The files on these patients are moved to a secure separate storage area, either onsite or offsite.

Tickler file: The tickler file is a reminder system. It's purpose is to "tickle" your memory.

With the advent of the computer came many progressive records management software systems. This eliminated the need for numerous file cabinets and the process of manual filing. At the time of publication, however, many medical environments dealing with patient information (e.g., private practices, hospitals) are still using manual filing systems or a combination of both manual and electronic. The reason for this is mainly the cost of the massive computer storage requirements for recording patient histories and test results, as well as government legislation (for example, the *Public Hospitals Act*) that requires the retention of a hard copy for all patient reports. Progress is being made in this area and facilities are moving toward or have implemented networked systems, optical disk storage, and voice recognition, or both. Some facilities have been more progressive than others in moving toward an electronic record system. Another reason many medical offices are still dependant on the manual system is the need for immediate access to the medical record. The electronic system needs to be 100 percent dependable, and this is not always possible.

ASSIGNMENT **3.1**

In order to determine the status of technological advancement in your community, research the following topic with your local healthcare facilities. Your instructor will direct this project.

In this chapter we will discuss the importance of good filing procedures, the typical patient file or chart, the most common filing system (alphabetical) used in private practice, the **tickler file**, and the charging-out of files, as well as a numerical filing system that may be used in larger clinical settings or facilities.

The patient's chart is a legal document, and maintenance of this record is extremely important. Correction fluid cannot be used on a medical record. If there is an error, you will need to cross it out, and date and initial the error. Information concerning transfer of files, release of information from files, and the length of time files must be retained is covered in a later chapter. Medical records management in a hospital setting will also be discussed in Chapter 11.

The doctor generally maintains a personal file folder (chart) for each patient. The chart provides a chronological history of the patient's care. This includes diagnostic tests, hospital visits, admissions, and consult visits with other providers. Information is filed in reverse chronological order, which means the most resent visit or test is on the top. The folders are usually filed in alphabetical order and colour-coded, or both for easy reference.

Since files are the backbone of the physician's practice, the administrative assistant must be precise when handling the files. Any office personnel responsible for filing charts and chart information must have accurate spelling skills. When multiple practitioners or physicians are using the same space, it is advisable to use different coloured file folders for each physician. For example Dr. Plunkett has beige files and Dr. Singh has grey files. They can all be filed together and they are easy to spot. Here are a few important things to keep in mind when you are handling files:

- A lost file could cause a disaster—be very careful to accurately file all documents. When files have been removed, be sure you use an "out-card" (discussed in more detail later in this chapter) and promptly return the files to their proper place when they are no longer needed.
- Do not leave files in open view of non-medical personnel in the office—remember the importance of maintaining confidentiality. If you leave your desk, even for a moment, cover the files or turn them face down.
- When colour-coding is used, a periodic scan for misplaced files can be accomplished quickly and ensures that each chart is in the correct location.
- Be sure to put all relevant material in the correct patient's file.
- All charts should be filed by the end of the day. If this is not possible, it is good practice to put them in the order in which they are to be filed, either alphabetical or numerically, and then place them in a storage area (a drawer or empty file area) where they can be locked up.

3.1

DO NOT try to do a large filing job at the end of the day when you are tired and anticipating going home. Errors are more likely to occur at this time.

Each doctor has preferences for the set-up of individual patient files. The outside and inside cover of the file folder, or both, can be utilized to provide patient information, thereby saving time when looking up patient details. (A rubber stamp can be designed and ordered to suit the physician's requirements, or a computerized label maker may be used—see Figure 3.1.)

FIGURE **3.1 Rubber Stamp/Label Format**

NAME _____	D.O.B. _____
HEALTH CARD # _____	VERSION CODE _____
PHONE # (HOME) _____	WORK _____
ALLERGIES _____	
EMERGENCY CONTACT _____	

Patient allergies may be written in red pen, or a coloured sticker (preferably red) may be placed beside the word "allergies" in order to alert the doctor that a patient has allergies. What the patient is allergic to should be easily visible on the chart. Each page that is added to the patient's history should also include an allergy notation.

In Quebec, patient charts must include a woman's maiden name—Mary Jane Belliveau (Brown).

A typical file may include the following:

1. A family medicine chart (also referred to as a progress note or a patient history note) (see Figure 3.2). This will provide all the details about the patient's past history up to and including the most recent illness. (This sheet should have the patient's name and medical billing number displayed at the top.)
2. Other relevant forms the doctor requires. This may include infant and child progress record forms (see Figures 3.3 and 3.4), prenatal or antenatal records, results of tests, X-rays, and so on. These forms should be filed following the family medicine sheet.
3. Correspondence. Correspondence is filed behind all pertinent medical information. This would include consult notes from other providers, operative notes, and hospital notes.

Special notations regarding allergies, medications, or serious illnesses may be noted on a form and attached to the left inside cover of the folder, so that they will be immediately noticeable.

Items (1), (2), and (3) would be filed on the right side of the folder with the history sheet on top, followed by reports in date order, and then correspondence in date order, with the most recent on the top.

Small forms and notes should be taped or stapled to a full-size ($8\frac{1}{2}$ inch × 11 inch) sheet of paper in order to avoid misplacement. Most lab results and other diagnostic reports are now printed on $8\frac{1}{2}$ × 11 paper. Some physicians prefer that all records concerning a specific illness be stapled together. Paper clips are not recommended because papers can pull away from the clip and become mixed with unrelated documents, or the clip may catch onto other documents.

FOLDERS

Letter-size manila file folders with $\frac{1}{5}$, $\frac{1}{2}$, or full cut tabs are generally used. The tab is the projection at the top or side of the folder. Fifth and half cuts would appear in a file drawer as shown in Figures 3.5 and 3.6.

FIGURE **3.2** **Family Medicine Chart**

FAMILY MEDICINE						
Name			Insurance #			S M W D
Address			Phones (H)		(O)	
Occupation			Date of Birth			Age
Medical Data	HT	WT	BP	PULSE	RESP	TEMP
Allergies			Drug Allergies			
DATE	HISTORY & PHYSICAL					

FIGURE **3.3** **Infant Progress Report**

INFANT PROGRESS RECORD
0 – 24 Months

Name _____

Date of Birth _____ Sex M/F

B.Wt._____ Kg_____ lb. Length_____ cm. Head_____ cm. Chest_____ cm. D.Wt_____ Kg_____ lb.

Maturity_____ wks. Apgar_____ /_____ Blood Gp._____ Rh_____ P.K.U._____ Thyroid_____

Problems: Prenatal_____ Labour_____ Neonatal_____

Defects: _____ Marks_____ Circ. _____

Breast until _____ Bottle until _____   Started juice _____ Started solids_____

Landmarks — 25th Percentile – 90th Percentile in months

Motor	Date	Mo	Social	Date	Mo
Prone lifts head 1.3 – 3.2			Blinks to clap		
Follows light 1.8 – 4.0			Smiles back – 1.9		
Rolls over 2.3 – 4.7			Laughs 1.4 – 3.3		
Grasps 2.5 – 4.2			Sleeps through night 6 + hours		
Reaches out 2.9 – 5.0			Turns to voice 3.8 – 8.3		
Sits unsupported 4.8 – 7.8			Things to mouth		
First tooth			Feeds self 4.7 – 8.0		
Stands holding 5.0 – 10.0			Says Dada or Mama 5.6 – 10.0		
Stands alone 9.8 – 13.9			Drinks from cup 10.0 – 14.3		
Walks 11.3 – 13.3			Uses spoon 13.3 – 23.5		
Kicks ball 15.0 – 24.0			Combine 2 words 14 – 23		

DPTp: 1 _____ 2 _____ 3 _____ 4 _____

O.T.T. _____ M.M.R. _____ Reactions _____ Allergies _____

Months	1	2	3	4	6	9	12	15	18	24
Date										
Wt. kg.										
Length/cm.										
Head circ.										
Heart sounds										
Breath sounds										
Abdomen										
Skin										
Legs										
Other	Hips	Hearing	PKU	Hips	Babbling	Hb				

FIGURE **3.4** **Child Progress Record**

CHILD PROGRESS RECORD
2 – 15 Years

Name _____

Date of Birth _____ Sex M/F

INFANT & HEREDITARY PROBLEMS _____

_____

LANDMARKS 25-90%ile in Yrs.	Date	Age
Testes Descended		
Clean at night		
Dry at night		
Throws ball 1.4 – 2.6		
Gives own name 2.0 – 3.8		
Does up buttons 2.6 – 4.2		
Recognizes 3 colours 2.7 – 4.9		
Hops on one foot 3.0 – 4.9		
Catches ball 3.5 – 5.5		
Ties shoelaces		
First menstruation		
Voice breaks		
Axillary hair		

ILLNESSES	Date	Age
Eczema		
Croup		
Bronchitis		
Allergies		
Tonsillitis		
Ear infections		
Pyrexia over 40°C		
Convulsions		
Chicken Pox		

IMMUNIZATIONS:

Pre School
DPTp x 3 + 1 _____
M.M.R. _____
DPTp _____
O.T.T. _____

10 Years
DPT _____
O.T.T. _____
Hb _____
Rubella Titre _____

15 Years
DPT _____
O.T.T. _____
Hb _____
ASOT _____

Years/Months	2	3	4	5	6	7	8	9	10	11	12	13	14	15
Height cm.														
Height %ile														
Wt. kg.														
Wt. %ile														
Vision Right														
Left														
Near														
Urine Albumin														
Glucose														
Blood Pressure														
Ears														
Eyes														
Nose														
Throat														
Teeth														
Neck														
Lungs														
Heart sounds														
Abdomen														
Legs														
Back														
Posture														
Other														

PUBERTY STATUS

Female
1. Flat
2. Breast buds
3. Enlargement – Slight raising
4. Separate breast contour

Male
1. Infantile
2. Testes enlarging, scrotum & coarse
3. Penis lengthening
4. Penis enlarging, scrotal skin pigmented

Pubic Hair
1. None
2. Sparse, downy
3. Pigmented, coarse, curling
4. Adult

FIGURE **3.5**   ¹/₅ **Cut Folders**

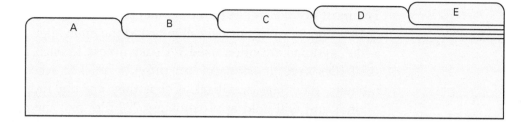

FIGURE **3.6**   ¹/₂ **Cut Folders**

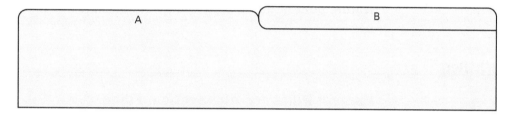

Some physicians prefer file folders that have inside fasteners embedded into the chart. All diagnostic tests are filed on the left side of the chart, with all visits and correspondence on the right side (see Figure 3.7). A special hole-punch is needed in order to prepare your information for filing in this type of chart. The benefit of this type of file is that it reduces the risk of information falling out of the chart. The downside is that it takes longer to file the information.

FIGURE **3.7**   **A, Chart Folders. B, Manila Folder**

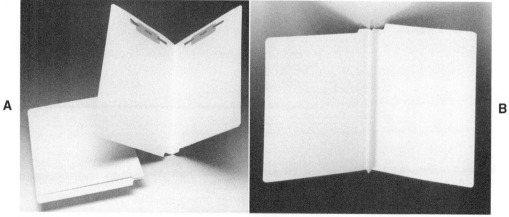

SOURCE: Courtesy Bibberro Systems, Inc., Petaluma, Calif. 94954, (800) 242-2376, http://www.bibbero.com.

CABINETS

The most popular types of file cabinets used in medical offices are the four- or five-drawer upright steel cabinets and the open-shelf file cabinets. "Hang-a-file" systems are often used for easy access to each file. Although open-shelf files save floor space and provide quicker access than drawer-type cabinets, their one drawback is that they are not fireproof. The 5-drawer cabinet unit will hold approximately 720 files and the open-shelf unit with seven 90-cm (36-inch) shelves will hold approximately 1000 files. A lock is essential on any type of medical record holder in order to maintain confidentiality.

If ordering new filing cabinets, also keep in mind how many people will be accessing the cabinets at the same time. Some cabinets have a safety feature built in that will not allow another drawer to be opened if one is in use.

FILING

General Rules for Alphabetical Filing

The following general rules should be applied when filing patient file folders:

1. A person's name is divided into separate indexing units, using the surname as the first unit, first given name as the second unit, and so on. Usually three indexing units are used in the average medical office (see Box 3.2). Always use the proper name and not a nickname. For example, use Robert even though the patient is known as Bob or Rob. It is important to ask the patient what their legal name is; Betty or Bette is not always a short form for Elizabeth.

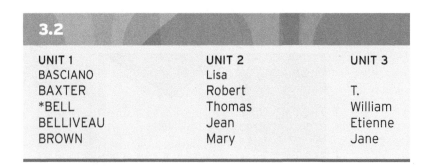

3.2		
UNIT 1	UNIT 2	UNIT 3
BASCIANO	Lisa	
BAXTER	Robert	T.
*BELL	Thomas	William
BELLIVEAU	Jean	Etienne
BROWN	Mary	Jane

NOTE: When identical names occur, the next consideration may be town or city, province, followed by street address. For example, Thomas Bell, 175 Park Street, Ottawa; Thomas Bell, 134 King Street, Ottawa; and Thomas Bell, 283 King Street, Ottawa, would be indexed as follows:

3.3				
UNIT 1	**UNIT 2**	**UNIT 3**	**UNIT 4**	**UNIT 5**
BELL	Thomas	Ottawa	King Street	134
BELL	Thomas	Ottawa	King Street	283
BELL	Thomas	Ottawa	Park Street	175

In some medical offices, when identical names occur, the next consideration may be date of birth.

2. Include the patient's health card numbers since they are now unique to each individual. This is the best way to ensure that you have the correct patient file.
3. Always remember the rule "nothing before something" when considering *all* alphabetizing; for example, N & S would precede Nothing & Something.
4. Surname prefixes and hyphenated names are considered to be one indexing unit; for example, St. John, MacDonald, and MacKenzie-King would all be indexed under Unit 1. When inputting hyphenated names or names with apostrophes into a computer, the hyphen and apostrophe are left out. For example MacKenzie-King would appear as MACKENZIEKING.
5. Abbreviated names should be considered in full; for example, Jas. is James, Chas. is Charles, and Wm. is William.
6. Titles and degrees such as Dr. or M.D. are not considered when indexing names.
7. When filing correspondence for medical facilities and other businesses, names are filed as they are written (introductory and connecting words such as "the," "and," and "A" are not considered when indexing). See Box 3.4. If a business name consists of a person's given name and surname, follow rule 1.

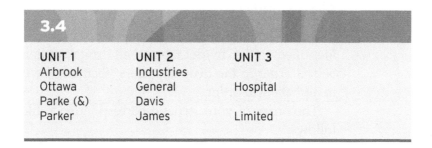

3.4		
UNIT 1	**UNIT 2**	**UNIT 3**
Arbrook	Industries	
Ottawa	General	Hospital
Parke (&)	Davis	
Parker	James	Limited

8. When a name consists of a title and either a given name or a surname, do not transpose the name; make the title an indexing unit (see Box 3.5). This can cause some confusion when filing so it is always good to ask the patient for their other name.

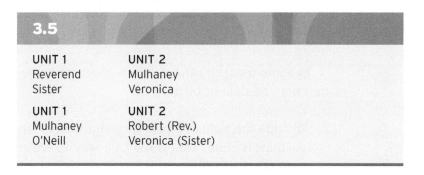

3.5	
UNIT 1	**UNIT 2**
Reverend	Mulhaney
Sister	Veronica
UNIT 1	**UNIT 2**
Mulhaney	Robert (Rev.)
O'Neill	Veronica (Sister)

General Correspondence

A doctor's private practice is classified as a small business. As a result, you will be dealing with records other than patient charts. Some general correspondence files would be kept separate from patient charts. The following are examples of files your general correspondence requirements may include

- Drug suppliers
- Travel agents
- Building and equipment maintenance
- Insurance companies
- Utilities, heat, and telephone
- Office supplies
- Medical supply companies

You may choose to file your general correspondence alphabetically, or you may use a subject filing system.

Subject Filing

In a subject filing system, the main subject (for example, drug suppliers) is identified on the divider tab and all drug suppliers' files are placed in alphabetical order in the drug suppliers' section. The main sections are also filed in alphabetical order.

The order of your general correspondence file system would appear as follows:

BUILDING AND EQUIPMENT MAINTENANCE—Main Subject Index
    Adams Carpentry Service
    Brintnell General Maintenance   Subsidiary Files
    Dynamic Maid Service

DRUG SUPPLIERS
　　Best Buy Drugs
　　Medicare Drug Company
　　Zanzibar Clinical Supplies
INSURANCE COMPANIES
　　Component Property Insurance
　　Friendly Automobile Insurance
　　Jackson Life Insurance
TRAVEL AGENCIES
　　Fly Safe Travellers
　　Plan-a-Trip Agencies
　　Quiet Vacations Limited
UTILITIES, HEAT, AND TELEPHONE
　　Bell Canada
　　Public Utilities Ltd.
　　Research Gas Company

Numerical Filing

Hospitals and large group practices generally use a numerical filing system. Doctors may choose to file by number for reasons of confidentiality. Each patient chart is assigned a special number and filed in numerical order. This number can be generated by the computer when the new patient information is entered. The same number is also used for accounting purposes. A **cross-reference** file is required where the patients' names are listed with their assigned numbers and filed in alphabetical order. The cross-reference system may be on cards (see Figure 3.8), on paper, or stored in a computer.

FIGURE **3.8   Cross-Reference File**

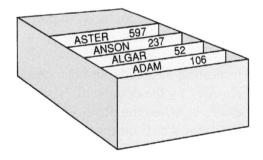

In most offices and other healthcare facilities the cross-referencing is computerized. When the patient information is accessed, the patient's assigned number also appears on the screen. If your files are numerical, you will need to look up each patient every time you need his or her chart or to file patient reports, etc. Most doctors' offices file alphabetically, which removes the need to look up every patient in the computer each time the chart is needed.

Soundex Filing

Soundex filing is generally used to overcome the problem of names that sound similar but are spelled many different ways, for example, Bare, Bear, Baher, and Bayer. The soundex system incorporates six basic phonetic sounds with coded numbers. Some computer systems have this built in as an additional patient search. Although not widely used, it is efficient and allows for rapid filing. Because it is fairly complex, it will not be discussed further in this text.

Tickler File

Every efficient medical administrative assistant has some type of reminder system. In a busy medical office, it is impossible to remember all the details for efficient patient health care. A reminder system is often referred to as a "tickler file," because the system is designed to "tickle" your memory. There are several ways to implement a tickler system. You may choose simply to record reminder notes on your daily calendar and asterisk them with a red pen. A more complex system is to have a small file box with twelve divisions for each month of the year. A subdivider for each day of the month is placed behind the month divider. Reminders are recorded on cards and placed behind the appropriate month/day division. Most computer programs have a built-in reminder system. It may be in the form of a calendar or a reminder beside your daily schedule. Some systems have reminders that appear as post-it notes when you turn on your computer.

It is important to refer to your tickler file each day, as soon after your arrival in the office as possible. This system will only work if you use it faithfully.

Filing Preparation

Offices use various methods to prepare documents for filing. Some routines include the following:

- Indicating by a code number, checkmark, or other means that action, as required by the document, has been taken and it is ready for filing. For example, when the physician has viewed the information he writes a "C" on it which means that you will need to pull the chart. If an "F" is written on it, it can then be filed. Charts that are returned for filing can be placed in a designated area that is identified as "To Be Filed."
- Using a coding system to indicate where the material should be filed (e.g., John T Parker—this indicates the document will be filed as PARKER, JOHN T).
- Preparing a cross-reference page to be filed with material that may be filed under a different heading. Cross-reference sheets should be coloured (for easy identification) and lightweight (to conserve space). Here are some situations that would require cross-referencing:

a. When names sound the same but are spelled differently (e.g., "Thompson" and "Thomson").

b. When it is difficult to distinguish between a given name and surname; (e.g., Lloyd George, when George is the surname). It is a good idea to capitalize or underline the last name.

c. When a woman retains her maiden name after marriage and you want to have a cross-reference to her husband's name.

- Sorting all material in preparation for filing. The documents to be filed are sorted in the order (alphabetical, numerical, by subject) of the system that is being used. This procedure generally takes place on a desk or by means of a collating rack. The sorted documents are then taken to the file area for quick and easy insertion into the appropriate file folders.

It is important that your filing take priority, even though it is the one responsibility that seems to get postponed. Inefficient filing will result in an inefficient office.

Charge-Out Systems

If a file is removed, an "out" card may be inserted in its place (see Figure 3.9). The card is generally made of heavy coloured cardboard and has lines on which to write the date of removal, the name of the person who has removed the file, and the file's present location. It would be very

FIGURE **3.9 Charge-Out Card**

FILE LOCATION				
Date Removed	By	Can Be Found	Date Returned	Initial When Ret.
Dec. 20/94	Jane Smith	In Business Office	Dec. 23/94	J.S.
Jan 1/95	Dr. Plunkett	My Desk	Jan 15/95	JEP
Mar. 18/95	Dr. Pelham	at my home	Mar. 22/95	C.J.P.

time-consuming for a medical administrative assistant to "charge-out" the files of patients visiting the office each day, so for regular patient visits you should not insert an "out" card in place of the patient's file, because it should either be on your desk or with the doctor. Removal of a patient's chart from the files for any other reason, however, requires a "charge-out."

Some offices may use a computerized chart location system to eliminate the need for a manual charge-out system. This is usually utilized by large facilities that share a central records department or a hospital records department.

Out-Folders

An **out-folder** is used for temporary filing of data. It is used in the same way as a **charge-out card**. The folder is placed where the chart should be, and test results or correspondence for the patient are placed in the folder. When the chart is returned, it is easy to file the information.

Purging Files

In order to maintain an efficient filing system, it is necessary to perform periodic **purging** of your records. This task may be done when the physician is absent from the office and your workload is not as heavy as usual. Files of patients who have moved out of town, have transferred to another physician, or are deceased would be removed from your active files and stored as inactive files in a storage area. (Note: An accurate and current list of stored files and their location must be maintained.) Some offices store their purged files in a secure off-site location, due to lack of space.

It is important that you scan your files regularly in order to detect any charts or folders that have been misfiled. It is often necessary to secure patient information on a moment's notice; misfiled charts may result in serious problems.

Colour-Coded Files

The use of colour-coded files is a very efficient system for identifying file folders and is used extensively in the medical environment. It is easy to find misplaced files in a colour-coded system: if a purple label is mixed in with the red labels, it is easily spotted. Colour-coding also makes filing records faster and easier.

There are many colour-coding systems produced by office supply companies. They consist of adhesive coloured tabs, with each colour stamped with a letter of the alphabet. However, if these tabs are not affordable, file folders may be colour-coded with coloured pencils or coloured file labels. The first two letters of the last name are identified with colours. For example, if your colour-coded system stipulated that the letter "A" would be red, the letter "G" would be blue, and the letter "U" would be pink, then the folder for "Agar" would have a red tab and a blue tab, and the folder for "Austin" would have a red tab and a pink tab. The folder tab would still have the full name typed on it, last name first.

FIGURE **3.10** **Colour-coding patient charts makes it easy to see a file that is misplaced.**

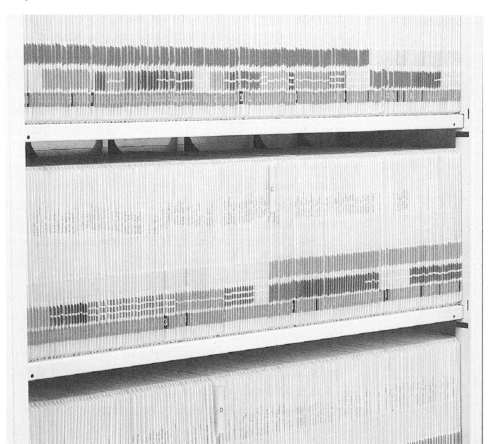

Courtesy Bibberro Systems, Inc., Petaluma, Calif. 94954, (800) 242-2376, http://www.bibbero.com.

In Figure 3.10 the coloured tabs are facing out. When colour-coding your charts, the first letter of the patient's last name should be on the outer edge of the chart, and the second letter should be placed beside it, followed by the name. When using this type of system, you can see at a glance where the charts are for patients with the last name beginning with an "A" as they have red tabs facing out. If you are looking for Elizabeth Austin's chart, for example, you simply go to where the charts show a red and pink tab and begin your search from there.

Numerical files can also be colour-coded.

123456—Each number would have a colour assigned.
123457-12345 would match the 12345 of the previous chart but 6 and 7 would be a different colour, and so on.

Suggestions for Efficient Filing

- File *behind* the guides. This is common practice because it is more efficient.
- Place the miscellaneous folder behind its matching primary guide so that it is the last folder before the next primary guide. For example, the

miscellaneous folder for accounting documents would be filed as the last folder in the "accounting" section. That section's primary guide is the divider at the beginning of the section labelled "accounting."

- Collect a maximum of five items for one firm or customer in a miscellaneous file. Miscellaneous files are not usually used in a patient file system. However, the doctor would have miscellaneous files in his or her business files.
- Arrange letters and other material in individual folders by date, with the most recent appearing at the front. Generally, you are dealing with current information, and using this system allows easier access.
- Allow 10 to 15 cm of working space in drawers to prevent jamming and tearing material.
- When removing folders from the file, always grasp them by the side or centre, never by the tab. When filing or removing papers, lift up the folders part way and rest them on the side of the drawer to avoid inserting papers between folders.
- Ensure that all headings of papers appear to the left as you face the file to facilitate correct placement and easy finding.
- In order to prevent injuries to staff, close all file drawers when not in use.
- To locate misplaced files, charts, or documents, do the following:
  a. Look immediately in front of and behind the place of the file folder—materials may not have been put in the folder.
  b. Look under names that have similar spelling or that sound alike.

ASSIGNMENT 3.2

For this assignment you will be required to purchase sixteen file folders.

Prepare file folders using the information found on the patient information forms (Figure 3.11). Use age, birthday, and current year to calculate each patient's year of birth. Code the folders using coloured pencils and the following colour key (see Figure 3.10). Also prepare a miscellaneous folder for documents that do not pertain to your regular patient files.

A = red	J = dark blue
B = light green	L = gold
C = light blue	M = dark green
D = orange	P = mauve
E = yellow	R = purple
G = black	S = pink
H = brown	T = tan

Blank stamp forms (as shown in Figure 3.1) are included in the CD and can be pasted on the front of each file folder. Alternatively, you can print off a computer label, or your instructor may have an ink stamp prepared for this assignment.

Text continued on p. 63.

FIGURE **3.11** Patient Information Forms

PATIENT INFORMATION

(Please Print Clearly)   Date _July 30 –_

NAME _Robert (Bob) Bastien_ AGE _27_ SEX _M_

ADDRESS _24 Stapleton Road_

CITY _Manotick_ PROV. _Ont_ CODE _K6Y 3T7_

Oct 7 Date of Birth ☑ Mar. ☐ Sing. ☐ Wid. ☐ Div.

PHONE: Home _652-3179_ Work _652-6643_

EMPLOYED BY _Town of Manotick_

CITY _Manotick_ PROV. _Ont_

OCCUPATION _Township Clerk_

SPOUSE'S NAME _Sylvia_

EMPLOYED BY _Self_

CITY _Ottawa_ PROV. _Ont_

PHONE _652-6643_ OCCUPATION _Boutique Owner_

REFERRED BY _____

HEALTH CARD NO. _4892608532_ VERSION CODE _____

ALLERGIES _____

SERIOUS ILLNESS _____

EMERGENCY CONTACT _Sylvia_ _Wife_ _652-6643_
                   Name   Relation   Phone

PATIENT INFORMATION

(Please Print Clearly)   Date _Aug. 31, 20 –_

NAME _Lisa Basciano_ AGE _42_ SEX _F_

ADDRESS _2796 Waycross Cres._

CITY _Ottawa_ PROV. _Ont._ CODE _J7X 2X9_

Nov. 19 Date of Birth ☑ Mar. ☐ Sing. ☐ Wid. ☐ Div.

PHONE: Home _742-2717_ Work _743-7776_

EMPLOYED BY _Government of Canada_

CITY _Ottawa_ PROV. _Ont._

OCCUPATION _Accountant_

SPOUSE'S NAME _Dino_

EMPLOYED BY _Government of Canada_

CITY _Ottawa_ PROV. _Ont._

PHONE _743-7776_ OCCUPATION _M.P._

REFERRED BY _____

HEALTH CARD NO. _2719278836_ VERSION CODE _____

ALLERGIES _____

SERIOUS ILLNESS _Rheumatoid Arthritis_

EMERGENCY CONTACT _Dino_ _Husband_ _243-7776_
                   Name   Relation   Phone

continued

PATIENT INFORMATION

(Please Print Clearly)   Date _June 23, 20-_

NAME _Melville Thompson_   AGE _75_ SEX _M_

ADDRESS _22 Edward Road_

CITY _Ottawa_   PROV. _Ont_   CODE _J7X 2t6_

Nov · 8   [✓] Mar. [ ] Sing. [ ] Wid. [ ] Div.
Date of Birth

PHONE: Home _427-5432_   Work _____

EMPLOYED BY _Retired_

CITY _____   PROV. _____

OCCUPATION _____

SPOUSE'S NAME _Laura_

EMPLOYED BY _____

CITY _____   PROV. _____

PHONE _____   OCCUPATION _____

REFERRED BY _____

HEALTH CARD NO. _6448417672_   VERSION CODE _____

ALLERGIES _____

SERIOUS ILLNESS _Emphysema_

EMERGENCY CONTACT _Laura_   _wife_   _427-5432_
Name   Relation   Phone

PATIENT INFORMATION

(Please Print Clearly)   Date _JULY 12, 20-_

NAME _AMELIA JACKSON_   AGE _57_ SEX _F_

ADDRESS _13 CROSS ST._

CITY _KEMPTVILLE_   PROV. _ONT_   CODE _KON 2L0_

APR. 29   [ ] Mar. [ ] Sing. [ ] Wid. [✓] Div.
Date of Birth

PHONE: Home _748-3192_   Work _748-5532_

EMPLOYED BY _KEMP HOSPITAL_

CITY _KEMPTVILLE_   PROV. _ONT_

OCCUPATION _NURSE_

SPOUSE'S NAME _____

EMPLOYED BY _____

CITY _____   PROV. _____

PHONE _____   OCCUPATION _____

REFERRED BY _DR. JAMES_

HEALTH CARD NO. _8806773712_   VERSION CODE _____

ALLERGIES _____

SERIOUS ILLNESS _____

EMERGENCY CONTACT _STEVEN_   _SON_   _427-0098_
Name   Relation   Phone

FIGURE **3.11** Patient Information Forms, cont'd

PATIENT INFORMATION (right form)

(Please Print Clearly)   Date April 12, 20—

NAME Hazel Davis   AGE 30   SEX F

ADDRESS 539 Cherryhill Lane

CITY Ottawa   PROV. Ont.   CODE KOW 3S5

Feb. 2.   ☑ Mar.   ☐ Sing.   ☐ Wid.   ☐ Div.
Date of Birth

PHONE: Home 427-7006   Work ____

EMPLOYED BY _____

CITY _____   PROV. _____

OCCUPATION _____

SPOUSE'S NAME Brent

EMPLOYED BY Ottawa College

CITY Ottawa   PROV. Ont

PHONE 426-0001   OCCUPATION Maint. Mech.

REFERRED BY _____

HEALTH CARD NO. 178 105 0552   VERSION CODE _____

ALLERGIES _____

SERIOUS ILLNESS _____

EMERGENCY CONTACT Brent   Husband   426-0001
                   Name   Relation   Phone

PATIENT INFORMATION (left form)

(Please Print Clearly)   Date March 12, 20—

NAME Mary Jane Brown   AGE 21   SEX F

ADDRESS 731 Hampole St.

CITY Ottawa   PROV. Ont.   CODE J8X 4X9

Jan. 1   ☐ Mar.   ☐ Sing.   ☑ Wid.   ☐ Div.
Date of Birth

PHONE: Home 427-3333   School/Work 427-5566

EMPLOYED BY _____

CITY _____   PROV. _____

OCCUPATION Student

SPOUSE'S NAME _____

EMPLOYED BY _____

CITY _____   PROV. _____

PHONE _____ OCCUPATION _____

REFERRED BY _____

HEALTH CARD NO. 3820703795   VERSION CODE _____

ALLERGIES Sulpha, Aspirin

SERIOUS ILLNESS _____

EMERGENCY CONTACT Bert   Father   Work 456-9321
                   Name   Relation Phone

FIGURE 3.11 Patient Information Forms, cont'd

continued

PATIENT INFORMATION

(Please Print Clearly)   Date _MARCH 11, 20—_

NAME _BELLIVEAU, JEAN_   AGE _22_   SEX _M_

ADDRESS _729 UPPERHILL DRIVE_

CITY _OTTAWA_   PROV. _ONT._   CODE _J8Z 4X7_

DECEMBER 26   ☐ Mar. ☑ Sing. ☐ Wid. ☐ Div.
Date of Birth

PHONE: Home _427-3899_   _SCHOOL_ ~~Work~~ _427-9987_

EMPLOYED BY _____

CITY _____   PROV. _____

OCCUPATION _STUDENT_

SPOUSE'S NAME _____

EMPLOYED BY _____

CITY _____   PROV. _____

PHONE _____   OCCUPATION _____

REFERRED BY _____

HEALTH CARD NO. _6910047635_   VERSION CODE _____

ALLERGIES _____

SERIOUS ILLNESS _____

EMERGENCY CONTACT _BARB_   _MOTHER_   _427-3665_
                    Name   Relation   Phone

PATIENT INFORMATION

(Please Print Clearly)   Date _Feb 13, 20—_

NAME _HEATHER SMITH_   AGE _18_   SEX _F_

ADDRESS _BEAVER CRES._

CITY _MANOTICK_   PROV. _ONT_   CODE _K6Y 3T7_

APRIL 4   ☐ Mar. ☑ Sing. ☐ Wid. ☐ Div.
Date of Birth

PHONE: Home _576-3225_   Work _____

EMPLOYED BY _GOVERNMENT OF CANADA_

CITY _OTTAWA_   PROV. _ONT_

OCCUPATION _FILE CLERK_

SPOUSE'S NAME _____

EMPLOYED BY _____

CITY _____   PROV. _____

PHONE _____   OCCUPATION _____

REFERRED BY _DR. JOHNSTON_

HEALTH CARD NO. _9086182038_   VERSION CODE _____

ALLERGIES _____

SERIOUS ILLNESS _____

EMERGENCY CONTACT _CHRISTINE_   _MOTHER_   _576-3225_
                    Name   Relation   Phone

FIGURE **3.11**   Patient Information Forms, cont'd

PATIENT INFORMATION

(Please Print Clearly)
Date: MAY 3, 20-

NAME: Robert ERIK SHULTZ   AGE 55   SEX M

ADDRESS: 17 BOND STREET

CITY: OTTAWA   PROV. ONT.   CODE J8Z 4H3

MAY 26   ☑ Mar.   ☐ Sing.   ☐ Wid.   ☐ Div.
Date of Birth

PHONE: Home 427-9977   Work 427-3456

EMPLOYED BY: TEXTILES LIMITED

CITY: PERTH   PROV. ONT.

OCCUPATION: PERSONNEL DIRECTOR

SPOUSE'S NAME: MARY

EMPLOYED BY:

CITY: PROV.

PHONE: OCCUPATION HomemAKER

REFERRED BY:

HEALTH CARD NO. 7819749313   VERSION CODE

ALLERGIES:

SERIOUS ILLNESS: CANCER, RIGHT THIGH -ON CHEM,

EMERGENCY CONTACT: MARY   WIFE   427-9977
                    Name   Relation   Phone

PATIENT INFORMATION

(Please Print Clearly)
Date: June 18, 20-

NAME: Peter John Scott   AGE 14   SEX M

ADDRESS: 16 Bonn St.

CITY: Ottawa   PROV. Ont.   CODE J7X 2X6

Aug. 18   ☐ Mar.   ☑ Sing.   ☐ Wid.   ☐ Div.
Date of Birth

PHONE: Home 727-2245   Work

EMPLOYED BY:

CITY: PROV.

OCCUPATION:

SPOUSE'S NAME:

EMPLOYED BY:

CITY: PROV.

PHONE: OCCUPATION

REFERRED BY:

HEALTH CARD NO. 9191807099   VERSION CODE

ALLERGIES: Morphine

SERIOUS ILLNESS: Epilepsy

EMERGENCY CONTACT: Glen   Father   work 372-7687
                    Name   Relation   Phone

FIGURE **3.11**   Patient Information Forms, cont'd

continued

PATIENT INFORMATION

(Please Print Clearly)   Date ___Sept. 26, 20—___

NAME ___LOIS ELLIOTT___   AGE __51__ SEX __F__

ADDRESS ___RR3___

CITY ___KARS___   PROV. __ONT.__ CODE __W9U4W9__

___MARCH 19___ ☐ Mar. ☐ Sing. ☑ Wid. ☐ Div.
Date of Birth

PHONE: Home __748-3355__   Work __427-3478__

EMPLOYED BY ___GLOUCESTER CLOCK WORKS___

CITY ___OTTAWA___   PROV. __ONT.__

OCCUPATION ___EXECUTIVE SECRETARY___

SPOUSE'S NAME _____

EMPLOYED BY _____

CITY _____   PROV. _____

PHONE _____   OCCUPATION _____

REFERRED BY ___DR. CARL ROLLINGS___

HEALTH CARD NO. ___L954154509a___   VERSION CODE _____

ALLERGIES _____

SERIOUS ILLNESS _____

EMERGENCY CONTACT ___LORRAINE___ ___DAUGHTER___ ___799-5473___
                        Name   Relation   Phone

PATIENT INFORMATION

(Please Print Clearly)   Date ___OCT 3. 20—___

NAME ___TIMOTHY PETERS___   AGE __36__ SEX __M__

ADDRESS ___10 LORD ST.___

CITY ___KEMPTVILLE___   PROV. __ONT.__ CODE __KOW 2W0__

___JAN 1___ ☑ Mar. ☐ Sing. ☐ Wid. ☐ Div.
Date of Birth

PHONE: Home __743-2525__   Work __743-5550__

EMPLOYED BY ___SMITH AND SMITH LIMITED___

CITY ___OTTAWA___   PROV. __ONT.__

OCCUPATION ___LABOURER___

SPOUSE'S NAME ___KRISTA___

EMPLOYED BY ___KEMPTVILLE COLLEGE___

CITY ___KEMPTVILLE___   PROV. __ONT.__

PHONE ___743-7557___   OCCUPATION ___TEACHER___

REFERRED BY _____

HEALTH CARD NO. ___7051381135___   VERSION CODE _____

ALLERGIES _____

SERIOUS ILLNESS _____

EMERGENCY CONTACT ___KRISTA___ ___WIFE___ ___WORK OR HOME ABOVE___
                        Name   Relation   Phone

FIGURE **3.11** Patient Information Forms, cont'd

PATIENT INFORMATION

(Please Print Clearly)   Date Jan. 20, 20-

NAME Thomas Bell   AGE 82   SEX M

ADDRESS 321 Adelaide St.

CITY Ottawa   PROV. Ont.   CODE J3Z 5X3

Date of Birth Sept. 25   ☑ Mar. ☐ Sing. ☐ Wid. ☐ Div.

PHONE: Home 427-5327   Work 427-3227

EMPLOYED BY Self

CITY Ottawa   PROV. Ont.

OCCUPATION Free Lance Writer (Retired)

SPOUSE'S NAME Janet

EMPLOYED BY —

CITY   PROV.

PHONE   OCCUPATION House Wife

REFERRED BY

HEALTH CARD NO. 6875231059   VERSION CODE

ALLERGIES Penicillin

SERIOUS ILLNESS

EMERGENCY CONTACT Janet   Wife   427-5327
                   Name   Relation   Phone

PATIENT INFORMATION

(Please Print Clearly)   Date Jan. 16, 20-

NAME Elizabeth Green   AGE 36   SEX F

ADDRESS 72 Hillcrest St.

CITY Ottawa   PROV. Ont.   CODE J3Z 5X4

Date of Birth Aug. 12   ☑ Mar. ☐ Sing. ☐ Wid. ☐ Div.

PHONE: Home 427-3774   Work

EMPLOYED BY

CITY   PROV.

OCCUPATION

SPOUSE'S NAME Gary

EMPLOYED BY ABC Deliveries

CITY Ottawa   PROV. Ont.

PHONE 427-4545   OCCUPATION Manager

REFERRED BY

HEALTH CARD NO. 3777220777   VERSION CODE

ALLERGIES Nil

SERIOUS ILLNESS Hypertension

EMERGENCY CONTACT Gary   Husband   427-4545
                   Name   Relation   Phone

FIGURE **3.11** Patient Information Forms, cont'd

continued

PATIENT INFORMATION

(Please Print Clearly)   Date __Nov 1, 20—__

NAME __William Harris__   AGE __2 mth__ SEX __M__

ADDRESS __362 BlueJay Cres.__

CITY __Ottawa__   PROV. __Ont__   CODE __J7K 2X9__

__Sept. 5__   ☐ Mar. ☑ Sing. ☐ Wid. ☐ Div.
Date of Birth

PHONE: Home __776-2367__   Work _____

EMPLOYED BY _____

CITY _____   PROV. _____

OCCUPATION _____

SPOUSE'S NAME _____

EMPLOYED BY _____

CITY _____   PROV. _____

PHONE _____   OCCUPATION _____

REFERRED BY _____

HEALTH CARD NO. __272257 5673__   VERSION CODE _____

ALLERGIES __Sulpha, milk, Penicillin__

SERIOUS ILLNESS _____

EMERGENCY CONTACT __Brad__   __father__   __427-0009__
                          Name   Relation   Phone

FIGURE **3.11** **Patient Information Forms, cont'd**

FIGURE **3.12** **File Folders**

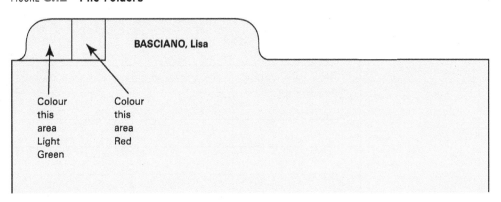

Print the patient's name (or place a file folder label with the name) on the tab of the folder, last name first in capitals, for example, BASCIANO, Lisa (see Figure 3.12). Insert a family medicine chart and a record form for allergies and medications in the appropriate place in each file. These, and any other forms your instructor wishes inserted in the file, will be provided. Extra forms are available on the CD. Samples of these forms include a patient information form (see Figure 3.11), a prescription record (see Figure 3.13), a family medicine chart (see Figure 3.2), and an infant and child progress record (see Figures 3.3 and 3.4). It is your responsibility to file all information pertaining to each patient in the appropriate folder and in the order indicated in this chapter.

ASSIGNMENT **3.3**

a. Index the following list of names.
b. Prepare an alphabetized list.

Indexing may be keyed or handwritten. Submit both the indexing exercise and the alphabetized list. For the purposes of this assignment *only*, consider all shortened names to be abbreviations of the full name; for example, Nick would be Nicholas.

Mary Shier-Sorrie
Don Bruce, 156 Park St., Ottawa
Dr. Rob T. Durin
Mrs. John L. Kingston (Rena)
Masie Shierman
Nicholas Maziotti, 223 George St., Virgil, B.C.
Delbert J. McCall
Robbin Durin
Nick Mazzioti, 107 George St., Virgil, N.S.
Jamie Dickens
Connato DiCarlo
Michael Terry Masters
Wm. Ainsworth
John Kingston
Mike T. Masterson

FIGURE **3.13** **Prescription Record**

NAME

# OF PRESCRIPTION	LONG TERM MEDICATION AND TREATMENT	DATE FILLED

Nicholas Mazziotti, 372 George St., Virgil, Alta.

Wilma Ainsworth

Nick Mazziotti, 315 George St., Virgil, Ontario

Donald Bruce, 101 Park St., Ottawa

D.J. MacCall

Mrs. Donalda Bruce, 96 Park St., Ottawa, Ont.

ASSIGNMENT **3.4**

a. File the following names alphabetically:

James Park

Sister Rosemary McManus

I.D.A. Drug Stores
Lois Armstrong, D.C.
Brother McCarrell
Dr. David Sneddon
Sister Veronica
Josie Iammancini

b. Colour-code these patient charts using the guide listed as follows:

A=Blue	**B**=Green	**C**=Yellow
I=Brown	**M**=Red	**N**=Purple
P=Pink	**R**=Orange	**S**=Dark Green

1. _____   5. _____

2. _____   6. _____

3. _____   7. _____

4. _____   8. _____

TOPICS FOR DISCUSSION

1. What may be the consequences of a misplaced file in the following environments:

   a. In an office setting?
   b. In a hospital setting?

2. Discuss the pros and cons of both an alphabetical and a numerical filing system.

3. What type of tickler file system would help you remember most easily, and why?

CHAPTER 4

The Telephone

CHAPTER OUTLINE

General Telephone Procedures
Types of Calls
Answering Services

The Telephone Directory
Equipment
Topics for Discussion

LEARNING OBJECTIVES

After reading this chapter, you will be able to describe

- Effective telephone usage including answering, triage, holding, and making outgoing calls
- How to handle calls regarding appointments, house calls, prescription requests, and emergencies

- How to use the telephone directory as a reference source
- Types of telephone equipment
- Methods of dealing with callers other than patients
- Good telephone etiquette

KEY TERMS

Primary care physician: The physician who is responsible for most of the patient's personal health care, which includes health maintenance, therapy during illnesses, and consultation with specialists. Source: Venes, D., Clayton , T.L., & Taber, C.W. (2005). *Taber's Cyclopedic Medical Dictionary* (20th edition). F.A. Davis Company.

Provisional diagnosis: What the physician suspects is wrong with the patient, based on presenting symptoms.

Triage: Screening and setting priorities for patient treatment as well as priorities for urgency of incoming telephone calls.

GENERAL TELEPHONE PROCEDURES

The telephone is the link between the physician and the patient. Do not let the phone ring while you finish adding a column of figures or chat with another patient. Answer it immediately (at least within three rings) but do not sound rushed or out of breath. If you put a smile on your face when you answer the phone, you will also put a smile in your voice. Your voice should sound pleasant and friendly, calm and professional. You cannot sound pleasant or friendly if you are distracted. Clear your mind and concentrate on the caller. Identify the doctor's office and then yourself: "Good morning. Dr. Pelham's office, Ann speaking." Then determine if you can accommodate the patient's needs, or answer a question. If not, inform the patient you will speak to the doctor and either you will return the call or have the doctor do so. If the doctor is to return the call, try to give the patient an approximate time at which the doctor will be calling. This will avoid having the patient wait at home unnecessarily for the phone call.

One of the most important aspects of telephone usage in a medical practice is to *record all incoming patient requests and inquiries (not appointment bookings)*. You should have a notebook and pencil beside the telephone at all times. When a patient calls, record the time, date, patient's name and telephone number, the message, and your initials or signature. After you have noted details of the call, it is good practice to repeat the message to the caller. This ensures the information is correct. Most offices use message pads similar to the one shown in Figure 4.1. (Note: If you receive an urgent message, highlighting "urgent" will indicate to the doctor that the message requires immediate attention.) There are message books available with NCR paper (see Figure 4.2). This enables you to give the doctor his message while retaining a copy for your own records.

When your message has been relayed and completed, or both, place a checkmark (√) through it and initial it if there is more than one person working in your office. Do not use scraps of paper to record messages, as they are easily lost or misplaced and there is no way to follow up.

4.1

Record everything in writing. Do not depend on memory.

Computer networks are a part of today's modern offices. If you work in an office where you have the responsibility of answering the telephone, and you have a computer network system in your office, you will no longer need to write telephone messages on paper. Your system will likely be equipped with electronic messaging capabilities. You will call up a preprogrammed message form (see Figure 4.3) on your screen, key in the details of the call, and forward the message using the computer. The terminal of the

FIGURE **4.1**   Telephone Message

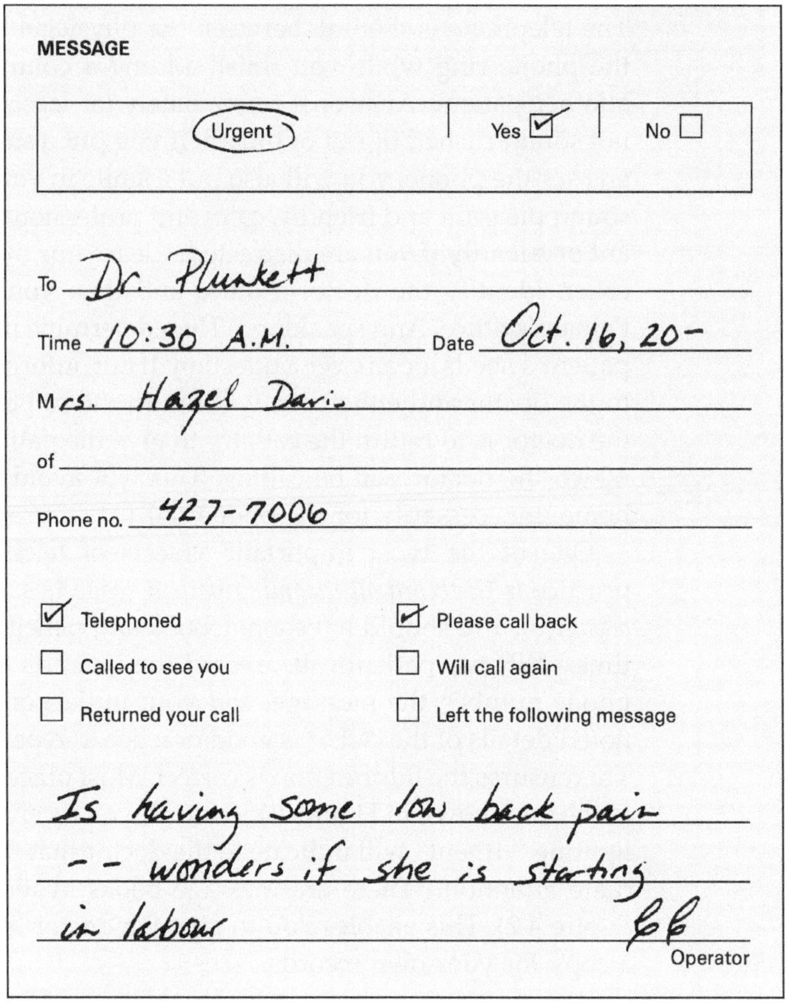

MESSAGE

| Urgent | | Yes ☑ | | No ☐ |

To _Dr. Plunkett_

Time _10:30 A.M._   Date _Oct. 16, 20–_

Mrs. _Hazel Davis_

of _____

Phone no. _427-7006_

☑ Telephoned   ☑ Please call back

☐ Called to see you   ☐ Will call again

☐ Returned your call   ☐ Left the following message

Is having some low back pain
-- wonders if she is starting
in labour   _CC_
                                    Operator

FIGURE **4.2**   Telephone Message Pad with NCR Paper

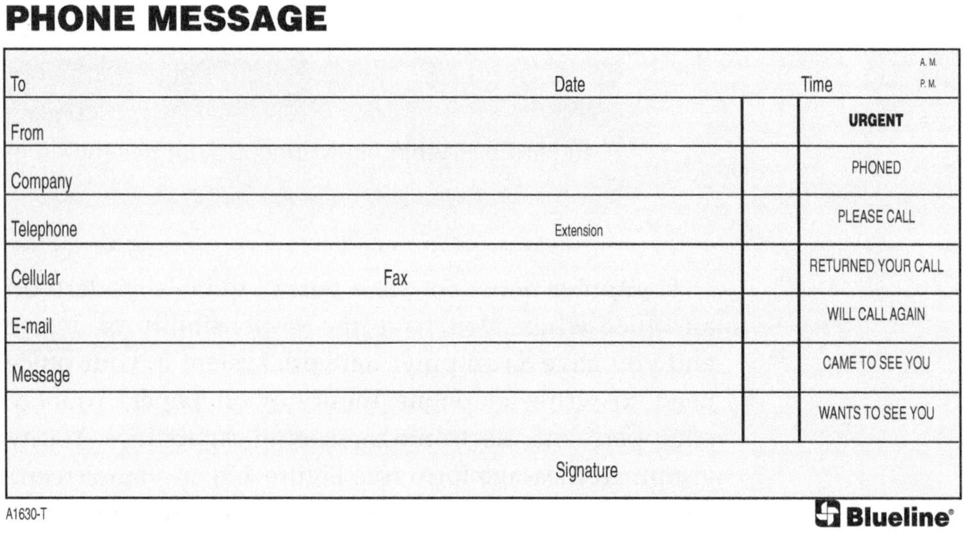

PHONE MESSAGE

To		Date		Time	A.M. / P.M.
From					**URGENT**
Company					PHONED
Telephone		Extension			PLEASE CALL
Cellular	Fax				RETURNED YOUR CALL
E-mail					WILL CALL AGAIN
Message					CAME TO SEE YOU
					WANTS TO SEE YOU
		Signature			

A1630-T

🔲 **Blueline**®

FIGURE **4.3**   **Preprogrammed Message Form**

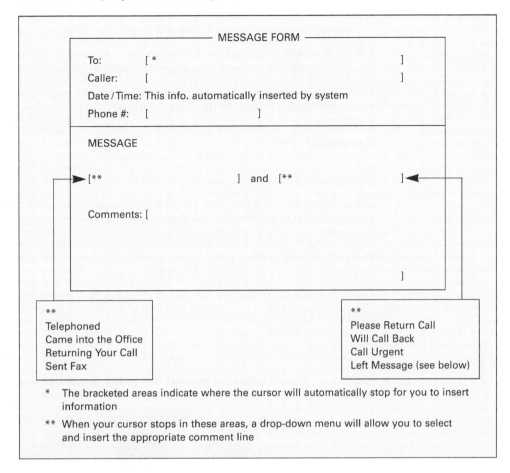

message recipient will display the message for perusal. Computers also enable you to send your messages by e-mail. This system is dependent on the receiver frequently checking for messages. (E-mail etiquette is discussed in Chapter 5.)

Be patient and courteous at all times. Remember, the people you are dealing with usually have medical problems. They are not like customers coming to buy a product. You must be sympathetic and empathetic; let them know you are listening to what they are saying and that you will do whatever is necessary to help. Your voice should be friendly, interested, expressive, calm, and natural. Try to speak in a normal tone and speak clearly and slowly. You need to present yourself as confident, knowledgeable, and professional. If the patient is in distress, be sympathetic and, most important, be reassuring.

How you listen is also very important. Be sure to get the caller's name and use it during the conversation to show that you are attentive. Do not allow your mind to wander while a patient talks to you. Some patients may want to discuss their problems at length. Because you work in a busy environment, it is important, without being rude, to encourage patients to be specific about their needs. You may say, "Do you wish to make an appointment, Mrs. Davis?"

A large percentage of your time in a busy office is spent on the telephone. Often you are required to listen as well as write or find information from a chart. A headset (as shown in Figure 4.4) is recommended, as it leaves both hands free and does not require you to hold your head and neck in an uncomfortable position for extended periods of time. If a headset is not available to you, position yourself as shown in Figure 4.5A when using the telephone.

Triage (Screening)

The administrative assistant is the barrier between the doctor and interruptive calls. **Triage** all calls. Do not interrupt the doctor unless absolutely necessary. Be careful not to give the impression that the doctor is never available. If the doctor is with a patient, relate that to the caller. Don't say, "The doctor is busy"; say, "The doctor is with a patient. May I give him a message?" Discuss with your doctor/employer the preferences regarding callbacks, and what calls will be accepted during the day.

FIGURE **4.4   A good telephone headset leaves the hands free and facilitates good body posture.**

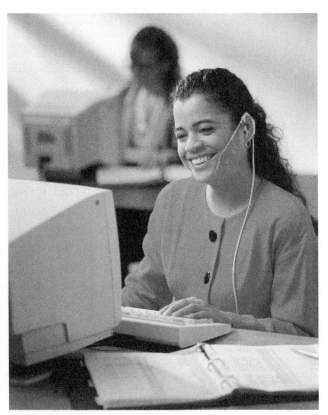

SOURCE: Eggers, D.A. & Conway, A.M. (2000). *Mosby's Front Office Skills for the Medical Assistant* (p. 144: Figure 6.7). St. Louis: Mosby.

FIGURE **4.5**   **A, Good posture when answering the telephone improves voice quality and prevents muscle strain. B, Leaning back in the chair and using the shoulder to hold the telephone results in poor voice quality and muscle strain.**

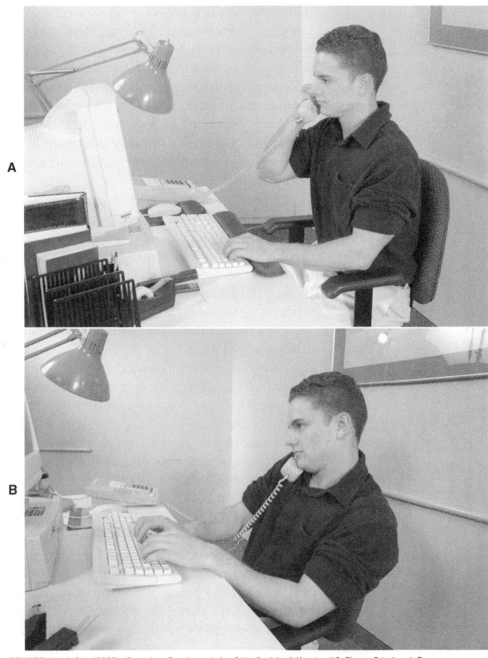

SOURCE: Hunt, S.A. (2002). *Saunders Fundamentals of Medical Assisting* (p. 113: Figure 7-1, *A* and *B*). Philadelphia: Saunders.

Most physicians will only return calls to other physicians or personal calls. Patients are encouraged to book an appointment to speak with the doctor. Of course there are always exceptions to the rule.

Many of the phone calls that come into the office can be handled by you without referring to the doctor. However, the Canadian Medical Protective Association recommends that you *do not give any medical advice at any time*. Phone advice *can* be given through Telehealth Ontario or another provincial health advice service, where patients can speak directly with a registered nurse or a nurse practitioner. Make sure you have these telephone numbers available for your patients. You may want to include them on the patient brochure or information sheet. You may also want to have them displayed in the waiting room. Encourage your patients to access this service when your office is closed.

Patients often explain their symptoms and then ask, "What do you think I should do?" Your only answer is to ask the patient to come in for an appointment or arrange for the patient speak to the doctor. If the doctor is not available, make complete and accurate notes concerning the patient's call; this will save time when the doctor makes the return call. In some circumstances you will need to pull the patient chart and attach the message to it. If the patient is calling about specific test results, check the chart to see if he or she arrived *before* giving the chart to the doctor. If the patient has not arrived, call the referral facility and request a fax of the results or get a verbal report.

The administrative assistant should use discretion when relaying test results over the phone. If you receive a call requesting tests results, it is absolutely essential that you know the caller; otherwise ask for the person's name and number and discuss the situation with the doctor. Of course, you should never release any results without checking first with the doctor. If test results indicate medical problems, you should make an appointment for the patient to see the doctor. When a lab calls your office with verbal results, be prepared to repeat the results back to the caller and give them your name. It is good practice to repeat *all* verbal test results.

Many physicians will not renew prescriptions (Rx) over the telephone—they will ask you to make an appointment for the patient. In some provinces, pharmacies will take telephone prescriptions from physicians only. Some physicians will charge the patient when prescriptions are called into a pharmacy without the patient seeing the doctor (i.e., repeat prescriptions). This is charged by individual call or by the patient paying a flat fee per annum that covers uninsured services.

"Holding" Callers

Do not answer the phone and say, "Dr. Plunkett's office, will you hold please?" and then immediately leave the line. In today's busy office, it is not uncommon to have two or three lines engaged at one time (see Box 4.2). If another line rings, make certain before you place the caller on hold that it is not an emergency. It is common courtesy to wait for an answer to the "will you hold?" question. If the call is not an emergency, and you cannot handle the call immediately, inform the caller that you are on the other line and give the caller a choice of holding or being called back. Some telephone systems have music playing or a beep at intervals that lets callers know that they are still on hold and have not been mistakenly cut off. If the caller is waiting to speak with the physician and the physician is on another call, check back frequently to assure the caller that he or she has not been forgotten. Inform the caller that the doctor is still on the other line, and ask whether he or she would like to continue holding or leave a message and have the doctor call back. If the caller is another physician, you can ask if there is a chart that your physician will need for this call. If so, pull the chart and have it ready.

4.2   Interrupting a Call to Answer Another Line

- Ask the person if he or she can hold while you answer the other line. Inform the person that you will be right back.
- When you answer the other line, ask the second caller if he or she can hold as you are on another call. If it is not an emergency, ask if the caller wants to hold or have you call back.
- Return to the first caller as soon as possible and thank him or her for holding.

Outgoing Calls

In the course of your working day, you will have many occasions to make calls on behalf of your employer. Ensure that you have all pertinent information organized before placing the call. For example, if you are scheduling a test, have available all the patient's sociological information, as well as the types of tests required, and the days and times the patient is available to have the tests performed (see Box 4.3). It would be helpful if you had some information about related tests previously performed and the names of the facilities where these tests were administered.

4.3   Information Needed for Diagnostic Testing/Physician Referrals

- Type of test or appointment
- Patient's name, date of birth, health insurance number, phone number
- Urgency of test
- When the patient is available
- **Provisional diagnosis** if possible

Most patients today have answering machines or voicemail. Many times you will need to leave a message for the patient. You must always remember patient confidentiality. The following guidelines are recommended if leaving a message on a patient's voicemail or answering machine.

1. Make sure you have reached the appropriate number.
2. If the patient is not identifiable do not leave a message. For example, a message that states "you have reached 555-1111" does not mean that the patient is still at that number.
3. Leave as little information as needed, e.g., "Please have Mr. Baxter call this number when he arrives."
4. Do not leave appointment times or test results in a recorded message.

Try to limit the number of outgoing calls you are required to make. Some you can control and others you cannot. Patients need to be able to access your office and you do not want to have your lines engaged unnecessarily. Do not commit to calling patients back unless absolutely necessary. Try to handle the situation on the first call. Personal calls are discouraged unless absolutely necessary.

If patients are continuously calling for directions to hospitals, labs, etc., have copies of maps available and attach them to their referral or requisition when needed.

TYPES OF CALLS

Appointments

Be sure to obtain all the necessary information in order to book the appointment properly: name, reason for appointment, phone number, time frame (how soon if urgent), and best time for the patient. After booking a date and time, repeat this back to the patient and give any further instructions, such as urine sample required or diet restrictions prior to lab tests. Be sure to always give this information both verbally and in written form. If someone is accompanying the patient, it is advisable to have that person hear the instructions as well (if the patient has given you permission to share this information with him or her).

Prescriptions (Rx)

If a prescription renewal is required, ask the patient for the name and number, or both, of the medication and at what pharmacy the prescription was purchased. If this information is not available from the patient, you can refer to the file. Of course, you must record the patient's name; ask for the telephone number as well to save time in case you have to call back.

At a convenient time, prescriptions should be transferred to a separate record. A steno pad is ideal if using a manual system, or you may utilize a computerized database. This information must also be recorded in the patient's file. All drug orders must be kept as part of the physician's records.

Ensure that hard copy or backed-up computer files are stored safely and securely.

Before calling the prescription in to the pharmacy, *you must always have approval from the doctor*. He or she should place his or her initials beside the entry in your book that lists the patient's name, date of order, medication name, dosage and/or number, and name of the pharmacy where the prescription is ordered.

Please note that the preceding information regarding prescriptions is for your consideration. In today's healthcare environment, from a risk management and quality care perspective, few physicians will consider renewing prescriptions over the telephone. They prefer to have the patient come into the office for an assessment, as discussed previously in this chapter.

Cancellations

If a patient calls to cancel an appointment, make a note in the patient's chart and on the appointment record. You may have a cancellation list in your office. If you are given enough notice, you can call another patient in to take the cancelled appointment time. Inform the doctor so he or she can update his or her daily schedule. Often the patient will arrange another appointment. If this does not happen and you feel it is important for the patient to be seen, discuss it with the doctor.

New Patient Inquiries

With the shortage of family practitioners in the country, many individuals do not have a **primary care physician**. If your practice is full and you are not accepting new patients, be firm but give them an alternative phone number to call. This could be the area Medical Society or the names of doctors who *are* accepting new patients. It is common practice for these physicians to set up interviews for potential patients.

Emergencies

The administrative assistant will at times be faced with panic situations or emergencies. Use *common sense* and *keep calm*. First, determine if it is a real emergency or just a patient overreacting. Get all the necessary information: the type of emergency, duration, and whether an ambulance is required. Where possible, the ambulance should be arranged by the person calling the doctor's office. If that person is unable to make the call, be sure to get all necessary information, such as location and directions, and call for the ambulance yourself. If you have more than one line, inform the caller that you will put the call on hold and then call the ambulance. After you have the instructions from the ambulance service, go back to the patient and report when the ambulance will arrive. In *most* areas, dialling 911 will give you immediate access to emergency services.

You should have guidelines that outline what is considered an emergency in your office for appointment scheduling. Sudden diplopia (double vision), severe headache, facial or limb paralysis, high fever, burning urination, or blood in urine or stool are some examples. In the healthcare field, circumstances and conditions can change momentarily. Such guidelines are only that—guidelines. You will need to use common sense. When in doubt always consult the physician.

Ordering Supplies

The administrative assistant will be responsible for keeping sufficient stock of all office supplies. Before calling your supplier, ensure that you have an accurate list of your requirements and follow your telephone order with a formal purchase order.

ANSWERING SERVICES

There are two types of answering services. One is a separate number (usually listed after the office number in the telephone directory), where messages can be left for after-hours callback. The most common type, however, is a direct connection with the doctor's office telephone so that when a call is made to the office, it is picked up by the answering service when the office is unavailable. Answering services are user-friendly to the caller in a world of automation. The patient can speak to a real person. The answering service will take messages and relay them to the office. If the physician is on call, the service will contact the doctor on his or her pager (beeper) or cell phone and relay the message directly. There are certain areas in the hospitals that prohibit the use of cell phones; therefore the service will usually call the pager number.

Answering services can be used after hours, at lunch time, or at peak periods to relieve the administrative assistant. If a service is used, you must check first thing every morning for all messages, and last thing before you leave to advise the service where the doctor may be reached (if on call) and when the office will be open again.

Answering Machines

In areas where telephone answering services are not available, many physicians use answering machines. Some physicians prefer to use answering machines rather than have the additional cost of an answering service. The administrative assistant will record a message on the machine informing the caller of the office hours and what to do in the case of an emergency. If you are in the office but unavailable, you can program a message that states, "I am in the office but either away from my desk or on the other line. Please leave a message and I will return your call as soon as possible. If this is an emergency please dial 911 or go the nearest emergency department." Some answering machines are for information only and the caller is unable to leave a message. Most telephone systems will have a flashing light that will prompt you that there is a message waiting. Other systems only have an interrupted dial tone when you pick up the receiver that indicates you have a message.

With this type of system, you will need to check frequently; in a busy office this is often inconvenient and may result in missed or delayed messages.

Voicemail

Individual staff members may have their own extension with their own messaging systems. This is separate from the main answering system. A call can be redirected to that extension and the caller can then leave a message for that individual only. Voicemail requires a password from the staff member to access his or her message.

4.4   Telephone Etiquette

- Answer the call within three rings.
- Clearly identify the doctors' office and then yourself.
- Answer your call with a smile.
- Speak clearly and slowly.
- Do not have candy or gum in your mouth.
- Concentrate on the call—do not let your mind wander.
- Listen actively.

THE TELEPHONE DIRECTORY

The administrative assistant's best reference source is the local telephone directory. Take time to go through it and note the wide variety of information available, not only about telephone services—local areas, long-distance charges, area codes, business hours—but for other available services such as government offices, yellow pages listings, and so on.

You should also set up your own office telephone directory, listing in it numbers you call frequently, such as drug stores, hospitals, laboratories, other doctors, ambulance and emergency services, the Victorian Order of Nurses or other home nursing services, social service/community agencies, and staff home telephone numbers.

A Cardex or Rolodex system is an efficient way to keep reference information such as referring physicians' names, addresses, identification numbers, and telephone numbers.

If you are using a computer, you can access alphabetized lists of frequently used information with one or two keystrokes.

If you have a speed dial feature on your telephone system, store the most frequently called numbers. Have an index of the stored numbers in a convenient location.

EQUIPMENT

Several companies offer sophisticated telephone equipment for business and industry. If you work in a private-practice setting with one or two physicians, you will probably have a telephone system with three or four incoming lines and a separate line and number for a fax machine. A hospital, clinic, or medical centre generally employs a receptionist/switchboard operator, and the equipment used in this type of setting is generally a multi-line device.

Modern telephones are programmed to allow you to do such things as dial a second number if the first number you called is busy; when the number you have called is free, your telephone will ring, at which time you can complete your call. Call waiting, redial, speed dial, caller identification, call forwarding, and call transfer are other telephone features that assist in the operation of an efficient office.

Fax Machines

Most medical offices have fax machines. In some cases these machines have replaced the use of the mail service. It is good practice to program frequently used numbers into the speed dial function. This will avoid confidential information being sent to the wrong location. Always use a cover sheet when sending anything over a fax machine. This sheet should have your doctor's name, address, phone number, and fax number clearly visible on it.

ASSIGNMENT 4.1

The following situations are designed for role play. Choose a partner, decide how you would handle the situation, and write the script. If possible, you should have a prop telephone for authenticity. You and your partner will then act out the scene, with one student playing the role of the administrative assistant and the other the role of the patient. The remainder of the class will observe, and a session to evaluate your performance should follow.

1. Mrs. Scott calls to inform you that Peter John has just rammed his head into a brick wall while pushing his brother on his bicycle. His head is bleeding profusely, and she thinks the child needs stitches. It is 4:30 p.m., and the doctor has just left to do rounds at the hospital.
2. Mary Shultz, who is extremely inebriated, calls and insists on speaking to the doctor. The office is full of patients, and the doctor is running behind schedule.
3. A woman calls and tells you her husband has locked himself in the bathroom and is threatening suicide. The doctor is out of town at a convention.
4. Thomas Bell calls and tells you his wife has just collapsed on the floor. He thinks she has had a stroke because her mouth seems to be twisted.
5. The doctor has asked you to take all calls because he is having a consultation with a patient who is on the verge of a nervous breakdown. Amelia Jackson calls and insists on speaking to the doctor.
6. Julie Harris calls and is at the point of hysteria. Her son, William, has a very high temperature and is convulsing. She lives 5 kilometres outside the city, her husband has taken the car to work, and she does not know any of the people who live in her neighbourhood. The doctor is not in the office.

7. The doctor's husband is on the phone wishing to speak with his wife. You know that he often calls without good reason, but he insists on speaking with the doctor.

8. Mr. and Mrs. Chang have recently arrived from Korea and their sponsor has asked Dr. Plunkett to take them into his practice. Mrs. Chang calls you to book an appointment; however, she is not fluent in English and you are having trouble understanding her.

9. A new patient (Rosa Geary) called two weeks ago and you booked her for an appointment. She did not come to the office for her appointment. She called the next day with an excuse and you booked her again. Again, she did not arrive for her scheduled appointment. She is now calling with an excuse and a request for another appointment.

10. Lori Brier (a single parent) was injured at work. Dr. Plunkett examined and treated her and sent the required forms to the Workplace Safety and Insurance Board (WSIB). Mrs. Brier calls. She is very anxious. She hasn't any money for rent and groceries. She has called WSIB and they have informed her that they haven't received the required documents from her doctor. You tell Mrs. Brier that you have sent the forms, but she doesn't believe you— she NEEDS MONEY NOW!

11. Dr. Plunkett has agreed to cover emergencies for Dr. Moore, who is going on vacation. Dr. Plunkett is doing rounds at the hospital when you receive a call from Tiffany Black, one of Dr. Moore's patients. (You don't know anything of her history.) She tells you she has attempted suicide twice in the past and is considering it again.

12. Gary Brown is schizophrenic and has been receiving treatment in the psychiatric ward of Ottawa Civic Hospital. You received a call from the hospital last week informing you that Gary had left the hospital and had not returned. Today you receive a call from Gary. He is in Florida. He doesn't have any money and he seems very confused.

ASSIGNMENT **4.2**

Appoint two members of your class to arrange to have a telephone equipment supplier in your area visit your classroom; or you may prefer to arrange a class tour of a telephone equipment supply office.

TOPICS FOR DISCUSSION

1. An institution calls stating they have admitted your patient and need information. You have no documented or prior knowledge of this admission. How would you handle the call?

2. You need to get in touch with a patient on an urgent basis but all you get is the answering machine that only gives the patient's phone number. What would you do?

3. A concerned mother calls and is sure that her daughter, who is 18, has an appointment with you today. She wants to leave a message for her. You know that the daughter does not want her mother to know about the office visit. How would you handle the call?

4. You have highly confidential information that a referral facility needs immediately. The only way to get it there is by fax machine. How would you ensure that the receiving facility gets the appropriate information?

5. Many phones have call display. You have called Mr. Baxter's home but the call went to the answering machine, which only identified the telephone number. You did not leave a message but his wife saw your number on the call display and is calling to see what the call was about. How would you respond?

CHAPTER 5

Office Correspondence: Mail, Memos, Letters, and Envelopes

CHAPTER OUTLINE

Mail
Postal Services
Courier Services
Electronic Equipment

Memos
Styles of Memo
Letters and Envelopes
Topics for Discussion

LEARNING OBJECTIVES

After reading this chapter, you will be able to outline

- How to handle incoming mail
- How to handle outgoing mail
- Confidentiality of electronic transmissions
- The varieties of delivery services

In this chapter, you will review

- The purpose of a memo
- Different styles of memo format
- Letter styles; block, modified block, and modified block with paragraph indentation
- Parts of a business letter
- Punctuation styles; all-point (closed), two-point (mixed), and no-point (open)
- Preparing envelopes

KEY TERMS

FRCPC: Designation used by licensed physicians that means Fellow of Royal College of Physicians in Canada. FRCSC stands for Fellow of Royal College of Surgeons in Canada. The "C" at the end of the designation signifies that the physician is a Fellow of the College in Canada.

Postage meter: Postage equipment that seals the envelope and stamps the appropriate selected postage on the envelope (upper right hand corner).

Proofreading: To review a written work for errors.

Salutation: The salutation is an act of greeting. Dear Dr. Plunkett, To Whom It May Concern, Dear Sir or Madam are the greetings extended from the letter writer to the recipient.

MAIL

One of your responsibilities as administrative assistant will be the handling of both incoming and outgoing mail (see Figure 5.1). Part of this responsibility is to prioritize the process. The physician wants to see only the mail that is pertinent to him or her. These are guidelines that should be discussed with your employer. It is essential that you become familiar with postal services, delivery services such as couriers, and electronic mailing equipment.

Much of the patient information that would previously have arrived in your office by mail or priority post is now being sent via the fax machine. Another mode of communicating information to your office is by the use of e-mail. Memos from medical organizations can be sent as an attachment and printed off when received if necessary. Many medical newsletters and journals are now available on the Internet, which eliminates the need to send them by mail.

FIGURE **5.1 Every medical office should have an established policy regarding the processing of incoming mail.**

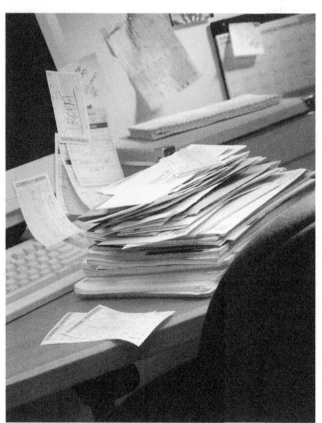

SOURCE: Eggers, D.A. & Conway, A.M. (2000). *Mosby's Front Office Skills for the Medical Assistant* (p. 195: Figure 8.2). St. Louis: Mosby.

Incoming Mail

Incoming mail consists of the following:

1. Correspondence (reports from consultants, legal claims, insurance claims)
2. Circulars
3. Magazines and medical journals
4. Medical information (from medical associations)
5. Cheques
6. Health insurance plan documents (supplies, updates, remittance advice information, diskettes, or medical consultants' inquiries)
7. Confidential mail
8. Laboratory, diagnostic imaging, other diagnostic reports and consultation reports
9. Hospital reports (admission, discharge, operative notes, etc.)
10. Advertisements and drug samples

On receipt of incoming mail, you should open all correspondence with the exception of envelopes specifically marked "confidential" or "personal." If any letters refer to previous correspondence, retrieve the relevant documents from the file and attach. The administrative assistant should date stamp each piece of mail, organize it in order of importance, and place it in the doctor's incoming mail tray or on his or her desk.

Prioritizing or sorting should be completed according to the importance or urgency with which the information should be handled. The following is an example of how you might prioritize:

1. Patient information (lab, X-ray, other diagnostic testing reports, and consultation reports)
2. Correspondence (special delivery, registered mail, or telegrams first)
3. Cheques, health insurance plan information, and supplies (disks)
4. Medical information
5. Drug samples
6. Medical journals, magazines, and circulars

All cheques must be stamped "For Deposit Only" (see Figure 7.8). Magazines (with the exception of the doctor's professional journals) can be placed in the waiting room, and inconsequential unsolicited mail goes in the wastebasket.

If a return address does not appear on the letter, check the envelope before discarding it. It is good practice to staple the envelope to any letters that arrive in the office. This eliminates the chance of the envelope being discarded, only to find that the return address is not on the correspondence when you are asked to respond to it.

Loose enclosures should be attached to the appropriate correspondence.

Enclosed cheques should be safely stored and a notation made on the accompanying letter to this effect.

After the doctor has read the mail, documents should be initialled to indicate they have been read and a notation made to indicate what action is required, e.g., file, discard, or reply. Patient information is usually flagged as "F" for file or "C" for chart to be pulled. By using this system there is no need to pull the charts for every piece of patient information when it arrives in your office.

5.1   Equipment Useful for Processing Mail

Letter opener
Date stamp
Stapler
Staple remover
Paper clips
Pen/pencil
Highlighter
In larger offices:
Postage machine with automatic sealer
Weigh scale
Postage guidelines

Outgoing Mail

Outgoing mail consists of the following:

1. Doctor's correspondence (replies to requests, doctor's inquiries, and information reports)
2. Health insurance submissions (disks)
3. Insurance information forms [Workplace Safety Insurance Board (WSIB), accident reports]
4. Referral letters
5. Referral requisitions
6. Supply requisitions and purchase orders
7. Patient account statements for uninsured services
8. Files of transferred patients (a photocopy of the complete chart or a résumé dictated by the doctor should be sent "confidential" by courier)

After the document is prepared, it should be appropriately assembled. A general rule of thumb is to place the original and enclosure, if any, on top of all copies together with an envelope. The completed mail pack should then be secured with a paper clip and placed on the doctor's desk for signature. In most medical offices it is the administrative assistant's responsibility to transcribe the physician's dictated letters and reports. Some physicians will use a voice recognition system. This system eliminates the need for a transcriptionist, as it formats the document as the physician dictates. Both require

proofreading before being mailed out, however. The spell-check option on your computer is not enough to ensure accuracy. The spell-check cannot differentiate between *ilium* and *ileum*, *through* and *threw*, or *to, too*, and *two*, for example. Proofread the document before giving it to the physician for final approval. After it has been read and signed, the completed correspondence will be returned to you for mailing.

Remember, it is essential that you retain a *dated copy* of *all* documents. It may be useful to keep general correspondence in a correspondence file or binder. All patient-related documents would be filed in the patient's chart.

Fold and insert documents in the appropriate size envelope (see Figure 5.10) and seal. Make sure that if an enclosure is part of the package, you remember to include it before sealing the envelope.

Stamps should be available in the office for regular mail. Some larger offices may use a **postage meter**. If using a postage meter you need to check daily the amount of postage available. The postage is added to the meter by the post office. This can be done electronically. Larger packages may require a visit to the post office. If you are in doubt about the mailing of any correspondence, consult your local postal authorities.

Pickup time at the nearest mailbox (or by internal mail in a large organization) should be investigated. It is your responsibility to ensure that urgent mail reaches the box or the internal mail room in time to be collected that day.

POSTAL SERVICES

Canada Post offers many types of mail-handling services. Important letters and other documents can be sent "registered" or by Priority Post, which gives overnight delivery; valuable parcels can be "insured"; sealed letters and postcards are sent "first class"; parcels may be sent "parcel post"; "second class" mail is used for some newspapers and periodicals; small parcels and printed matter would be sent "third class." Because Canada Post's services and rates are extensive, and subject to frequent change, we will not elaborate any further. Most administrative assistants, if they are uncertain about the method to use in forwarding material by mail, will consult the local postal authorities or access the Canada Post web site (http://www.canadapost.ca.).

COURIER SERVICES

To ensure prompt and safe delivery of special letters and parcels, many businesses use courier services. Although using a courier is more expensive than regular mail services, it guarantees prompt delivery—often overnight. When using couriers, such as Purolator or FedEx, each package is given an identification number. This allows you to trace your package if it does not arrive within the required time frame. It is important that you keep a log of mail that is delivered by one of these services. Courier services are listed in the yellow pages of the telephone directory. It is important for the efficient administrative assistant to be aware of the cost of courier services and to use them with discretion.

Most communities have intercity courier and lab services that will pick up correspondence, specimens and drugs to be transported between physicians' offices and laboratories, and hospitals. Medical administrative assistants should know the names and scope of service of such courier services in their locality. If it is necessary to send specimens or drugs by mail, there are specific rules that must be followed. Check with your local postal authorities before placing such materials in the mail. The courier services will also have guidelines for transporting these materials.

ELECTRONIC EQUIPMENT

More and more medical professionals are utilizing computer network systems that allow communication of medical information among offices and hospitals. Many large medical offices have computer networks that allow communication from office to office. Letters, memos, and reports are keyed into a computer terminal and can be received by another user within the same network. Messages and memos can be sent by e-mail to one individual or a large number of individuals in the time it takes to key the information and have it transmitted to the receiving terminal—a matter of minutes (see Box 5.3).

Hospitals and large medical clinics may have a transcription department or designated transcription employees for each physician or diagnostic service. All the transcription is done within the clinic/hospital and is accessible via the individual office computers. This eliminates the need to mail or send out this information. The administrative assistant needs only to identify the patient and choose the note or report required. In some medical clinics, all external correspondence and reports received are scanned into the computer system by the administrative assistant at the discretion of the physician they are addressed to. Any office within the clinic can access this information, therefore creating an almost paperless office environment.

Hospital departments can access required lab, diagnostic imaging, admission, discharge, and operative/procedure reports through the departmental computers. This eliminates the need to call the departments for results or for the department to use the internal mail. In some areas, two or more hospitals may be linked by the same computer network, therefore making it possible to retrieve information from each facility in the same way. Confidentiality checks are run frequently to ensure that patient information is not being accessed by unauthorized personnel.

ASSIGNMENT 5.1

This assignment is designed as a group project. Choose one of these three delivery services—the post, electronic mail, or courier—and write a report outlining all aspects of the service. Assign specific duties to each student; for example, two students may be responsible for gathering the material, two may be responsible for organizing and writing the information, and one or two may be responsible for keying. Prepare the information in an attractive form and have copies produced for each member of the class. Students responsible for gathering the information will contact a courier service or visit the post office to determine details of regular mail and electronic mail services. Prepare a summary of the service, including points such as the name of the service, how it is provided, where the service extends (intercity/country to country), the cost of the service, preparations necessary before using the service, and so on.

ASSIGNMENT **5.2**

Research how medical environments in your community handle incoming and outgoing mail, and prepare a report on your findings.

In order to accomplish this, form into groups, develop a simple questionnaire, and distribute it to your target audience.

Don't forget to request information on the current use of mail technology, such as e-mail and fax.

Insert your report in your portfolio.

The purpose of the next two sections of this chapter is to provide a reference and instructional guide, or both, for producing memos, letters, and envelopes. It is assumed that students have had previous instruction on the appropriate formats for these documents. If you have not received such instruction, however, we have provided practice exercise assignments. Some of these assignments contain deliberate errors, which you are expected to correct.

Tasks that were once performed on a typewriter are now prepared using computer software, such as word processing programs and integrated packages that include spreadsheets, word processing, data base, medical billing, appointment scheduling, and others.

MEMOS

The most informal type of written communication is a memo. Three acceptable memo styles will be reviewed below. A memo can be a handwritten note scribbled on a piece of paper. Producing the note with the date, name of the sender, and receiver formalizes the message.

Most business organizations send informal messages in a memo form. The most common mode of relaying these messages is through departmental e-mail. Another option is to produce the memo, photocopy it, and then distribute either through internal mail or the postal service. Either way, a copy is kept by the sender for future reference and filing.

Although there are several acceptable styles for memo headings, most headings consist of the elements that appear in Box 5.2.

5.2

To (the name of the recipient)
From (the name of the sender)
Date (the date the message is produced)
Subject (what the message is about)

The body of the memo is generally single-spaced, but can be double-spaced if the message is short. (If double-spaced, indent the beginning of each paragraph five spaces.) Initials of the person who produced the memo appear at the left margin, a double-space below the last line of the message.

If four or five people are to receive the memo, key all names on the memo beside "To" and place a check mark or an arrow opposite the appropriate name or highlight the name with a marker when distributing or mailing the finished memo.

In today's medical office environment, most memos are created and distributed by e-mail. Multiple recipients can be selected from the e-mail address book. The memo can be produced and distributed to all recipients with one key stroke. When the recipient has opened the memo the program can then notify you of receipt of the e-mail. Proper language and spelling are to be used when sending memos. The memo should look professional.

5.3   E-Mail Etiquette for the Professional Office

MIND YOUR MANNERS
- Remember the basic rules of please and thank you
- Address people you do not know as Mr., Mrs., Dr., etc.

WATCH YOUR TONE
- You want to come across as respectful and friendly. You do not want to sound curt or demanding. Using ALL CAPS indicates shouting.

BE CONCISE
- Get to the point of your e-mail quickly without leaving out important details.

BE PROFESSIONAL
- Do not use abbreviations or emoticons (i.e., those little smiley faces ☺). **Use correct spelling and proper grammar.**
- Use a dictionary or spell-checker.
- Pay attention to basic rules of grammar.

ASK BEFORE SENDING AN ATTACHMENT
- Many people will not open an attachment unless they know the sender, due to the proliferation of computer viruses. Before sending an attachment, ask the recipient for permission.

WAIT TO FILL IN THE "TO" E-MAIL ADDRESS
- To prevent accidentally sending your e-mail before it is completed, fill in the "TO" e-mail address last. It is very easy to accidentally click on the "Send" icon when you really intended to click on the "Attachment" icon.

STYLES OF MEMO

Headings and body styles of the following memo forms can be interchanged to produce a style that is appealing and acceptable to your employer/physician.

Style I

The headings are placed flush with the left margin with enough space allowed for the rest of the information (names, date, and subject) to be blocked as well. Double-space between heading lines and triple-space before the memo message. Single-space the body (double-space if the message is short) and double-space between paragraphs. Initials are typed at the left margin, a double-space below the last line of the message.

Note that there is no formal signature line on a memo because the sender's name appears in the memo headings. A memo produced on 21.5-cm (8½-inch) paper usually has approximately 4-cm (1½-inch) margins.

Style I is shown in Figure 5.2.

Style II

Headings are placed as in Style I, except the longest line (subject) is keyed flush with the left margin and the last letters of the heading titles are aligned. The body is single-spaced with five-space paragraph indentation.

Style II is shown in Figure 5.3.

Style III

"To" and "Subject" are placed flush with the left margin; "From" and "Date" begin at the centre point. The headings can be rearranged, for example, "To" and "From" at the left margin and "Subject" and "Date" at the centre. Note that, depending on its length, a memo can be double-spaced. Paragraphs would then be indented five spaces at the beginning (see Figure 5.4).

FIGURE **5.2**   **Memo Style I**

TO: Dr. J.E. Plunkett

FROM: Dr. M.C. Scott

DATE: (current date)

SUBJECT: Mrs. Hazel Davis

Thank you for referring Mrs. Davis, who certainly appears to have an epidermoid cyst behind the right ear.

I will be making an arrangement for the removal of this, under general anaesthesia as an outpatient at the Ottawa General Hospital.

/ti

FIGURE **5.3** **Memo Style II**

> TO: Dr. E.J. Pelham
>
> FROM: Dr. M.C. Scott
>
> DATE: (current date)
>
> SUBJECT: Mrs. Hazel Davis
>
>   Mrs. Davis is scheduled to have an epidermoid cyst removed from behind her right ear. Surgery is scheduled for September 30, 20___ at 9 a.m. in operating room 4 at Ottawa General Hospital.
>
>   I would appreciate it if you would administer the anaesthetic during surgery. Please advise if the date and time fit in with your schedule.
>
> /ti

FIGURE **5.4** **Memo Style III**

> TO: Dr. M.C. Scott   FROM: Dr. E.J. Pelham
>
> SUBJECT: Mrs. Hazel Davis   DATE: (current date)
>
>   I will be pleased to administer anaesthetic on Mrs. Hazel Davis during surgery and will be in
>
> operating room 4 at O.G.H. on September 30, 20___ at 9 a.m.
>
> /ti

ASSIGNMENT **5.3**

Produce the following memo using each of the three different styles mentioned previously. Check for correct spelling and paragraphing.

   Dr. Plunkett has asked you to send a memo to the Ottawa Hospital Board of Directors informing them that the annual board dinner meeting will be on December 1, 20__, at the Holiday Inn in the Wilfrid Laurier Room. Dinner will be served at 6 p.m.; meeting at 8 p.m. Members are asked to be prepared to present their annual reports.

   Compose the memo and present it in an appropriate style. Submit the assignment for assessment.

Produce the following memos using Style I for the first memo, Style II for the second, and Style III for the third.

Memo to JEP From Dr. W. Parks Subject: Bob Baxter.

Thank you for referring the above named patient who certainly appears to have an infected chilagion on the right upper eyelid. I have as of the present time treated him with antibiotics and will be reviewed in a week's time. ~~P~~ He also has been booked for some cutanery excisional surgery as an outpatient at O.G.H.

To. Dr ESP From Dr. T Hicks Sub. L. Elliott

Mrs. Elliott was reviewed in my off. today after being referred by Dr. ~~John~~ Elmer Plunkett. At this time she has a large ulceration on the lateral aspect of her left leg, just above the lateral malleous. I will arrange to have her admitted for surgery next week. ~~for~~ Will you be available to administer anaesthetic?

Write a memo to above stating I will be available any day next week except. Wed.

ESP.

LETTERS AND ENVELOPES

We will now review letter styles, punctuation styles, parts of a business letter, envelope addressing, and folding and inserting. The material used will allow you to observe how medical correspondence is composed in the medical office environment and how medical terminology is applied to communication documents.

Inappropriate format, misspelled words, and improper use of grammar will reflect on your office. Your professional reputation as well as your physicians' office expectations can be judged on the type of correspondence that is distributed by your office. Be sure to proofread all correspondence before it is sent out. Do not depend on your computer's spell-check function for accuracy.

Letter Styles

Several styles of letters have been used over the years. At one time, the very formal indented style was used extensively. Since the advent of the computer, letter styles have become more simplified and the indention of paragraphs is seldom used.

Block Style—This is the easiest style to remember. All lines begin at the left margin. Figure 5.5 is an example of the block format.

Modified Block Style—The body, inside address, and **salutation** of the letter are identical to the block style. But the date, complimentary closing, writer's name, and title all begin at the centre of the page (see Figure 5.6).

Modified Block Style with Paragraph Indentation—This style is the same as modified block but the first line of each paragraph is indented five spaces. This can either be done with the space bar or by simply using the tab function.

Spacing

A letter properly arranged on the page should resemble a picture in a frame. This effect is achieved by using proper line lengths and by correctly spacing between parts of the letter.

The letterhead usually occupies the first ten to twelve lines of the paper. Depending on the length of the letter, you may prefer to begin the date on the fourteenth or fifteenth line and adjust your spacing between the date and the inside address, or you may adjust the position of your letter by always leaving five or six spaces between the date and inside address and placing the date according to the length of the letter.

FIGURE **5.5** **Block Letter Style–Open Punctuation**

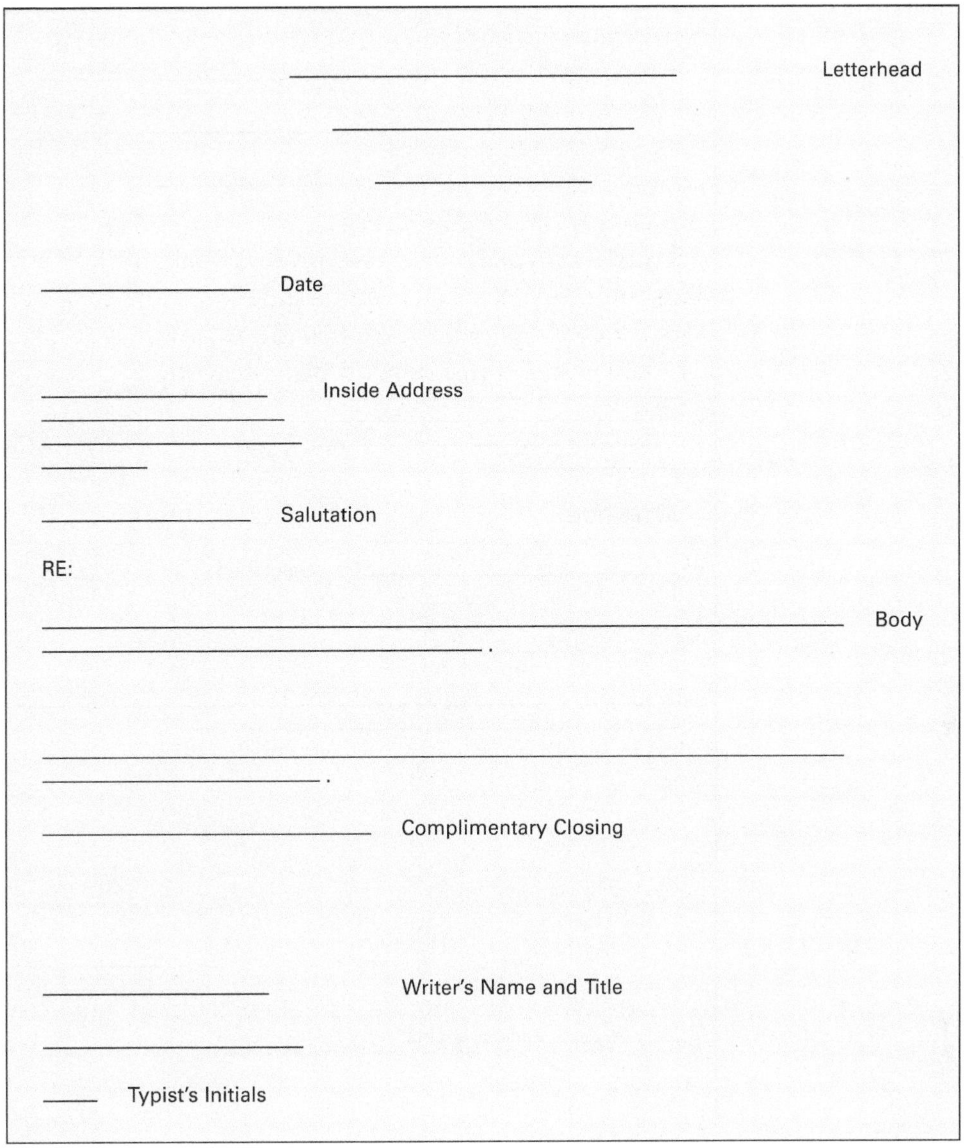

_____ Letterhead

_____

_____

_____ Date

_____ Inside Address
_____
_____
_____

_____ Salutation

RE:

_____ Body
_____ .

_____
_____ .

_____ Complimentary Closing

_____ Writer's Name and Title

_____

_____ Typist's Initials

Box 5.4

An efficient administrative assistant does not spend time calculating line lengths and spaces. You should assess the letter to be produced and position it according to your assessment.

Computer programs will allow you to view the whole document on your screen before printing. You can then assess your work and make appropriate adjustments.

FIGURE **5.6 Modified Block Style–Mixed Punctuation**

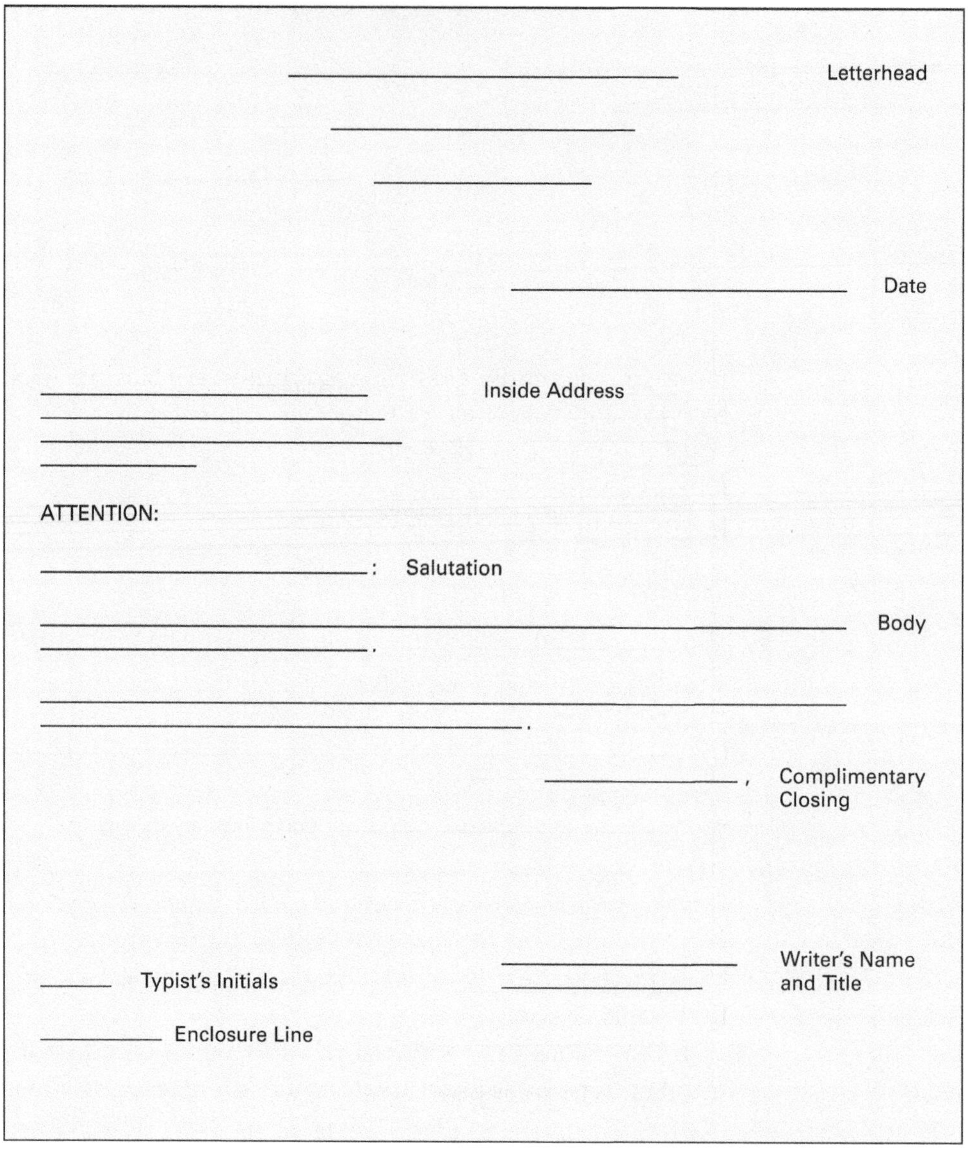

_____   Letterhead

_____

_____

_____   Date

_____   Inside Address
_____
_____
_____

ATTENTION:

_____: Salutation

_____   Body
_____.

_____
_____.

_____,   Complimentary
Closing

_____   Writer's Name
_____   and Title

___   Typist's Initials

_____   Enclosure Line

Punctuation Styles

The two accepted styles of punctuation are open (no-point) and mixed (two-point). Punctuation styles do not pertain to the body of the letter. They deal only with the date, inside address, salutation, complimentary closing, and the writer's name and title lines (all short lines).

Open Punctuation—This is also referred to as no-point because there is no punctuation after any short line. This style is generally used with the block style shown in Figure 5.5.

Mixed Punctuation—Mixed punctuation style, or two-point punctuation, means there is punctuation at two points in the letter: a colon after the salu-

FIGURE **5.7**   **Second Page—Block or Modified Block Style**

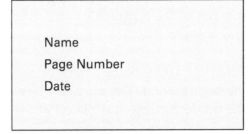

> Name
>
> Page Number
>
> Date

tation and a comma after the complimentary closing. Mixed punctuation can be used with any style of letter (see Figure 5.6).

While it is acceptable to use any style of punctuation with any style of letter, general practice is to use the simplest style (open) with block style letters and mixed with the modified block styles.

Two-Page Letters

When producing letters with more than one page, place the name of the recipient, the page number, and the date at the top of the second and succeeding pages. If referring to a patient, replace the recipient's name with "Re (patient's name)" or keep both names. When you are producing a medical note (Consultation Note, History, and Physical Note) include the type of note on the second and any succeeding pages under the patient name. If the second page is preprinted with a company name, begin keying three or four lines below the heading. If plain paper is used for the second page, begin keying on line six or seven. Triple-space before continuing with the body of the letter. Most letters will only have letterhead information on the first page.

If the block or modified block style is used, place the name, page number, type of note, and date at the left margin, single-spaced, as shown in Figure 5.7.

Parts of a Business Letter

Letterhead—The essential parts of the letterhead are the name and address of the office, and should also include the telephone number, and fax number, as well as other physicians in the clinic. Many offices use good-quality bond paper on which the letterhead is preprinted. Medical offices usually use ordinary bond paper for their correspondence (this is physician preference), with the letterhead only on the first page. Many companies have preprinted second-page stationery. (The second page is usually preprinted with only the firm's name.)

Date—The date is generally placed three or four lines below the letterhead and includes the month, day, and year. Most computer programs will insert the date automatically when producing a letter.

Inside Address—This is placed at least four and as many as ten or twelve lines below the date, depending on the length of the letter. The inside address consists of the recipient's name, title (if any), street address, city, province, and postal code.

Attention Line—Some letters are sent to the attention of a specific person in the organization. The attention line is double-spaced below the last line of the inside address and placed at the left margin. The position of the attention line is shown in Figure 5.6. The attention line is often in bold font.

Salutation—The salutation is double-spaced after the last line of the inside address or attention line, if used. When a letter is addressed to a company and contains an attention line, or both, the salutation is usually Gentlemen, Ladies and Gentlemen, or Dear Sir or Madam. When the letter is addressed to an individual, the salutation is Dear Dr. Plunkett, Dear Mr. Smith, Dear Ms. Jones, or Dear Jim.

Subject or Reference Line—Some writers identify the letter's subject in a reference line, which appears a double space below the salutation. The reference line is placed at the left margin (see Figure 5.5). In the medical environment, letters contain the patient's name and date of birth in the reference line. Any other pertinent identifying information, for example, a health insurance number or a workers' compensation claim number, should follow the date of birth.

Body—The body of the letter begins a double space below the reference line (or the salutation if there is no reference line). The body is generally single-spaced with a double-space between paragraphs. The body of the letter should contain at least two paragraphs.

Complimentary Closing—The closing is placed two spaces below the last line of the body of the letter. "Yours truly" and "Sincerely" are the most commonly used closings for business letters. Only the first word of the closing is capitalized.

Signature Block—This contains the writer's name and title. A space (not less than three or more than five spaces) after the complimentary closing is left for the signature, and the writer's name is placed below this space. The title line(s) should be single-spaced after the writer's name. A doctor's name is usually followed by his or her degree but not preceded by "Dr," e.g., "J. Plunkett, M.D., **FRCPC**."

Reference Initials—There are several styles used when keying reference initials. At one time, the writer's initials followed by the typist's initials was the preferred style, as in ABC/DEF or ABC:def. However, since the writer's name is already at the end of the letter, the initials of the person producing the letter are all that are required (/def, :def, or def.). Initials are placed at the left margin, usually two spaces below the signature block. In large transcription departments (or even in a multiple employee office) where many individuals are producing the documents, the initials help to identify the transcriptionist if any follow up is needed.

Enclosures—If a document is enclosed with the letter, a reference to the enclosure is made either single- or double-spaced below the reference initials. If more than one document is enclosed, the number may appear after the word "enclosures." Some styles of enclosure lines follow:

> Enclosure
> Encl.
> Enclosures (3)
> Enclosures—Policy
> Cheque
> Questionnaire

Copy Notations—If copies of a letter are being sent to people other than the addressee, a copy notation must be included. Copy notations are placed a double-space below the last line of a letter, that is, the producer's initials or enclosure line. The copy notation comes before the postscript.

Figure 5.8 shows an example of the method for making copy notations.

Postscript (P.S.)—The postscript can be used to express an important afterthought. The postscript appears at the very end of the letter, a double space below the last keyed line.

5.5   Parts of a Business Letter

Letterhead
Date
Inside address
Attention line (if applicable)
Salutation
Subject or reference line (if applicable)
Body
Complimentary closing
Signature block
Reference initials
Enclosure (if applicable)
Copy notations (if applicable)
Postscripts (if applicable)

FIGURE **5.8** **Copy Notations**

lbp
Enclosure

c: J.E. Smith – Accounting Dept.
      R.S. Green – Bell Clinic

bc: Dr. M.R. Dantzer – Psychiatric Department

ASSIGNMENT **5.5**

Produce the following letters on appropriate letterhead. For Letter 1 use block style, open punctuation; for Letter 2 use modified block style, mixed punctuation; and for Letter 3 use block style with open punctuation.

Letter 1

From Doctor Pelham to Dr. H.A. Schmidt, 33 Block Avenue, Ottawa, Ontario, J5Z 3Y7. Reference Mrs. Lisa Basciano. Mrs. Basciano whom we thought had an acute carpal tunnel syndrome on the right wrist was reviewed in my office today. I presume you have the E.M.G. report with you and those indicate normal tracing with no evidence of any compression of the median nerve at the wrist. Also, clinically today, when I examined her, she seems to have normal sensation but with the occasional pain and tenderness whenever she lifts heavy objects. I think she should be left alone and periodically reviewed.

Letter 2

From Doctor Plunkett to Dr. R.J. Mahon, Bell Clinic, 377 Unger Street, Ottawa, Ontario, J5Z 5X8. Subject Peter J. Scott. Thank you for referring me to see Peter John who certainly has a lesion on his upper lip, as well as a possible intradermal naevus on the temporal areas. I will be making an arrangement for the removal of this under local anaesthesia (Loc. or L/A) as an out-patient at the O.G.H. I am enclosing a reference report on this patient.

Letter 3

From Doctor Pelham to Heavenly Haven Home for the Aged, R.R. 3, Kars, Ontario A7W 5S3. Attention: Mr. R.J. Seymour, Administrator. Re: Mr. Mel Thompson. Mr. Thompson was reviewed in my office today, regarding his persistence of having an operative procedure of blepharoplasty done on his lower eyelids. I certainly appreciate the bagginess of his bilateral lower eyelids, and he tells me they are impairing his vision because they are dragging his lower eyelids down. Dr. Blenkan, medical consultant for MOH, did phone me that it has been approved in May 20__ and I could carry out the procedure of bilateral lower blepharoplasty with this approval. I will be making an arrangement for him to be admitted to the Ottawa General Hospital and carry out the procedure of bilateral blepharoplasty and reconstruct the orbital septum.

Letters 4, 5, and 6

Produce Letter 4 using modified block style and mixed punctuation, Letter 5 using block style and open punctuation, and Letter 6 using block style and mixed punctuation. Use proper sentence structure and paragraphing. Correct *all* spelling errors.

Keep Letters 1 to 6 for use in Assignment 5.6.

Letter 4

Dear Dr. Pelham

→Subject latent Syphilis

It has been brought to my attention by the Ont. Min. of Health that many cases of latent syphilis are becoming evident in your people. These are persons who have been treated for

Insert * →gonorrhaie but without having blood taken for possible syphilis being present concurrently. By doing syphilis serology (when positive) adequate doseges of antibiotics can be administered which will control together both gonorrhaea and syphilis. This will prevent the later fatal complications of syphilis, including neurosyphilis. It will also prevent the further spread of syphilis which is increasing each year.

Your cooperation will be of great assistance.

*Insert - treatment for gonorrhaea above is at a level which temporarily can mask syphilis but not control it

JN Brownd MDCN
DDH
Med. Off. of Health

Letter 5

From Med. Off. of Health as above to Dr. Plunkett. Re. Birth Control Clinics. Recently it was suggested to us by the Ont. Min. of Health that we open a birth control clinic with spec. emphasis on our teenage pop. The abortion rate in Ontario arising at an alarming rate. Since ab. as ~~togi~~ a failure of birth control the best method of avoiding abortion is to give instr. on b.c. At its last meeting our Bd. of Health approved the opening of a b.c. Since in our health unit. This clinic will open in ~~Sept~~ Oct. We shall be asking our physicians to man this clinic since it will be on Wed. afternoon. There is remuneration for each case attended. For full details will you please call Elizabeth Myles at 745-7677.

Letter 6

To: Kenmar Ins.
Co. Ltd.

327 Crown Dr.
Ottawa

Re: Lois Elliott
Accident Feb. 9,
20___

(This letter was
actually mailed by a
medical secretary)

Thank you for your letter dated May 6, 20___ regarding _____ _____. I had seen her in the Emergency Department at the Ottawa General Hospital on February 9, 20___, at the request of Dr. _____. She was involved in a motor vehicle accident with crush avulsion injury involving the forehead along with multiple pieces of glass (foreing bodies) in the skin and subcutaneous tissues. She was taken to the operating room the same day and the procedure of debridement and plastic reconstruction along with removal of the foreing

She was kept in the hospital from February 9, 20___ to February 13, 20___. During this period, she did well, with good recovery, along with good wound healing. She was reviewed after being discharged from the hospital in my office for a follow-up. The sutures were removed, the wound was healing well and naturally the scars were visible. She had a palpable, tender, painful foreign body in the form of a glass piece in the forehead and she was taken to the O.R. on September 12, 20___ and this was removed under general anaesthesia (G/A) as an out-patient at the O.G.H. Since then, she has been followed up and her progress has be satisfactory.

She was reviewed in my office on May 28, 20___ for the purpose of this information to you. Mrs. _____ says that _____ complains of headaches, dizziness, occassionally. To my knowledge, she did not have any head injury at the time of the accident. I attribute this headache and dizziness symptoms are probably due to the lacerations she had sustained to the forehead. However, if the symptoms persist and she continues to have problems and a neurological consultation is necessary. The scars are visible and she likes to have the forehead scars covered by a type of hairdo.

continued

She feels the scars are rough and visible. On examination she has a visible scar which is irregular and almost resembles a hockey stick running from right side forehead hairline and obliquely towards nose and then turning horizontally above the nose in the center of the forehead then again up toward the scalp. The whole area approximately measures 7-8 cm in oblique pattern. There is still marked roughness and irregularity on her forehead. The area is hyperaemic and and certain parts break open due to the instability of the epithelium. This, I think, will gradually epithelialize in time. The irregularity of the area may be improved by the way of dermabrasion in about 6 months or 1 year's time. She does not appear to have numbness or a tingling sensation distal to the laceration indicating that the nerves on her forehead are intact and injuries were mostly superficial in the way of abrasion of skin and subcutaneous tissue only.

The skull bones and facial bones are all intact and normal. The maxilla and mandibles are also intact and with good occlusion of the teeth.

In summary, this young lady was involved in a motor vehicle accident and injuries were confined to her forehead. There were abrasions and lacerations which were treated and repaired. There were foreign bodies removed and repaired. She is still left with a visible, irregular, rough, scar on her forehead. I think in 6 months to a year's time, she needs to be re-assessed and if I thing she needs to have any dry skin surface abrasion surgery, I will be considering it. The disability at the resent time is a visible, irregular, roughened scar on the forehead. There will be some of this persistent for a long time.

I hope this report will be of help to you and accompanied is the account in the amount of $_____.

Letter 6, cont'd

Envelopes

The two sizes of envelopes most commonly used are no. 8 and no. 10. A no. 8 envelope measures approximately 16.5 cm x 9 cm ($6\frac{1}{2}$ inches x $3\frac{5}{8}$ inches), and a no. 10 envelope is approximately 24 cm x 10.5 cm ($9\frac{1}{2}$ inches x $4\frac{1}{8}$ inches).

The address on the envelope should duplicate the letter both in name and address and in punctuation style.

FIGURE **5.9**   **Envelope Set-Up**

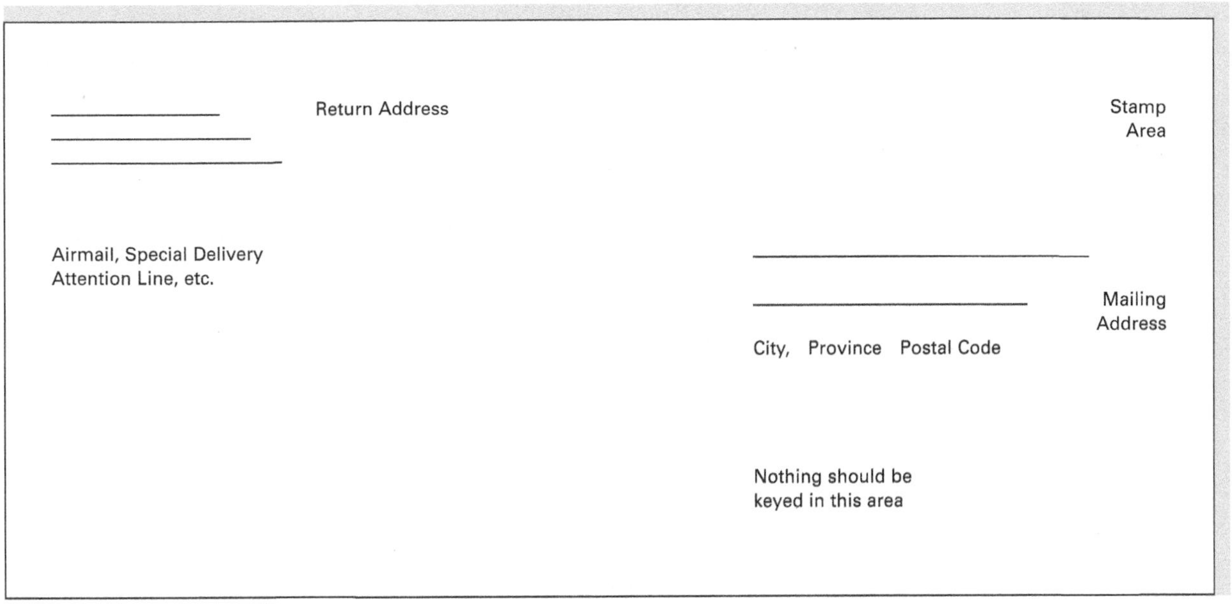

Return Address

Stamp
Area

Airmail, Special Delivery
Attention Line, etc.

_____

_____   Mailing
Address

City,   Province   Postal Code

Nothing should be
keyed in this area

Computer programs have a label function. Some programs can produce the labels to a pre-programmed label printer. Others will allow you to create the label free text.

Most addresses are single-spaced. The address consists of the name of the recipient, the title (if any), street address or post office box number, city or town, and province. The postal code is keyed two spaces after the province on the same line. Regardless of the style of punctuation used, there is no punctuation after the postal code. Nothing should be placed opposite, or in the space below, the postal code. Special mailing instructions, attention lines, and so on are usually placed two or three spaces below the return address (see Figure 5.9).

When folding a letter for insertion into a no. 8 envelope, place the letter on the desk facing you and fold from bottom to top to within roughly 0.5 cm ($\frac{1}{4}$ inch); fold from the right one-third to the left and fold from the left to within roughly 1 cm ($\frac{1}{2}$ inch) of the right edge. With the envelope opening facing you, insert left creased edge first with the open side facing toward you.

When folding a letter for insertion in a no. 10 envelope, you may do as follows: with the letter on the desk facing you, fold from bottom to top one-third of the way and from top to bottom to within roughly 1 cm ($\frac{1}{2}$ inch) of the first creased edge. Insert the last creased edge toward the bottom of the envelope. Or, with the letter on the desk facing you, fold from bottom to top one-third of the way, turn the letter over, and fold the top edge down over the first crease approximately 1 cm ($\frac{1}{2}$ inch). Insert with the overlap to the top of the envelope.

The second method of folding eliminates the risk of the recipient cutting the letter in two with a letter opener.

When folding a letter to fit a window envelope, bring the bottom third of the letter up and make a crease, then fold the top of the letter back to the crease. The inside address should be facing you. Insert the correspondence. The inside address should appear in the window. (See Figure 5.10 for folding instructions.)

Remember to insert any required enclosures before sealing the envelope.

FIGURE **5.10   Correct Methods of Folding Letters**

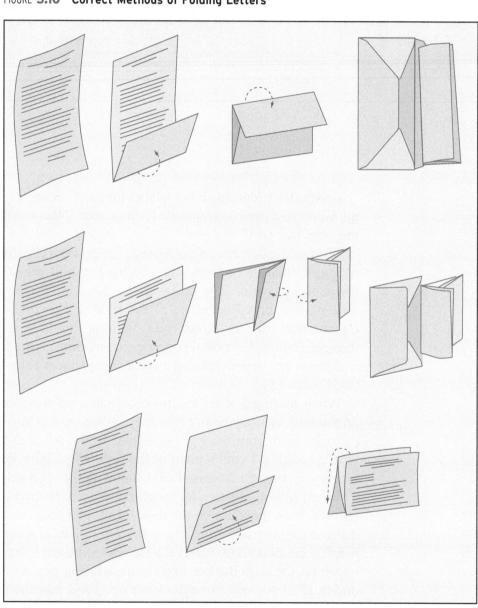

SOURCE: Young, A.P. (2003). *Kinn's The Administrative Medical Assistant: An Applied Learning Approach* 5th ed. (p. 215: Figure 12-6). St. Louis: Elsevier/Saunders.

ASSIGNMENT **5.6**

Dr. Plunkett has sent the following letter to Mr. Ronald Gilmour, 3279 Circle Square, Ottawa, J5X 7W4. Mr. Gilmour is about to be discharged from the hospital following a heart attack. Dr. Plunkett has asked you to send a copy of the letter to Dr. Pelham and to Dr. E.S. Langan at the heart clinic. Produce the required copies.

Once you are discharged from the hospital, you should continue to add activities according to the schedule I have given you. It would be helpful to yourself if you established realistic weekly goals of activity or other alternatives of lifestyle that are important for your heart's health. For example, make a contract with a family member that you will lose one kilogram each week for a month, or you will walk a set distance every day, reduce cigarette consumption by one cigarette per day until you stop. You may help someone else besides yourself! Continue with your activity program even after complete recovery. Whatever form of activity you choose, remember, it must be performed a minimum of three times a week to be of any benefit. You are well on the way to recovery and if you follow the instructions I have given you, a full recovery and resumption of normal activities is expected.

TOPICS FOR DISCUSSION

1.   You have mail that arrives in your office stamped "URGENT/CONFIDENTIAL." Your employer is at a conference and will not return to the office for a week. The letter looks important. What would you do?

2.   You suspect that someone has accessed confidential information from your computer while you were assisting the physician with a procedure. You had not signed off your terminal, therefore it will appear under your sign-on, which then makes you responsible if the information was not related to your position. What would you do?

CHAPTER 6

Health Insurance Plans

CHAPTER OUTLINE

LEARNING OBJECTIVES

After reading this chapter, you will be able to

- Understand provincial eligibility for a health-care plan.
- Appreciate the similarities and differences between provinces.
- Understand the format of the physician's fee schedule and how to use the information it provides.
- Demonstrate knowledge of submitting health claims.
- Develop the ability to interpret remittance advice and understand the reprocessing of returned claims.

- Understand the implications of error codes.
- Understand physician responsibility, employee responsibility, employer responsibility, and medical administrative assistant's responsibility when processing a Workers' Compensation Board (WCB) claim.
- Understand the process for out-of-province claim submissions.
- Develop an awareness of grants or assistance that may be available for patients.

KEY TERMS

Diagnostic code: The diagnostic code identifies the reason the patient is seen by the provider. The code is usually three to four numeric characters. Most services require a diagnostic code when processing a healthcare claim.

Physician registration number: The physician registration number is a unique number assigned to each physician by the Ministry of Health in the province in which they are practising. This number is also known as the physician billing number.

Remittance advice: The remittance advice is an itemized statement of the individual payments made by the Ministry of Health for insured services.

Service code: The service code identifies the service that was provided by the physician or healthcare provider to the patient. It is found in the provincial fee schedule and must be submitted when processing a healthcare claim.

INTRODUCTION

Adequate medical care can be very costly, especially for accident victims, the chronically ill, and those needing surgery. In order to minimize these expenses, Canada has instituted a universal healthcare plan. This protection came about through the enactment of the *Medical Care Act*, introduced by Prime Minister Lester B. Pearson during the 1966/67 session of Parliament. This Act was replaced by the *Canada Health Act* of 1984.

Each province has its own government-sponsored plan, for example, Nova Scotia's Medical Services Insurance (MSI) program, British Columbia's Medical Services Plan (MSP), the Alberta Health Care Insurance Plan (AHCIP), and Ontario's Health Insurance Plan (OHIP).

Most features—eligibility and enrollment, out-of-province benefits, payment options, and the fact that the plan pays only for *medically necessary* services—are almost identical.

Complete information on processing of claims, physician and subscriber registration, and eligibility can be obtained through your provincial Ministry of Health (MOH) office or through each province's government Web site.

Pertinent information to complete a billing (claim) includes physician identification, patient identification (including registration number), date of service, service codes, service fee, **diagnostic codes** (where applicable), admission date, and facility number. If the patient has been referred by another provider, that providers' number is also included.

ELIGIBILITY

As mentioned previously, eligibility for most provinces is similar. The following are some of the provincial guidelines and Web sites:

Ontario (OHIP–Ontario Health Insurance Plan)

An applicant must meet the following criteria:

- Must be a Canadian citizen or have immigration status as set out in Ontario's *Health Insurance Act*
- Must have a permanent and principal home in Ontario
- Must be physically present in Ontario 153 days in any 12-month period

Coverage normally becomes effective three months after the date of established residency in Ontario. (See http://www.gov.on.ca for further details.)

British Columbia (MSP–Medical Services Plan)

An applicant must be a resident of British Columbia and meet the following criteria:

- Must be a Canadian citizen or be lawfully entitled to Canada for permanent residence
- Must make his or her home in British Columbia
- Must be physically present in British Columbia at least six months in a calendar year.

All dependants of MSP beneficiaries are eligible for coverage if they are residents of British Columbia

Coverage normally becomes effective after a waiting period which normally consists of the balance of the month of arrival plus two months. (See http://www.gov.bc.ca for further details.)

New Brunswick (Medicare)

An applicant must meet the following criteria:

- Must be a Canadian citizen or be legally entitled to remain in Canada
- Must have a permanent residence in New Brunswick

- Must physically reside in New Brunswick for at least 6 months (183 days—consecutive or not) during a 12-month period

Coverage becomes effective after a three-month waiting period, which is legislated under New Brunswick's *Medical Services Payment Act*, and no exemption can be made. (See http://www.gov.nb.ca for further details.)

Saskatchewan (Saskatchewan Health Benefits)

An applicant must meet the following criteria:

- Must have a permanent residence in Saskatchewan
- Must ordinarily live in the province for at least six months a year
- Must be registered with Health Registration at Saskatchewan Health to be eligible for benefits

As a general rule, coverage will begin on the first day of the third calendar month. (See http://www.gov.sk.ca for further details.)

Alberta (AHCIP—Alberta Health Care Insurance Plan)

The Alberta Health Care Insurance Plan is available to all residents of Alberta and their dependants. This excludes tourists, transients, and visitors.

The coverage will normally be effective the first day of the third month following the date of arrival. (See http://www.gov.ab.ca for further details.)

Newfoundland and Labrador (MCP—Medical Care Plan)

Eligible applicants are classified into three groups:

- Canadian citizens—must present documents confirming citizenship status.
- Landed immigrants—must present Record of Landing documents from Immigration Canada.
- Foreign workers—must present an Employment Authorization (work visa), which must be issued before coming to Canada. This must be for a named Newfoundland and Labrador employer and for a specific job within the province. It must also be valid for at least twelve months (except foreign healthcare workers).
- Must reside in Newfoundland or Labrador for at least four consecutive months in each twelve-month period.

The coverage will normally be effective the first day of the third month following the date of arrival. (See http://www.gov.nf.ca for further details.)

The previous provincial Web sites and the provincial MOH also provide patients with the following information:

- Services that are not covered
- Coverage if travelling to another province
- Travelling outside of Canada
- Moving within Canada
- Instructions for registering for coverage
- Instructions for applying for a new card (i.e., name change, lost or stolen card, address change)

NOTE: It is the patient's responsibility to report an address change to the Ministry of Health; not the physician's).

The following individuals are *not* eligible for provincial coverage:

- Native Canadians living on reserves
- Regular members of the R.C.M.P. and the Canadian Armed Forces (however, their family members *are* eligible)
- Inmates of federal penitentiaries
- Tourists and visitors to the province
- Transients
- Students from other provinces or on student visas

The federal government is responsible for Native Canadians, regular members of the R.C.M.P., the Canadian Armed Forces, and inmates of federal penitentiaries.

REGISTRATION

In order to receive a health number, a provincial registration form must be completed by the patient and submitted to the MOH. Forms for registration are available on-line as well as through the nearest provincial MOH office.

Newborn Registration

In Ontario, the hospital or midwife is provided with pre-assigned health numbers by the MOH. At birth the newborn is given a health number. A tear-off sheet at the bottom acts as a temporary health card until the parent receives the actual health card. The new card usually arrives within three months of receipt of the completed top portion of the form.

In British Columbia, the hospital provides a Baby Enrollment Form. This is to be completed by the parent and submitted as soon as possible to the group plan.

In Alberta, coverage is provided to the newborn from the date of birth if notification is received within one year. Otherwise, coverage begins on the first day of the month in which notification is received.

One parent must have a valid provincial health registration number in order for a newborn to qualify for a health number. All newborns must be registered in order to receive a birth certificate. In Ontario, when a newborn's health card expires, a birth certificate is required before a new card can be assigned.

INSURANCE PREMIUMS

Alberta, British Columbia, and Ontario are the only provinces where residents pay health insurance premiums. Health care in the remainder of Canada is paid through tax money.

Premium payments for Ontario residents were re-implemented in 2004 after being eliminated in 1990. This premium is based on individual or family income. Some employers deduct the premium from the individual's pay.

In Alberta all persons registered with the AHCIP must pay premiums directly or have their premiums submitted by an employer, union, or organization. There are two regular premium rates: one for single persons with no dependants and one for families. There are also premium subsidies available for low-income residents who qualify. Senior citizens may also qualify for a full or partial reduction of premiums under the Alberta Seniors Benefit program.

British Columbia premiums are paid either individually or through an employer, union, or pension plan. These premiums vary according to family size.

> ### 6.1
>
> No one will be refused access to necessary health care due to non-payment of premiums.

HEALTH CARD

Each province provides eligible residents with a health card that displays their registration number (see Figure 6.1). Some cards have an expiry date, and in Ontario, a card may show a version code.

In Ontario the MOH has converted from a family-based OHIP number to an individual health number. There are still several versions in use at present. Some residents have red and white cards, which were issued before 1991. These cards have the old OHIP number on the bottom right-hand corner. Red and white cards issued after 1991 do not have the old OHIP number. These cards are gradually being replaced with a new green photo identification health card. Children under 16 years of age do not have their pictures on their cards.

In Alberta each family member is given a personal health number. For billing purposes, family members are covered on the same account.

FIGURE **6.1** **Sample health cards from Nova Scotia, Quebec, Ontario, and Manitoba.**

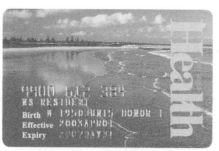

Reproduced with permission of
Nova Scotia Department of Health

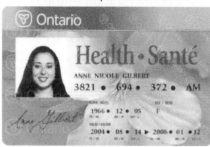

© Queen's Printer for Ontario
Reproduced with permission.

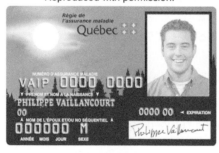

Régie de l'assurance maladiedu Quebec.

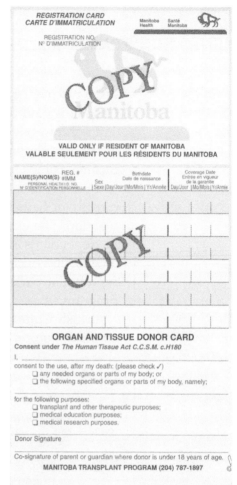

Reproduced with permission of Manitoba Health.

PRIVACY AND CONFIDENTIALITY

A valid health card shows that the individual has the right to healthcare services in that province. The card is for healthcare services only. Under the *Health Cards and Numbers Control Act, 1991* (Ontario), no person, business, or organization may make someone show their health card to get goods or non-health services. The health card number cannot be collected for credit checks, databanks, or identification. Senior citizens may choose to use their cards to prove they are over 65 to qualify for seniors discounts, but the law prohibits a business from "requiring" that the cards be shown. The business may ask to see a Health 65 card (Ontario) as proof of age but does not need to see the number.

The MOH in each province collects information for the following reasons:

- To be sure of eligibility for health coverage and drug benefits, or both
- To process payments for insured services
- To process payments for prescription drugs

Each ministry has security measures to protect all the personal information it collects (see Figure 6.2).

FIGURE **6.2**   **Medical Card Security Features, Canadian Provinces and Territories, March 2003**

Province	Expiry Date	Term Re-registration	Unique Identifiers
British Columbia	No	No	Birth date, signature, and information on electronic strip – Note 3
Alberta	No	No	Birth date
Saskatchewan	Yes	3 years	Birth date and information on electronic strip – Note 3
Manitoba	No	No	Birth date, address, and family members – Note 4
Ontario	Yes	5 years	Birth date, signature, address, digitized photo, and information on electronic strip – Note 3
Quebec	Yes	4 years	Birth date, signature, and digitized photo
New Brunswick	Yes	3 years	Birth date and signature
Nova Scotia	Yes	4 years	Birth date, signature, and magnetic strip – Note 5
Prince Edward Island	Yes	5 years	Birth date and magnetic strip – Note 5
Newfoundland and Labrador	No – Note 1	None	None
Nunavut	Yes	2 years – Note 2	Birth date and signature
Northwest Territories	Yes	2 years	Birth date, signature, and address
Yukon	Yes	1 year	Birth date, signature, and address

Source: Websites for Medical Care Plans and correspondence with provincial medical care plan officials.

Note 1: Expiry dates on temporary beneficiary cards issued for immigrants or students with visas and for residents who require out-of-province coverage for a maximum of 12 months.

Note 2: Beneficiaries re-register every 2 years with term to be extended to 5 years.

Note 3: The strip allows for the information printed on the front of the card to be read electronically.

Note 4: All health cards include the registration number and all the personal health care numbers for each individual family member who is registered under that registration number.

Note 5: No electronic information is maintained on the strip at the present time.

PHYSICIANS' FEE SCHEDULE

As mentioned in Chapter 7 (Financial Records), physicians bill for their services using the fees which are outlined in their provincial schedules. Each province may use a different name for this schedule and the schedule format may be different, but it serves the same purpose. In Ontario it is referred to as the Schedule of Benefits and in Alberta it is the Schedule of Medical Benefits. These fees are established through negotiations between the profession and the provincial MOH. The schedule is divided into sections. In the general preamble *(Ontario)* or general rules *(Alberta)*, the definitions and guidelines as well as premiums payable for services and the circumstances under which they may be paid out are outlined. Another section outlines the codes and fees for each service. Some services are calculated by time units (i.e., every half hour or major part thereof) and specific guidelines are found in this section. This section may also include the basic units to be used by anaesthetists and assistants. Diagnostic codes are not included in the MOH Benefits Schedule.

Each physician receives a copy of his or her provincial fee schedule. Whenever new fees are negotiated, providers receive the new updates, which can conveniently be replaced in their schedule. New diskettes (or electronic data transfer) will also be distributed from the MOH in order to update the computer software. This can take time, so it is good practice to let the download take place over the lunch hour or overnight so the computer will not be tied up during working hours.

As a medical administrative assistant you will require extensive knowledge of the fee schedule and will be required to pay close attention to the regulations and definitions in the preamble. Familiarity with these rules is a prerequisite for accurate billing.

PHYSICIAN REGISTRATION

In order to bill for services provided, all eligible physicians and groups, or both (if applicable), must be registered with their provincial MOH. The Ministry assigns a unique **physician registration number** to the physician to be used when practising in that province. This number is also known as the physician billing number. A physician who moves to another province to practise medicine must apply for registration in that province.

In Ontario this number is a twelve-digit number, with the first four digits identifying the group, the following six identifying the physician, and the last two identifying the specialty. In Alberta, the physician number is nine digits and divided into two segments. There is no special identification assigned to each segment.

Example (Ontario physician billing number)

1. Registration number 0000-123456-00

    0000   The provider is not in a group practice.

    123456 Indicates the provider's identification number. This number is unique and belongs to the provider for a lifetime. (It does not change if the provider changes option type or specialty.) This number should be quoted on any correspondence with the MOH.

    00   The specialty is general practice.

2. Registration number 9999-123456-13

    9999   This is the identification number of the group with which the provider is affiliated. A provider may be affiliated with more than one group, each of which will have a unique four-digit identification number.

    123456 Individual identification number as above.

    13   The specialty is internal medicine.

Once registered, the physician will receive a supply of MOH computer diskettes. The location of the practice will determine the MOH district office to which claims should be submitted. An introductory kit will be sent by the district office to each newly registered provider.

Any changes to registered information (such as specialty changes) must be submitted to the MOH in writing.

EXPLANATION OF PROVIDER SPECIALTY CODES

The following is a list of specialty services recognized by the Royal College of Physicians and Surgeons of Canada relevant to services covered by the MOH.

Physicians

Specialty Code	Explanation
00	Family practice and practice in general. This provider is not a specialist in any field, although he or she may limit his or her practice to a particular field.
01	Anaesthesia Specialist in anaesthetics.
02	Dermatology Specialist in diseases of the skin.
03	General surgery Specialist in general surgery.
04	Neurosurgery Specialist in surgery of the nervous system.

06   Orthopedic surgery
Specialist in the preservation and restoration of the skeletal system.

07   Geriatrics
Specialist in all problems peculiar to old age and aging.

08   Plastic surgery
Specialist in repair of skin and underlying tissues.

09   Cardiovascular and thoracic surgery
Specialist in surgery of the heart and chest.

12   Emergency medicine
Specialist in emergency department medicine.

13   Internal medicine
Specialist in diseases of the internal structures of the body.

18   Neurology
Specialist in diseases of the nervous system.

19   Psychiatry
Specialist in mental and emotional problems.

20   Obstetrics and gynecology
Specialist in two fields: pregnancy and childbirth, and the female genital organs.

23   Ophthalmology
Specialist in diseases of the eye.

24   Otolaryngology
Specialist in diseases of the ear, nose, and throat.

25   Pediatrics
Specialist in child care and diseases of children.

28   Pathology
Specialist in structural and functional changes in tissues of the body caused by disease.

29   Microbiology
Specialist in study of micro-organisms.

30   Clinical biochemistry
Specialist in the practice of chemical pathology.

31   Physical medicine
Specialist in the field of diagnosis and treatment of disease by physical methods (manipulation, massage, exercise).

33   Diagnostic radiology
Specialist in the taking and interpretation of X-rays.

34   Therapeutic radiology
Specialist in the treatment of disease by radiotherapy (radium, X-ray therapy).

35   Urology
Specialist in the urinary system (kidneys and bladder) in both male and female, and genital organs in the male.

41	Gastroenterology
	Specialist in the field of diseases of the gastrointestinal tract.
47	Respiratory disease
	Specialist in the field of diseases of the respiratory system.
48	Rheumatology
	Specialist in the field of rheumatic disease.
60	Cardiology
	Specialist in the field of heart and circulatory disease.
61	Haematology
	Specialist in the field of blood disease.
62	Clinical immunology
	Specialist in the field of immunity (producing immunity by natural or artificial stimulation).
63	Nuclear medicine
	Specialist in the clinical evaluation of a patient diagnosed or treated by unsealed sources of radionuclides.
64	General thoracic surgery
	Specialist in surgery of the chest.

Dentists

Specialty Code	Explanation
49	Dental surgery
	The dentist in general practice; not a specialist.
50	Oral surgery
	Surgical specialist (the surgical treatment of diseases of, and injuries to, the teeth, jaws, and associated structure).
51	Orthodontics
	Specialist in the field of malocclusion of the teeth, including developmental abnormalities of the jaws.
52	Pedodontics
	Specialist in the field of dentistry for children.
53	Periodontics
	Specialist in the field of treatment of the diseases of the supporting tissues of the teeth.
54	Oral pathology
	Specialist in identification and diagnosis of diseased tissue after it has been removed from its normal site.
55	Endodontics
	Specialist in treating diseases involving the pulp of teeth and periradical tissues.
70	Oral radiology
	Specialist at interpreting X-rays of the teeth.
71	Prosthodontist
	Specialist in the making of crowns, bridges, and dentures.

Other Providers

Chiropractors, chiropodists, osteopaths, optometrists, and physiotherapists are not certified in specialties. However, to avoid including these healthcare providers' statistical data with that of general healthcare providers, individual specialty codes have been assigned.

Specialty Code	Explanation
56	Optometrist
57	Osteopath
58	Chiropodist (Podiatrist)
59	Chiropractor
80	Private physiotherapy facilities approved to provide home treatment only.
81	Private physiotherapy facilities approved to provide office and home treatment.

A specialty code is also assigned to the non-medical laboratory director:

27	59993

Nonmedical laboratory directors are always registered under this number.

Additional copies of the schedule may be available from your local Ministry of Health office or, for a nominal fee (to cover printing and handling), from the Ontario Government Book Store, 880 Bay Street, Toronto M7A 1N8, or call toll free 1-800-668-9938.

INTRODUCTION TO CLAIMS SUBMISSION

The medical administrative assistant is responsible for sending claims (billings) to the Ministry of Health for all patients seen on a daily basis by the physician. It is advisable to do the billings the same day as the encounter (visit). The physician can bill for the patient's visit, including any procedures or tests that may be performed at the same time, such as a suture of laceration or a Pap smear. (Note: If the patient is at the office for an annual physical exam, the Pap smear is included in the service code and cannot be charged separately.) In most circumstances the physician will provide the medical administrative assistant with the appropriate service codes and diagnosis for each visit. This information is usually found in the patient's chart or on the physician's day sheet.

A provider can only bill the MOH for medically necessary services. Providers include physicians, healthcare providers, and private medical laboratories.

A claims submission will include the following:

• **Provider Registration Number:** Identifies the provider of the service. This is the unique number that the provider is given by the MOH in their province.

- **Health (Registration) Number:** Number that is assigned to eligible residents of a province that covers the individual for medically necessary health services. In Ontario, there may also be a version code.
- **Date of Birth:** Usually as day/month/year format but each billing software has its own format.
- **Accounting Number:** Computer generated and usually consists of eight alpha-numeric characters.
- **Payment Program:** Identifies if the payment is to be made by the Ministry of Health (HCP), the Workers' Compensation Board (WCB), or your province's equivalent, or the billing is to another province [Reciprocal Medical Billing (RMB)].
- **Payee:** Identifies who is to be paid for this service. Payment to the provider is identified by "P." This is the usual mode of payment. If the payment were to be made to the patient, it would be identified as "S."
- **Referral Provider:** Identifies the healthcare provider/physician (registration number) who has referred the patient for the service. This section must be completed for *all* types of consultations in any location, for *all* physiotherapy services, and for any referred diagnostic or laboratory services.
- **Facility Number:** Identifies the facility (not physician's office) where the service is performed (four digits). This component must be completed for all in-patient, out-patient, and emergency services performed in hospitals and long-term care facilities (including special-visit premium) and for all insured dental services.
- **In-Patient Admission:** Identifies the date the patient was admitted to the facility. The services include all hospital services and special-visit premiums to a patient who has been admitted to the hospital (referred to as a hospital in-patient).
- **Service Code:** Identifies codes for all insured services. These codes are listed in the provincial fee schedule.
- **Fee Submitted:** Amount the provider claims for the service rendered. This amount is found in the provincial fee schedule.
- **Number of Services (Price per Unit):** Claims are submitted by the number of services provided. Most services (units) are claimed as one service but for time-based services, a service or unit is the amount designated by the fee schedule. For example, some services may be for every 15 minutes or part thereof. This may also apply for consecutive visits to an in-patient.
- **Service Date:** Identifies the date the service was provided.
- **Diagnostic Code:** Identifies the reason the patient is being seen by the provider. If more than one diagnosis is involved, use the code for the primary diagnosis. Most, but not all, services require diagnostic codes. Some services that do not require diagnostic codes are newborn baby care in hospital and home, all immunizations and vaccinations, as well as several others.

SERVICE CODES

Service codes are in alpha-numeric format. In Ontario it consists of five alpha-numeric characters (e.g., i.e., A001A). An explanation of the Ontario code follows:

1. The first character is alpha and is an indicator of the service: Prefix alpha A indicates services listed under the general listing (consultations, assessments) or special visits to the office; B is for special visits to the patient's home; G is for diagnostic and therapeutic procedures; P is for obstetrical care; X is for radiology services, and so on.
2. The three middle characters are numeric service identifiers: for example, 001 is for a minor assessment.
3. The last character is alpha and identifies who renders the service.
    A = Provider rendered the service
        Combination of hospital technical and professional components
    B = Assistant rendered the service
        Hospital technical component
    C = Anaesthetist rendered the service
        Professional component

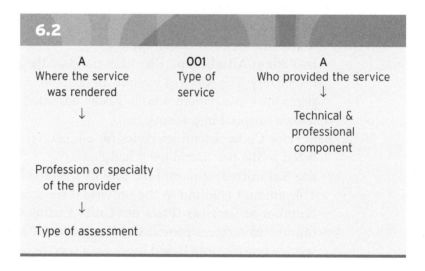

The most common service codes used in general practice (Ontario) follow:

1. **General Assessment (A003)**—the patient presents the provider with a complaint and the provider investigates all systems to make a diagnosis.
2. **General Reassessment (A004)**—The patient returns within one year with the same complaint (two per year per diagnosis may be charged).
3. **Intermediate Assessment/Well Baby Care (A007)**—The provider examines a specific system for a diagnosis (less time than a general

assessment), or sees an infant for periodic health assessment and progress up to two years.

4. **Annual Health Examination (K017 = child after two years of age; A003 = adolescent, adult)**—The patient visits the doctor for a yearly review of physical well-being with no complaint (one visit per year can be charged).

5. **Minor Assessment (A001)**—The diagnosis is fairly simple and less time-consuming than for an intermediate assessment.

The above service codes would have the alpha suffix "A" (A003A) because a provider renders the service.

DIAGNOSTIC CODES

The computer billing software contains the provincial fee schedule as well as the diagnostic codes. The provider diagnoses the patient's condition after performing an examination. For the purposes of healthcare billing, the diagnosis is identified by a three- or four-digit numeric code (i.e., 110 identifies athlete's foot, 850 identifies concussion, 303 identifies alcoholism, and 917 is the diagnostic code used for adolescent and adult annual health examinations). In most software the diagnostic code can be identified by simply keying in the actual diagnosis (i.e., key in cold, a pop up will appear and the appropriate diagnosis can be chosen). The computer will then supply the code of (460).

METHODS OF SUBMITTING CLAIMS

Health Claim Cards

Less than one percent of physicians submit their claims on health claim cards (see Figure 6.3). These are usually submitted by physicians who see only a few patients (i.e., semi-retired practitioners). Their practices are too small to warrant the expense of investing in a computer software system. The patient and visit information is written in the appropriate spaces on the card. A copy is kept for the office record and the cards are sent (usually by courier) to the MOH. The Ministry discourages this type of submission and applies a financial charge to the practitioner for using this method. Some MOH offices will not accept the cards at all.

Diskette

Submitting claims on diskette is one of the most popular delivery methods. The diskettes are couriered (usually weekly or bi-weekly) to the appropriate MOH office. These should be packaged securely to avoid damage.

Electronic Data Transfer (EDT)

In Prince Edward Island, electronic data transfer is the only method of claims submission used. It is becoming more popular provincially. British

FIGURE **6.3**   **Health Claim Card**

PROVIDER NUMBER	

HEALTH NUMBER	VERSION	DATE OF BIRTH YEAR MONTH DAY	ACCOUNTING NUMBER	PAYMENT PROGRAM	PAYEE

REFERRED BY	FACILITY NUMBER	IN-PATIENT ADMISSION YEAR MONTH DAY

SERVICE CODE	FEE SUBMITTED	NUMBER OF SERVICES	SERVICE DATE YEAR MONTH DAY	DIAGNOSTIC CODE	SERVICE CODE	FEE SUBMITTED	NUMBER OF SERVICES	SERVICE DATE YEAR MONTH DAY	DIAGNOSTIC CODE

Ministry of Health Ontario   ♲   HEALTH CLAIM   220-84 (03/91) 7530-4579 CONFIDENTIAL WHEN COMPLETED

SOURCE: © Queen's Printer for Ontario, 1981. Reproduced with permission.

Columbia sends 98 percent of claims by this method. Electronic data transfer is as simple to use as e-mail and can be sent daily. As with diskette submission, a system backup is always needed.

CLAIMS SUBMISSION

As mentioned previously, familiarity with the format of the provincial schedule is important. Preambles that precede the various sections in the schedule contain pertinent information necessary to the accurate process of medical billing. This information includes special-visit premium payments and service codes, calculation of time unit, and fees for anaesthetists and assistants. It is also important for the medical administrative assistant to understand the billing process and the importance of accuracy in both billing and records maintenance.

Billing software will vary in appearance and commands. The required fields for billing, however, will be the same. Software is designed specifically for the province or territory using it (see Figure 6.4).

Only one billing per patient per day is permitted. If a second billing is attempted, a flag will pop up on the screen inquiring if another billing for that patient is to be completed. If billing for a duplicate service code on the same patient, for the same day, but different time, a manual review needs to be flagged and a form completed to accompany the claim (see Figure 6.5).

When billing is completed it can be saved to diskette or electronically transferred to the MOH. If using diskettes, the weekly (or bi-weekly) billing is couriered to the Ministry. The MOH will send you information in the same

FIGURE **6.4**   **Computer Billing Screen**

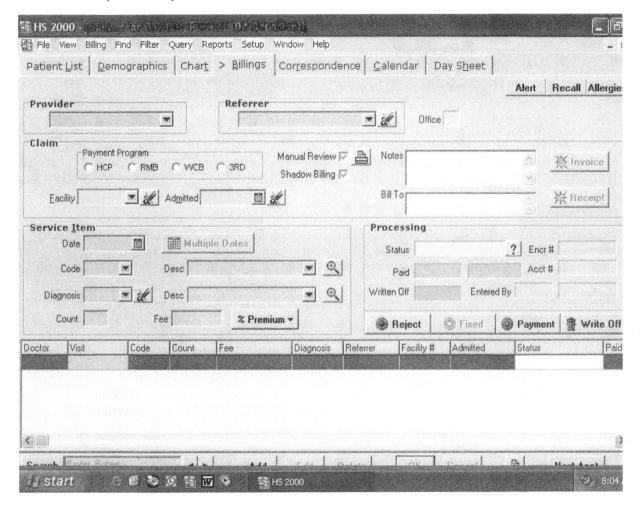

format in which you submit it. If you submit by diskettes, for example, the
Ministry will supply you with diskettes to resubmit.

CODING EXAMPLES (ONTARIO CODES)

Example 1

Mary Jane Brown came to Dr. Plunkett's office on January 16, 20__, with a
rash on her toes. The diagnosis was "tinea pedis."

The procedure for completing the health claim is as follows:

1. The provider name is usually shown on the billing screen (see Figure
   6.6). If billing for more than one physician it will be applied when the
   appropriate physician is identified.
2. Mary Jane's health number and date of birth will be inserted into the
   billing screen from the registration screen.

FIGURE **6.5** **Manual Review Form**

| ⊗ **Ontario** | Ministry of Health and Long-Term Care | **Claims Flagged for Manual Review** |
| | Ministère de la Santé et des Soins de longue durée | **Demandes de règlement à traiter manuellement** |

This form is for manual review only. DO NOT use this for inquiries. Submit the completed form(s) with your disk/tape.
*Cette formule porte uniquement sur le traitement manuel des demandes. Veuillez **ne pas** l'utiliser pour demander des renseignements. Remettez les formules dûment remplie accompagnée de votre disquette/cassette.*

A. Provider Information / Renseignements sur le/la fournisseur(euse)

Provider/Group number / N° du/de la fournisseur(euse) / du groupe	Provider's name / Nom du/de la fournisseur(euse)

Office contact name / Nom de la personne contact du bureau	Office contact phone no. / N° de tél. de la personne contact
	( )

B. Patient Information / Renseignements sur le/la patient(e)

Health Number / Numéro de carte Santé	Patient's name / Nom du/de la patient(e)	Date of birth / Date de naissance yyaa mm dj

Service date / Date du service	Service code / Code du service	Account number *(if available)* / N° de compte *(si disponible)*

C. Detention time *(including report and time spent with patient)*
Temps consacré exclusivement au cas *(Detention time) (y compris le temps passé à la rédaction d'un rapport et en compagnie du/de la patient(e))*

K001A: Time spent exclusively with the patient including the consultation/assessment. Refer to the Schedule of Benefits, General Preamble for conditions and limitations.
K001A : Temps passé exclusivement avec le/la patient(e) y compris de la consultation ou l'évaluation. Les conditions et les restrictions sont indiquées dans le préambule général de la liste de prestations (Schedule of Benefits, General Preamble).

Start time / Heure du début Hr. / h	End time / Heure de la fin Hr. / h

K101A: Time of departure patient(s) / Heure du départ du (des) patient(s) Hr. / h	Time of arrival / Heure d'arrivée Hr. / h

K111A: Boarding time patient(s) / Heure d'embarquement du (des) patient(s) Hr. / h	Disembark time / Heure de débarquement Hr. / h

K102A: Time of departure / Heure de départ Hr. / h	Time of arrival / Heure d'arrivée Hr. / h

K102A (Return) / (Retour) : Time of departure / Heure de départ Hr. / h	Time of arrival / Heure d'arrivée Hr. / h

Critical care with report including time spent with patient when providing resuscitation *(indicating actual beginning and ending time)*
Soins d'urgence avec rapport, y compris le temps passé à réanimer le/la patient(e) *(indiquer les heures exactes de début et de fin)*

Start time / Heure du début Hr. / h	End time / Heure de la fin Hr. / h

D. Independent Consideration *procedures or complex medical procedures, include an operative report and comparision with a listed service in terms of scope, difficulty and value.*
Interventions prises en considération *séparément (Independent Consideration) ou interventions complexes, y compris un rapport sur l'opération et une comparaison avec un service faisant partie de la liste sur le plan de l'étendue, de la difficulté et de la valeur.*

For other fee schedule codes requiring additional documentation, please refer to the Schedule of Benefits, General Preamble.
Pour d'autres codes du fichier des honoraires nécessitant des documents supplémentaires, se reporter au préambule général de la liste de prestations.

E. Multiple visits same day: *(state clinical reason)* / **Visites multiples le même jour :** *(indiquer la raison d'ordre clinique)*

Code	Time of 1st visit / Heure de la 1re visite Hr. / h	Reason / Raison
Code	Time of 2nd visit / Heure de la 2e visite Hr. / h	Reason / Raison
Code	Time of 3rd visit / Heure de la 3e visite Hr. / h	Reason / Raison

F. Other: / Autre :

Instructions on reverse / Instructions au verso →

2404–84 (00/03)   7530–5248

SOURCE: © Queen's Printer for Ontario, 2003. Reproduced with permission.

FIGURE **6.6**   **Billing Example for Mary Jane Brown**

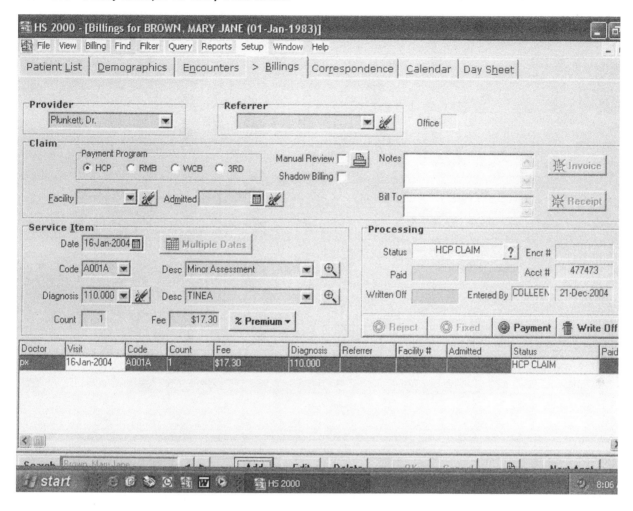

3. The payment program is the healthcare plan (enter HCP), and the provider is to be paid (enter "P"). Most billing software will default to "HCP" and "P."

4. Because the complaint is isolated and fairly simple to diagnose, Dr. Plunkett would charge for a minor assessment. Dr. Plunkett will provide the service code and the fee will be inserted when the service code field is completed. The service code would be obtained from the Schedule of Benefits under the appropriate section for that provider. Dr. Plunkett would bill under "Family Practice" and "Practice in General," as he is a general healthcare provider.

5. One service has been performed. This would be entered in the "Number of Services" or "Price per Unit" field.

6. The service date is the day Mary Jane presented her complaint.

7. The diagnostic code would be inserted into that field once the appropriate diagnosis is keyed in or the numeric code is inserted. Dr. Plunkett would provide the diagnosis.

FIGURE **6.7**   **Billing Example for Bob Baxter**

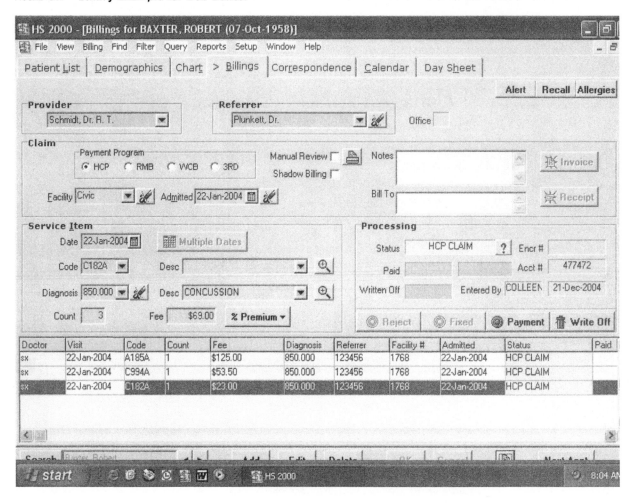

Example 2

While Bob Baxter was cleaning windows, he fell off the ladder, banged his head on a rock, and was knocked unconscious. His wife called an ambulance to take him to the hospital. Dr. Plunkett admitted Bob and then called in a neurologist, Dr. R.T. Schmidt, for consultation. Dr. Schmidt's diagnosis was concussion. He visited Bob on three consecutive days after the admitting date. The accident happened on Saturday, January 22, 20__.

The procedure for completing the health claim is as follows:

1. The provider number is usually shown in the billing screen (see Figure 6.7).
2. Patient's health number and birth date will be inserted from the registration screen.
3. Because Dr. Plunkett referred Bob to Dr. Schmidt, Dr. Plunkett's personal registration number would be entered in the field "Referred By."

4. Because Bob was admitted to hospital, the "Facility Number" and "In-Patient Admission" fields must be completed.
5. The service codes are as follows:
   a. A185A—The service is a consultation performed in the hospital by a specialist in neurology. When a provider makes a special trip, the billing code for the assessment component of the visit is taken from the general listing for the applicable specialty. In the fee schedule under neurology (18) you will find A185—Consultation. Service codes used for special trip billings *must* be taken from general listing's Office Service Codes. A consultation can only be charged when the provider is seeing a patient who has been referred by another provider.
   The suffix for each service code is "A" because the service was rendered by the provider.
   b. C994A—Providers can charge a premium if they respond to calls outside of office hours, on weekends and holidays, or if they sacrifice office hours. The appropriate codes are listed in the preamble under "Premiums." If the special visit is to the emergency department, the alpha prefix would be "K"; for a visit to a patient's home, the alpha prefix would be "B." However, in this instance, the alpha prefix is "C" because Dr. Schmidt rendered the service to a non-emergency hospital in-patient.
   c. C182A—This is the code used when a neurologist makes subsequent hospital visits to a patient; it is found just below the C185 consultation code.
6. The appropriate service fees will be applied and totalled from the relevant service codes.
7. Note that, under "Number of Services," the number "03" is entered opposite "C182A." This is because Dr. Schmidt visited the patient for three consecutive days. The service date entered is the date of the first visit. (If the visits run consecutively without a break, you can put them together.)
8. The diagnostic code for concussion is 850.

Figures 6.8 and 6.9 are examples of a Patient Billing History for the previous two patients. This is another feature available in billing software programs. Before the use of computers for billing, collecting a patient billing history could be very labour intensive for the medical administrative assistant. It is now available by using a couple of key strokes. Note that in this software, the "Number of Services" is identified as "Count."

TIME UNITS

As mentioned previously in this chapter, some services are billed by time units. An example would be a physician seeing a patient for a psychotherapy visit. The physician would bill "per half hour, or *major* part thereof" (as

FIGURE **6.8**   **Patient Billing History—Mary Jane Brown**

17-Dec-2004
8:38 AM

Patient Billing History

Mary Jane Brown

Patient: **Brown, Mary Jane**   Home Tel: **(613)427-3333**   Health #: **3820 703 795**   Ver:

Work Tel: Born: **01-Jan-1958**

Admitted: Facility:

Visit Date: **16-Jan-2004**   Encounter #:

Service	Count	Fee	Diagnosis	Paid	Amount	Acct #	Status
A001A	1	$17.30	110.000			476878	HCP CLAIM

Total for Visit: $17.30

Total for Patient: $17.30

FIGURE **6.9**   **Patient Billing History—Robert Baxter**

17-Dec-2004
9:02 AM

Patient Billing History

Robert Baxter

Patient: **Baxter, Robert**   Home Tel: **(613)652-3179**   Health #: **4892 608 532**   Ver:

Work Tel: Born: **07-Oct-1957**

Admitted: **22-Jan-2004**   Facility: **1768**

Visit Date: **22-Jan-2004**   Encounter #:

Service	Count	Fee	Diagnosis	Paid	Amount	Acct #	Status
A185A	1	$125.00	850.000			476879	HCP CLAIM
C182A	3	$69.00	850.000			476879	HCP CLAIM
C994A	1	$53.50	850.000			476879	HCP CLAIM

Total for Visit: $201.50

Total for Patient: $247.50

outlined in the fee schedule). If the appointment was for one hour, the number of services would be two. If the appointment was for 40 minutes, the number of services would be 1. Therefore, if the fee for service was $50.00, the physician would receive $100.00 for the 1-hour appointment and $50.00 for the 40-minute appointment.

An anaesthetist bills for "every 15 minutes *or* part thereof." If the procedure was 1 hour long, the number of services would be 4. If the procedure was one hour and five minutes, the number of services would be five. A physician assisting in surgery also bills by time units (the guidelines will differ from the anaesthetist—this information can be found in the preamble of the fee schedule). The time units may increase depending on the length of the service. For example, one time unit may be for every fifteen minutes (or part thereof) during the first hour or less. It then increases to two time units for every fifteen minutes (or part thereof) after the first hour but on or before the eighth hour, and then three time units for every fifteen minutes (or part thereof) after the eighth hour. Some service codes are assigned base units as well. In order to calculate the number of services, the base units are added to the calculated time units. The base units are found in the service code and fee section of the schedule.

BILLING PREMIUMS

As mentioned previously, premiums are available under specific circumstances. If a visit or surgery occurs after 1700 hours but before 2400 hours, a premium can be billed as well as the service. This also applies to services provided after 2400 hours but before 0700 hours, services provided on weekends or holidays, and special visits to a hospital, etc. The premiums are found in the preamble of the fee schedule.

6.3 Example of an Anaesthetic Claim (time units, base units, and premium) (Ontario Codes)

PROCEDURE: 10 hours anaesthesia for Craniotomy and Excision of an Infratentorial Tumour on a Sunday
FEE SCHEDULE CODE: N153C–Surgery - Including basic and time units
FEE SCHEDULE CODE: E400C–Premium - Increase the total anaesthetic fee by 50 percent

Fee code is calculated in the following way:
BASIC UNITS: 15 Units (assigned by the fee schedule for this surgery)

First hour	4 Units
Next 7 hours	56 Units (28 × 2 = 56)
Next 2 hours	24 Units (8 × 3 = 24)
No. of Services = 99	

The service fee would be multiplied by 99 to calculate the total for the surgery.
 The total would then be increased by 50 percent as the surgery was performed on a Sunday and a premium has been billed as well.

Remember the following 5-W's when submitting a claim:

WHAT?—Type of assessment/procedure is being billed.
WHEN?—The time the procedure is performed to determine the premium codes and to record correct date.

WHERE?—The location that the procedure/visit was carried out (i.e., office, hospital) (use facility number), other.

WHY? —The reason for visit/procedure to ascertain correct diagnostic code.

WHO? —Which physician is billing the procedure (i.e., attending physician, surgical assistant or anaesthetist).

6.4   Basic Steps for Completing a Claim

1. Identify the provider (if billing for more than one provider)
2. Identify referral provider (if applicable)
3. Identify appropriate patient from database
4. Identify type of billing if different than HCP
5. Insert facility number (if appropriate)
6. Insert admission date (if appropriate)
7. Insert service code (software will generate appropriate fee from the service code)
8. Insert number of services
9. Insert diagnostic code
10. Check completed billings with appointment day sheet to avoid any omissions
11. Save to diskette for submission or submit electronically

ASSIGNMENT 6.1

Using the personal data information provided in Chapter 3 (see Figure 3.9), complete health claims for the following procedures performed by Dr. Plunkett (0000-123456-00):

Mr. Mel Thompson, minor assessment on February 28, 20__ (diagnosis: influenza).

Mr. Jean Belliveau, two minor assessments on February 24 and 27, 20__ (diagnosis: (1) URI; (2) tension headache).

Mr. Thomas Bell, annual health exam, February 24, 20__.

Erik Shultz, special trip to hospital (no. 1100) during office hours on February 25, 20__ (sutured 4.5-cm laceration on head).

Peter John Scott, entered Ottawa General Hospital (no. 1179) on February 18, 20__. (Dr. Plunkett performed an emergency appendectomy, which involved complications such as gross perforation and peritonitis.)

Amelia Jackson, intermediate assessment and Pap smear, February 20, 20__ (diagnosis: vaginitis).

Dr. Plunkett (0000-123456-00) has referred patients in the following situations. Complete health claims for each service. (It is not necessary to complete the consulting physicians' data.)

Mr. Thomas Bell was seen by an internal medicine specialist (first visit) on admission to Ottawa General Hospital (no. 1220) on February 16, 20__. The specialist made four subsequent visits on February 17, 18, 19, and 20 (diagnosis: cirrhosis).

Mrs. Hazel Davis delivered a baby by caesarean section in hospital no. 1220 on February 18, 20__. She was attended by an obstetrician.

Lisa Basciano was attended by a urologist on February 20, 20__, in Ottawa City Hospital (no. 2463). Three consecutive visits were made (diagnosis: urethritis).

Erik Shultz's wife, Mary (born June 6, 19__), had individual psychotherapy with a psychiatrist on February 23, 20__ for one hour (diagnosis: alcoholism).

After your work has been evaluated, insert a copy of the billings for Peter John Scott, Thomas Bell, Hazel Davis, Lisa Basciano, and Mary Shultz in your portfolio.

SUPPORTING DOCUMENTATION

Certain services, e.g., independent consideration (IC), must include supporting documentation. IC may be given when a set fee is not listed in the fee schedule. Claims rendered under this heading should contain an explanation of the fee claimed. It is helpful to the medical consultant if claims for IC include an operative or consultation report and a comparison of the scope and difficulty of the procedure with other procedures in the schedule. (Note: The medical consultant, or provincial equivalent, is a provider assigned to each MOH district office to provide advice and guidance on medical and payment policy.) When submitting this claim, the field "Flag for Review" or "Manual Review" (field will differ with each software) must be identified. This ensures the Ministry of Health will be aware that there is supporting documentation for this claim, and that it may need an independent review by the medical consultant or equivalent. A manual review form (see Figure 6.5) is to be completed and submitted for all flagged claims.

SUBMISSIONS AND PAYMENTS

Claims must be submitted by a specific date to ensure payment by the next billing cycle. Most claims are submitted on a monthly basis (Newfoundland and Labrador have a two-week billing cycle). In Ontario claims need to be submitted by the eighteenth of the month. Payment is then made by the middle of the following month. Claims can be sent weekly or bi-weekly when made by diskettes. Rejected claims are re-submitted in the next billing cycle if there is not enough time for them to be identified, returned, corrected, and resubmitted within the current billing cycle. If sending claims by electronic data transfer on a daily basis, there is usually time to resubmit most rejected claims within the current billing cycle.

All claims must be submitted to the MOH within six months of the service date. Only under extreme circumstances will the MOH consider making payments for claims submitted six months after the date of service.

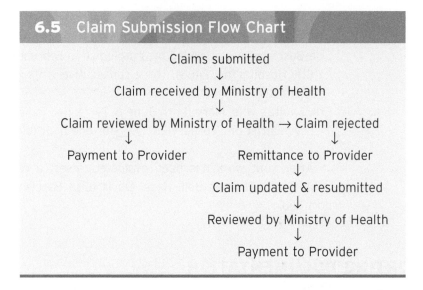

6.5 Claim Submission Flow Chart

Claims submitted
↓
Claim received by Ministry of Health
↓
Claim reviewed by Ministry of Health → Claim rejected
↓   ↓
Payment to Provider   Remittance to Provider
↓
Claim updated & resubmitted
↓
Reviewed by Ministry of Health
↓
Payment to Provider

VERIFICATION LETTERS

As part of a random audit, a letter may be sent to a patient asking for verification that the patient was seen on a certain date, for a specific reason by a physician. Private services such as abortion, organ retrieval, or treatment of sexually transmitted infections (STIs) would not be included.

It is extremely important that the medical administrative assistant ensure that appointment schedules, billing information, and chart documentation are up to date and accurate.

RECIPROCAL CLAIM

All provinces (except Quebec) have entered into an agreement to compensate residents who require medical attention outside of their home province. This compensation is compatible with the provincial fees. It is physician preference as to whether to bill the province or bill the patient directly. If billed directly, the patient is responsible for submitting the claim to his or her home province upon return. If this is the billing preference, the medical administrative assistant will need to provide the patient with an invoice detailing the date of visit, reason for visit, and fee amount. This type of billing is known as RMB. If the physician prefers to bill the province, the HCP field will be replaced with RMB.

Patients who move from another province or territory who require medical treatment before their new province's coverage comes into effect are usually covered by their previous health plan.

All areas of the reciprocal claim are identical to the health claim except for the additional required information:

> **6.6**
>
> PROVINCE: AB (Alberta), MB (Manitoba), BC (British
>   Columbia), NS (Nova Scotia), etc.
> REGISTRATION NUMBER: Ranges from six to twelve digits in
>   length
> PAYMENT PROGRAM: For *all* reciprocal billing claims enter
>   RMB in place of HCP
> PAYEE: *Must* be the provider "P"
> SEX: Enter "F" for female or "M" for male

TRAVEL GRANTS OR ASSISTANCE

Many Canadians are required to travel long distances to access appropriate health care. In some circumstances they can be reimbursed for part of the cost. This does not cover meals or accommodation.

The Northern Health Travel Grant is an Ontario Ministry of Health program that helps northern residents of the province pay for travel to receive medically necessary care that is unavailable locally. The program provides grants to help reimburse the transportation costs of residents who must travel more than 300 kilometres (one way) from their residence to visit a medical specialist or receive a medical specialist's services at a hospital in Ontario or Manitoba.

The amount of the grant is based on the distance travelled to the closest appropriate medical specialist, as determined by the referring provider. There may be a deductible distance applied.

Application forms and booklets detailing who is eligible and how a grant works are available for your patients through the provincial Ministry of Health or on the provincial or territory Web site.

VISITORS FROM OUTSIDE OF PROVINCE

While working as a medical administrative assistant you may encounter patients who are visitors from outside your province. As discussed earlier in this chapter, for Canadian residents (excluding Quebec) you will complete a reciprocal claim (unless otherwise directed by the physician) and submit it to the MOH. If the patient does not have a health card with him or her, the patient pays at the time of service and is given an invoice to submit to his or her provincial MOH.

OUT-OF-PROVINCE BENEFITS

The provincial MOH pays for insured medical and hospital services received in any part of the world by residents who have a valid health number. In Ontario, providers' services are paid at the rates listed in the MOH Schedule of Benefits for comparable services performed in Ontario. Hospital charges are reimbursed based on the level of care received. For example the Ontario health insurance will cover the following:

- $400 (Canadian) per day paid for complex hospital care such as surgery or coronary, neonatal, paediatric, or intensive care
- $200 (Canadian) per day paid for less intensive medical care
- Emergency and out-patient services (with the exception of dialysis) paid to a maximum of $50 (Canadian) for all out-patient services provided on any one day
- $210 (Canadian) per treatment for out-of-country dialysis

An itemized bill should be sent by the patient to the local MOH office. To avoid delays in payment, the bill should also state the patient's name, address, and health number.

It is advisable to get private insurance if travelling outside of Canada, as many health services outside of Canada charge much more than the provincial ministry pays.

PATIENTS FROM OUTSIDE OF CANADA

A visitor from another country may require medical attention. If he or she is staying with one of your patients, your physician may be asked to see the visitor. Out-of-country visitors are required to pay for the medical service at the time of the appointment. You will then provide them with an itemized statement that they can submit to their health insurance for reimbursement when they return to their home country. Some out-of-country visitors will not have any health insurance at all. In the United States, it is the individual's responsibility to obtain his or her own health insurance, unlike Canada, which has a universal healthcare system.

Billing out-of-country patients follows the same procedure as billing for uninsured services, which is discussed in detail in Chapter 7.

REMITTANCE ADVICE

The **Remittance Advice** is an itemized statement of the individual payments made by the Ministry of Health for insured services. Payments made for Workers' Compensation Board–related services will be identified in the payment identification column.

The Remittance Advice has the following three basic divisions:

1. Header information
2. Claim information
3. Total payment information

Figure 6.10 is an example of a Remittance Advice from a provincial MOH.

FIGURE **6.10**   **Remittance Advice**

勞	ACCT'G NUMBER	PATIENT'S NAME LAST	FIRST	PROV INCE	REGISTRATION NUMBER	VER- SION	CONVERTED HEALTH NO.	PAY PGM	CLAIM NUMBER	SERVICE DATE	NO. OF SERV'S	SERV. CODE	ELIG IND	FEE SUBMITTED	AMOUNT PAID	EX CD
01	57079111	Shaw	Olga	On	1234567899	L		HCP	B9876543342	910320	01	G310A		6.55	6.55	
02	78956624	Bradford	John	On	9877779933	Q		HCP	B1234577772	910620	01	G303A		8.80	8.80	
03	57085125	Andrews	Geof	On	8933340421	M		HCP	B1440823495	910326	01	G700A		4.60	4.60	
04	57009812	Arnold	Anit	On	9725356729			HCP	B1440701277	910408	01	J201A		103.00	103.00	
05	57092378	Kline	Robe	On	8945990023			HCP	B1356788841	910218	01	0310A		6.55	6.55	
06	57081321	Altas	Keit	On	7779356211			HCP	B5668932195	910421	01	J201A		103.00	103.00	
07	56912355	Quick	Glen	On	9921456144	Q		HCP	B4162889211	910506	01	G313A		8.80	8.80	
08	57092264	Jones	Ralp	On	7753219432	M		HCP	B6132115664	910423	01	G310A		6.55	6.55	
09	57699022	Bland	Sus	On	5558210036			HCP	B4442172561	910302	01	G313A		8.80	8.80	
10	55532144	Night	Zera	On	8832921443			HCP	B1440823178	910318	01	G310A		6.55	6.55	
11	57082166	Archibal	Marg	On	9727315693			HCP	B1663233997	910222	01	J210A		103.00	103.00	
12	59011125	Anthony	Edwi	On	7772457123			HCP	B1992123339	910210	01	G313A		8.80	8.80	
13	57781234	Crisp	Har	On	4321145679			HCP	B2133451677	910108	01	J201A		103.00	103.00	
14	53334891	Brown	Gai	On	7899332145			HCP	B1992347892	910307	01	G310A		6.55	6.55	
15	51782311	Lake	Gwe	On	9342322431			HCP	B2347891234	910523	01	G313A		8.80	8.80	

MINISTRY OF HEALTH Ontario

Dr. J.J.Jones   Oshawa (I) B 0000-123456-01

Page 3

REMITTANCE ADVICE FOR 10 MAY 91

PAGE TOTALS   493.35   493.35

4,096.50   4,045.60

CHEQUE # 301

INQUIRES REGARDING OVER-PAYMENTS, UNDER-PAYMENTS OR NON-PAYMENT MUST BE MADE WITHIN 6 MONTHS OF SERVICE DATE.
FOR LABORATORIES ONLY, FEE SUBMITTED IS TOTAL FEE PAID PER CLAIM

SOURCE: © Queen's Printer for Ontario, 1991. Reproduced with permission.

Header Information

The header information appears at the top of the form and includes the following:

A. Provider's name.
B. District office—the name of the district to which the group/provider has been allocated and a district identification code. In Ontario, it is a one-letter identifier where:

A is Mississauga   L is London
B is Oshawa   M is Toronto (Metropolitan Toronto)
C is Ottawa   S is Sudbury
H is Hamilton   T is Thunder Bay
K is Kingston

C. Group/provider's registration number.
D. Payment date.
E. Page number.

Claim Information

The claim information is the main part of the form and relates all data relevant to each claim submission as follows:

F. Provider accounting number—Number assigned by a provider to the patient for accounting purposes. Maximum of eight alpha-numeric characters. May or may not be present according to whether the allotted space was filled on the original claim.
G. Patient's last name—Maximum of fourteen alpha characters.
H. Patient's first name—Maximum of three alpha characters.
I. The patient's province of residence.
J. Ministry of Health registration number.
K. Version code—Each time a patient's registration card is revised, one alpha character is added beside the ten-digit number on the registration card (Ontario only).
L. The type of payment identification (e.g., HCP, WCB, or RMB).
M. The MOH claim number—A unique number assigned by the Ministry to identify each claim, eleven characters in length.
N. Initial service date—The date the service was performed.
O. Number of services.
P. Fee schedule code—Obtained from the MOH Fee Schedule.
Q. Fee submitted—The fee submitted by the provider.
R. Amount paid—The amount actually paid to the provider for the service. The fee allowed is usually 100 percent of that specified in the provincial Fee Schedule.
S. Explanatory codes—The explanatory code will appear in cases in which zero payment, or payment less than 100 percent of the fee allotted, is being issued. An example of explanatory codes is listed later in the chapter. More complete or detailed descriptions may be obtained from your MOH claims clerk.

Total Payment Information

T. Page totals—The total amounts billed and paid per page.
U. An aggregate total of previous pages.
V. Cheque number—A cheque number is given if payment is made by cheque. Deposits are usually made directly to the provider's account.

The last page will state the total claims payable to the provider and any accounting adjustments or interim payments.

A diskette or EDT will be sent by the MOH. The above information will be divided into claims paid, claims partially paid, and claims rejected.

It is important to check the remittance advice with the office records to make sure all claims are accounted for.

ERROR CODES

The Claims Error Code Report, or provincial equivalent, contains error codes to explain why the claim has not been accepted. As mentioned previously, this information is available through the provincial MOH. The following are examples of error codes for Ontario, Alberta, and British Columbia:

ONTARIO

EH5	Service date not in eligible period
*EJ1	Before effective date
EK3	Surname mismatch
ENB	Unregistered newborn
EQ2	Specialty mismatch
AD3	Not allowed with visit
A2A	Outside of age limit
A36	Claimed by other practitioner
VH4	Invalid version code
VK1	Invalid OHIP number

ALBERTA

05B **Unregistered WCB claim**—The patient is not eligible for Alberta Health Care coverage for the date(s) of service. Submit your claim directly to the Workers' Compensation Board.

05E **E.H.B. Coverage**—Payment has been refused as the service(s) were provided when the patient did not have coverage under the Extended Health Benefits Program.

01 **Not Registered**—We have no record of this person registered with this Personal Health Number.

01B **Non Resident**—We cannot confirm that this patient is a resident of Alberta. Please contact the patient to obtain the correct billing information.

02 **Registration Number/PHN Conflict**—The Health Registration Number and the Personal Health Number used are not for the same person.

03 **Newborn**—The claim was refused as the Plan is unable to contact the parent(s) of this child to confirm registration.

BRITISH COLUMBIA

*F Patient has opted out of MSP. Patient should be billed directly.

*H Our records indicate the patient requested coverage to be cancelled.

*1 Date of service is prior to coverage effective date.

AB PHN is not on our records.

A1   Dependant is not registered.

AK   Coverage for this dependant has been cancelled.

REMITTANCE ADVICE INQUIRIES

MOH staff attempt to minimize the necessity for inquiries concerning claims payment. However, sometimes discrepancies do occur.

If, after examining the Remittance Advice, you find a discrepancy, the first step is to verify that you have submitted the claim correctly. If this is the case, and you feel that you have been incorrectly paid for the service(s), the next step is to complete a Remittance Advice Inquiry form (see Figure 6.11).

The forms are self-explanatory. Assistance in completing the forms may be obtained from your MOH claims clerk. Forms may be ordered from your local MOH office or can be accessed on-line.

APPEALS

If the provider still disagrees with the payment of a claim after submitting an inquiry form, the unit supervisor should be consulted. Appeals of complicated claims may be directed to the ministry's medical consultant, or provincial equivalent, in a district office.

WORKERS' COMPENSATION BOARD

Every province has its own Workers' Compensation Board (WCB) or equivalent. The provincial boards raise money from the provincial employers in order to provide compensation to workers who are injured on the job or who contract an occupational disease or illness. The illness can also include acute psychological trauma resulting from work. In some provinces it is optional for small businesses, including small physicians' offices, to pay WCB premiums (see the following list).

- Ontario—Workplace Safety and Insurance Board (WSIB)
- Newfoundland and Labrador—Workplace Health, Safety and Compensation Commission
- Yukon—Yukon Workers' Compensation Health and Safety Board
- Nova Scotia—Workers Compensation Board
- Manitoba—Labour, Workplace Safety and Health Division
- Saskatchewan—Workers' Compensation Board
- Alberta—Workers Compensation Board
- British Columbia—Workers Compensation Board
- Prince Edward Island—Workers Compensation Board

Employers who pay WCB premiums are protected from lawsuits in exchange for financing the provincial program. In retrospect, employees also give up their right to sue for work-related injuries, irrespective of fault, for guaranteed compensation for accepted claims.

FIGURE **6.11**   **Remittance Advice Inquiry Form**

Ontario

Ministry of Health and Long-Term Care
Ministère de la Santé et des Soins de longue durée

**Remittance Advice Inquiry
Demande de renseignements
(Avis de règlement)**

Confidential when completed
Renseignements confidentiels

Important

A. State your Provider and Group number.
B. State your name and address.
C. Retain pink copy for your records.
D. Send white and yellow copies to your **Ministry of Health and Long-Term Care Office.**

A. Inscrivez votre numéro de fournisseur et votre numéro de groupe.
B. Inscrivez votre nom et adresse.
C. Gardez la copie rose pour vos dossiers.
D. Envoyez les copies blanche et jaune à votre bureau du ministère de la Santé et des Soins de longue durée.

Date of Remittance Advice
Date de l'avis de règlement

Provider / Group number
Numéro de fournisseur/groupe

Provider/Group name / Nom du fournisseur groupe

Address /Adresse

Postal Code / Code postal

Telephone number / N° de téléphone

Date of inquiry / Date de la demande

Instructions

1. Use this form to itemize **under** or **over** payments ONLY.
2. Claims outstanding for two payment cycles (remittances) after submission should be re-submitted if no advice received.
3. Inquiries on claim payments should be made within **one** month of receipt of remittance advice.
4. Submit all inquiries from one remittance advice at the same time.

1. N'utilisez cette formule **QUE** pour dresser la liste des paiements **insuffisants ou excédentaires.**
2. Les demandes de règlement toujours en souffrance après deux périodes de paiement doivent être soumises à nouveau si on n'a reçu aucun avis.
3. Les demandes de renseignements sur les paiements doivent être faites **moins** d'un mois après réception de l'avis de règlement.
4. Soumettre en une seule fois les demandes relatives au même avis de règlement.

Under review – you will be advised
À l'étude – on vous avisera — U.R. / À.É.

Paid correctly according to our records
Payé correctement selon nos dossiers — P.C.

Adjustment required – being processed
Redressement requis –présentement en cours — A.R / R.R.

U.P. – underpayment   O.P. – overpayment
P.I. – paiement insuffisant   P.E. – paiement excédentaire

Claim information Renseignements (demande de règlement)	U.P. O.P. P.I. P.E.	Provider/group remarks Observations du fournisseur/groupe	Office use only Réservé au bureau	Code
Health No. / N° de carte Santé				
Claim No. / N° de la demande de règlement				
Fee schedule code / Code du barème des droits				
Date of service / Date du service Y/A M/M D/J				
Fee submitted / Droits présentés				
Surname / Nom de famille First name / Prénom				
Date of birth / Date de naissance Y/A M/M D/J				
Accounting No. / N° de compte				
Health No. / N° de carte Santé				
Claim No. / N° de la demande de règlement				
Fee schedule code / Code du barème des droits				
Date of service / Date du service Y/A M/M D/J				
Fee submitted / Droits présentés				
Surname / Nom de famille First name / Prénom				
Date of birth / Date de naissance Y/A M/M D/J				
Accounting No. / N° de compte				
Health No. / N° de carte Santé				
Claim No. / N° de la demande de règlement				
Fee schedule code / Code du barème des droits				
Date of service / Date du service Y/A M/M D/J				
Fee submitted / Droits présentés				
Surname / Nom de famille First name / Prénom				
Date of birth / Date de naissance Y/A M/M D/J				
Accounting No. / N° de compte				

Name of clerk (print)
Nom du commis
(Lettres moulées)

Telephone
Téléphone

Date returned to provider/group
Retournée au fournisseur/groupe le

0918–84 (00/01)

7530–4240

SOURCE: © Queen's Printer for Ontario, 2001. Reproduced with permission.

Compensation includes payment for loss of wages that may result from the injury, disease, or condition; future economic loss and non-economic loss awards, or both, for permanent/partial disability; payment of healthcare expenses; a wide range of vocational and medical rehabilitation services; retraining programs; and survivor benefits in the case of a fatality.

Employers are now much more proactive in finding an employee modified work in their area or moving them temporarily to another more suitable job in another area within that company due to the education and promotion provided by the WCB.

If a worker is not satisfied with the decision rendered by any of the operating divisions at the WCB, the injured worker may appeal the decision to the Appeals Branch, which is the final level within the board.

MAKING A CLAIM

Employee's Responsibilities

1. Get first aid immediately. (By law, the employer must have a first-aid station available and a person trained in first aid on duty at all times.)
2. Notify a staff member trained in first aid.
3. Report the details of the accident to the employer, even if no further medical treatment is required.
4. Ask the employer for a Treatment Memorandum, and take it to the doctor or hospital if medical attention is required (see Figure 6.12). (Note: Read the Treatment Memorandum form for your information.)
5. Some employers require an Incident Form to be completed (this form should be available at your workplace).
6. Choose the physician or other qualified healthcare provider you want to administer treatment. (Note: Once you have made your choice, you must receive permission from the WCB before changing to another doctor. It may be necessary to change doctors because you are moving, for instance; or you may be dissatisfied with the treatment you are receiving. If you find it necessary to change doctors for whatever reason, remember to get permission from the WCB *before* making a change.)
7. Complete and return quickly any forms received from the WCB (for example, Figure 6.13). Be sure all forms are legible (in some provinces you will need to use black ink), that all information is exact and complete (including postal code), and that you sign all forms. When an accident is reported to the WCB, the injured worker is assigned a claim number. This number *must* appear on *every* form or letter that is sent to the WCB.

Employer's Responsibilities

1. Make sure first aid is administered immediately.
2. Complete and give a Treatment Memorandum to the employee if further medical treatment is required.

FIGURE **6.12**   **Treatment Memorandum**

WSIB ONTARIO **CSPAAT**	Workplace Safety & Insurance Board · 200 Front Street West · Toronto ON M5V 3J1 · Commission de la sécurité professionnelle et de l'assurance contre les accidents du travail · 200, rue Front Ouest · Toronto ON M5V 3J1 · **Treatment Memorandum** *Avis de traitement*

Practitioner/Hospital: The worker claims to have been injured in our employ and requests treatment. We, the employer, are sending a report to the Workplace Safety and Insurance Board (WSIB).

Praticien/Hôpital : *Le travailleur affirme avoir subi une lésion pendant qu'il travaillait pour nous et demande des traitements. En tant qu'employeur de ce travailleur, nous ferons parvenir un rapport à la Commission de la sécurité professionnelle et de l'assurance contre les accidents du travail (CSPAAT).*

Worker Identification / *Identification du travailleur*	Last Name/ *Nom de famille*		First Name/ *Prénom*	Initials/ *Initiale*	S.I.N./*N° d'assurance sociale*
	Address (no.,street,apt. no.)/ *Adresse (n°, rue, app.)*	City,Town/ *Ville*		Province	Postal Code *Code postal*

Identification / *Identification de l'employeur*	Firm Name/ *Nom de l'entreprise*			WSIB Firm No./ *N° d'entreprise à la CSPAAT*
	Address/ *Adresse*	City,Town/ *Ville*	Province	Postal Code *Code postal*

Accident Information *Renseignements sur l'accident*	Date and hour of accidental injury *Date et heure de l'accident* dd/jj mm/mm yy/aa time/heure am pm	Date and hour accident reported *Date et heure où fut signalé l'accident* dd/jj mm/mm yy/aa time/heure am pm	Nature of Injury/*Nature de la lésion*

Important: Please retain and file this document for future reference and submission to the WSIB if requested.

Veuillez conserver ce document pour référence future et pour présentation à la CSPAAT sur demande.

Name of Company Officer/ *Nom du dirigeant de l'entreprise*	Date (dd/mm/yy) (jj/mm/aa)

Please see other side/ *Voir au verso.*

Please submit your account to the WSIB/ *Veuillez envoyer votre compte à la CSPAAT.*

0156C (01/98)

SOURCE: Reprinted with permission of the Workplace Safety and Insurance Board.

3. Record the details of the accident (date, time, place, type of injury, medical aid given).
4. If necessary, provide transportation to doctor's office, hospital, or home (within reasonable distance of workplace).
5. Complete an Employer's Report of Injury/Disease (Figure 6.14) and send to the WCB immediately (completed within three days of the injury and received by the WCB within seven working days) if injury requires medical treatment. (Note: Read report details for your information.)
6. Supply any other information required by the WCB.
   All forms are available on the provincial WCB Web site.

Physician's Responsibilities

In all cases in which an injured worker has been treated for a work-related injury, complete and send to the WCB a Health Professional's First Report (Figure 6.15) as soon as the injured patient has been examined. Reports should be submitted within a 48-hour period. All reports can now be submitted on-line by employers, physicians, chiropractors, and physiotherapists.

Text continued on p. 152.

FIGURE **6.13** **Functional Abilities Form**

WSIB ONTARIO
CSPAAT

Workplace Safety &
Insurance Board
Commission de la sécurité
professionnelle et de l'assurance
contre les accidents du travail

200 Front Street West
Toronto ON M5V 3J1

200, rue Front Ouest
Toronto ON M5V 3J1

Health Professionals
Cannot Initiate
the Completion
of this Form

**Functional Abilities Form
for Timely Return to Work**

The following information should be completed by the employer or the injured worker. Please read the information on the following page.

Health No.

Claim No.

☐ Initial form   ☐ Follow-up form

Date of Accident
day   month   year

Employer Telephone No.
Area Code   Telephone
(   )

Worker's Last Name   First Name

Full Address (No., Street, Apt.)

City/Town   Province

Employer's Name

Full Address (No.. Street. Apt.)

Postal Code   Area Code   Telephone No.
(   )

City/Town   Province   Postal Code

Social Insurance No.   Date of Birth
day   month   year

Accident Information(*This information should be completed by the employer or the injured worker.*)

Type of Job at Time of Injury (Where available, attach description of job activities)   Area of Injury

The following information should be completed by the Health Professional:

1 Date of examination on which the report is based   Area of Injury

2 Rehabilitation/Treatment Required? ☐ yes ☐ no   Is the worker capable of returning to work immediately without restrictions? ☐ yes ☐ no   If no, please complete the next section.

Please complete where capabilities are known or limitations recommended. Note: `as tolerated' implies that restrictions are recommended but must be quantified in the workplace.

General Comments/Specific Limitations

3

Capabilities

Walking: short distance only ☐ ; as tolerated ☐ ; other (eg. uneven ground) ☐ _____

Standing: less than 15 min ☐ ; less than 30 min. ☐ ; as tolerated ☐ ; other ☐ _____

Sitting: less than 30 min ☐ ; less than 1 hour ☐ ; as tolerated ☐ ; other ☐ _____

Lifting floor to waist: less than 10 Kg. ☐ ; less than 25 Kg. ☐ ; as tolerated ☐ ; other ☐ _____

Lifting waist to shoulder: less than 10 Kg. ☐ ; less than 25 Kg. ☐ ; as tolerated ☐ ; other ☐ _____

Stair climbing: none ☐ ; 2-3 steps only ☐ ; short flight ☐ ; own pace ☐ ; as tolerated ☐

Ladder climbing: none ☐ ; 2-3 steps only ☐ ; 4-6 steps only ☐ ; own pace ☐ ; as tolerated ☐

Limited ability to use hand to: hold objects ☐ ; grip ☐ ; type ☐ ; write ☐

Limitations

☐ Bending or twisting of   ☐ Repetitive movement of

☐ Chemical exposure to   ☐ Environmental exposure to

☐ Operating motorized equipment   ☐ Restrictions related to medications: (specify)

☐ Above-shoulder activity   ☐ Below-shoulder activity

Exposure to vibration: high frequency ☐ ; low frequency ☐

Limit physical exertion to: mild ☐ ; moderate ☐ ; as tolerated ☐

4 Recommendation for Work Hours
☐ Full-time hours ☐ Modified hours ☐ Graduated hours

5 Complete Recovery Expected?
☐ no ☐ yes

Estimated Duration of Limitations

Health Professional - please complete section below for payment and send ONE copy by fax or mail to the WSIB.

Health Professional's Name (Please print)   Health Profession   Date of Next Appointment for Review of Capabilities
day   month   year

Full Address   City/Town   Province   Postal Code

Date (dd/mmm/yyyy)   Area Code   Telephone
(   )   Signature

Are you registered with the WSIB? ☐ Yes ☐ No   If yes, please enter the WSIB Provider Billing number in box provided below:

WSIB Provider Billing No.   Your own invoice No.   Service date
d d m m y y y y   Fee code
9 0 1

2647A (11/00)   **Copy 1 - WSIB**

What You Need to Know

To receive benefits under *The Workplace Safety and Insurance Act* , the injured worker is required to apply for benefits within six months of the time of work-related injury or disease. At the time of filing a claim for benefits, the injured worker must also consent to the disclosure of functional abilities information provided by a health professional to his or her employer for the sole purpose of facilitating return to work. Failure to file a claim or provide consent for the release of the functional abilities information can result in no benefits. The injured worker is also required to provide a copy of the claim and the consent to his or her employer.

Employers, workers and health professionals who have questions about the completion of this form may call 1-800-387-0750.

Worker

- This form is to be completed by your treating Health Professional who will discuss the information with you, once completed.

- You should contact your employer immediately to review the information on the completed form together to plan a return to work.

Employer

- This is the information that you need about this worker's physical capabilities and limitations to plan return to work.

- When you provide this form to the treating health professional, ensure that you have attached the worker's signed consent to the release of functional abilities information. This signed consent will either be on your Form 7, the copy of the Form 6 that the worker must give you after filing directly with the WSIB or on the Worker's Consent Form #1492. Where available, also attach a description of the worker's job activities to assist the health professional in completing the form.

- If you have a form that is specific to your workplace and have the co-operation of the injured worker in providing consent for the release of information on your form, you are able to use your own form. The prescribed form that is available from the Board is a generic form developed to assist employers with general functional abilities information and consent by the injured worker. The WSIB will pay the health professional to complete the prescribed form only. A charge will appear on your Accident Cost statement or Schedule 2 Invoice which reflects the cost of payment for each form completed.

- Do not send a copy of the completed Functional Abilities Form for Timely Return to Work to the WSIB. The Health Professional is responsible for submission of the form.

Health Professional

- The worker has signed a consent for the release of the functional abilities information to the employer when s/he applied for benefits. The employer will provide the worker's signed consent.

- The employer and worker will use this information to return the injured worker to suitable and available work. Their return to work plans will reflect the physical capabilities and limitations you have noted and presume that no clinical contraindications exist for other work activities, **therefore it is crucial that both the capabilities and limitations sections be completed in full.**

- The completion of this form is based on your examination of the injured worker and does not require a specialized Functional Abilities Evaluation.

- Diagnostic information **must not** be included.

- If you are able, please add more specific information on the duration of temporary precautions or maximum times or weights to be considered, in section 3 under General Comments/Specific Limitations. If necessary, please attach an additional page to this completed form to describe physical capabilities and limitations.

- **This does not replace clinical reporting requirements to the WSIB.**

- Once you have received the form, promptly complete it and give the worker and the employer their copies.

- To avoid delays or non-payment of the form insure that sections 1 through 4 and the billing section have been fully completed.

- When faxing a completed form for payment, do not also mail the original.

The Workplace Safety and Insurance Board will pay you for this completed form when a copy is received and you have filled in the billing sections.

Workplace Safety and Insurance Board	**WSIB Fax: (416) 344-4684**
Simcoe Place	1-888-313-7373
200 Front Street West	
Toronto ON M5V 3J1	

FIGURE **6.13**   **Functional Abilities Form, cont'd**

FIGURE **6.14** **Employer's Report of Injury/Disease**

WSIB ONTARIO **CSPAAT**

Mail To:
200 Front Street West
Toronto ON M5V 3J1

OR Fax To:
416-344-4684
OR 1-888-313-7373

Please PRINT in black ink

7

**Employer's Report
of Injury/Disease (Form 7)**

Claim Number

A. Worker Information

Job Title/Occupation (at the time of accident/illness - do not use abbreviations)

Length of time in this position while working for you

Social Insurance Number

Please check **if** this worker is a: ☐ executive ☐ elected official ☐ owner ☐ spouse or relative of the employer

Worker Name

Address (number, street, apt., suite, unit)

City/Town   Province   Postal Code

Is the worker covered by a Union/Collective Agreement?
☐ yes ☐ no

Worker Reference Number

Worker's preferred language
☐ English ☐ French
☐ Other

Date of Birth   dd   mm   yy

Telephone
( )

Sex ☐ M ☐ F

Date of Hire   dd   mm   yy

Fold here for #10 envelope

B. Employer Information

Trade and Legal Name (if different provide both)

Check one: ☐ Firm Number **OR** ☐ Account Number

Provide Number

Mailing Address

Rate Group Number

Classification Unit Code

City/Town   Province   Postal Code

Telephone
( )

Description of Business Activity

Does your firm have 20 or more workers? ☐ yes ☐ no

FAX Number
( )

Branch Address where worker is based (if different from mailing address - no abbreviations)

City/Town   Province   Postal Code

Alternate Telephone
( )

C. Accident/Illness Dates and Details

1. Date and hour of accident/Awareness of illness   dd   mm   yy   ☐ AM ☐ PM

2. Who was the accident/illness reported to? (Name & Position)

Date and hour reported to employer   dd   mm   yy   ☐ AM ☐ PM

Telephone
( )   Ext.

3. Was the accident/illness:
☐ Sudden Specific Event/Occurrence
☐ Gradually Occurring Over Time
☐ Occupational Disease
☐ Fatality

4. Type of accident/illness: **(Please check all that apply)**
☐ Struck/Caught ☐ Fall ☐ Slip/Trip
☐ Overexertion ☐ Harmful Substances/Environmental ☐ Motor Vehicle Incident
☐ Repetition ☐ Assault
☐ Fire/Explosion ☐ Other

5. Area of Injury (Body Part) - **(Please check all that apply)**

☐ Head	☐ Teeth	☐ Upper back	Left	Right	Left	Right	Left	Right	Left	Right
☐ Face	☐ Neck	☐ Lower back	☐ Shoulder		☐ Wrist		☐ Hip		☐ Ankle	
☐ Eye(s)	☐ Chest	☐ Abdomen	☐ Arm		☐ Hand		☐ Thigh		☐ Foot	
☐ Ear(s)		☐ Pelvis	☐ Elbow		☐ Finger(s)		☐ Knee		☐ Toe(s)	
☐ Other			☐ Forearm				☐ Lower Leg			

6. Describe what happened to cause the accident/illness and what the worker was doing at the time (lifting a 50 lb. box, slipped on wet floor, repetitive movements, etc. . .). Include what the injury is and any details of equipment, materials, environmental conditions (work area, temperature, noise, chemical, gas, fumes, other person) that may have contributed. **For a condition that occurred gradually over time, please attach a description of the physical activity required to do the work.**

0007A (07/05)   **A guide to complete this form is available at** www.wsib.on.ca   Page 1 of 3

SOURCE: Reprinted with permission of The Workplace Safety and Insurance Board.

WSIB ONTARIO
CSPAAT

7 **Employer's Report**
of Injury/Disease (Form 7)

Claim Number

Please PRINT in black ink

Worker Name	Social Insurance Number

C. Accident/Illness Dates and Details (Continued)

7. Did the accident/illness happen on the employer's premises (owned, leased or maintained)?   ☐ yes ☐ no
Specify where (shop floor, warehouse, client/customer site, parking lot, etc..).

8. Did the accident/illness happen outside the Province of Ontario?   ☐ yes ☐ no
If **yes,** where (city, province/state, country).

9. Are you aware of any witnesses or other employees involved in this accident/illness?   ☐ yes ☐ no
If **yes,** provide name(s), position(s), and work phone number(s).
1.
2.

10. Was any individual, who does not work for your firm, partially or totally responsible for this accident/illness?   ☐ yes ☐ no
If **yes,** please provide name and work phone number

11. Are you aware of any prior similar or related problem, injury or condition?   ☐ yes ☐ no
If **yes,** please explain

12. If you have concerns about this claim, attach a written submission to this form.   ☐ submission attached

D. Health Care

1. Did the worker receive health care for this injury?   ☐ yes ☐ no   If **yes,** when :   dd mm yy

2. When did the employer learn that the worker received health care?   dd mm yy

3. Where was the worker treated for this injury? **(Please check all that apply)**
☐ On-site health care   ☐ Ambulance   ☐ Emergency department   ☐ Admitted to hospital   ☐ Health professional office   ☐ Clinic
☐ Other:

Name, address and phone number of health professional or facility who treated this worker (if known)

E. Lost Time - No Lost Time

1. Please choose one of the following indicators.   **After the day of accident/awareness of illness, this worker:**
☐ Returned to his/her **regular job** and **has not** lost any time and/or earnings. **(Complete sections G and J).**
☐ Returned to **modified work** and **has not** lost any time and/or earnings. **(Complete sections F, G, and J).**
☐ **Has lost time and/or earnings. (Complete ALL remaining sections).**

▶ Provide date worker first lost time   dd mm yy   ▶ Date worker returned to work (if known)   dd mm yy   ☐ regular work   ☐ modified work

2. This Lost Time - No Lost Time - Modified Work information was confirmed by:
☐ Myself   ☐ Other   Name   Telephone ( )   Ext.

F. Return To Work

1. Have you been provided with work limitations for this worker's injury?   ☐ yes ☐ no

2. Has modified work been discussed with this worker?   ☐ yes ☐ no

3. Has modified work been offered to this worker?   ☐ yes ☐ no

If **yes,** was it :   ☐ Accepted   ☐ Declined
☐ If Declined please attach a copy of the written offer given to the worker.

4. Who is responsible for arranging worker's return to work
☐ Myself   ☐ Other   Name   Telephone ( )   Ext.

0007A (07/05)   Page 2 of 3

FIGURE **6.14**   **Employer's Report of Injury/Disease, cont'd**   *continued*

WSIB ONTARIO **CSPAAT**

7 **Employer's Report of Injury/Disease (Form 7)**

Claim Number

Please PRINT in black ink

Worker Name

Social Insurance Number

G. Base Wage/Employment Information - (Do not include overtime here)

1. Is this worker **(Please check all that apply)**

- [ ] Permanent Full Time
- [ ] Permanent Part Time
- [ ] Temporary Full Time
- [ ] Temporary Part Time
- [ ] Casual/Irregular
- [ ] Seasonal
- [ ] Contract
- [ ] Student
- [ ] Unpaid/Trainee
- [ ] Other
- [ ] Registered Apprentice
- [ ] Optional Insurance
- [ ] Owner Operator or (Sub) Contractor

2. Regular rate of pay $ _____ per [ ] hour [ ] day [ ] week [ ] other

H. Additional Wage Information

1. Net Claim Code or Amount   Federal _____   Provincial _____

2. Vacation pay - on each cheque? [ ] yes [ ] no   Provide percentage ____ %

3. Date and hour last worked

dd   mm   yy   [ ] AM [ ] PM

4. Normal working hours on last day worked

From ____ [ ] AM [ ] PM   To ____ [ ] AM [ ] PM

5. Actual earnings for last day worked $ _____

6. Normal earnings for last day worked $ _____

7. Advances on wages: Is the worker being paid while he/she recovers? [ ] yes [ ] no   If yes, indicate: [ ] Full/Regular [ ] Other

8. Other Earnings (Not Regular Wages): Provide the **total of additional earnings** for each week for the 4 weeks before the accident/illness.

> * For Rotational Shift workers - If the shift cycle exceeds 4 weeks, please attach the earnings information for the last complete shift cycle prior to the date of accident/illness.

Use these spaces for any other earnings ▼ (indicate Commission, Differentials, Premiums, Bonus, Tips, In Lieu %, etc..).

Period	From Date (dd/mm/yy)	To Date (dd/mm/yy)	Mandatory Overtime Pay	Voluntary Overtime Pay				
Week 1			$	$	$	$	$	$
Week 2			$	$	$	$	$	$
Week 3			$	$	$	$	$	$
Week 4			$	$	$	$	$	$

I. Work Schedule (Complete either A, B or C. Do not include overtime shifts)

- [ ] **(A.) Regular Schedule** - Indicate normal work days and hours.

Sunday	Monday	Tuesday	Wednesday	Thursday	Friday	Saturday

▶ **Example:** Monday to Friday, 40 hours

S	M	T	W	T	F	S
	8	8	8	8	8	

or,

- [ ] **(B.) Repeating Rotational Shift Worker** - Provide

NUMBER OF DAYS ON	NUMBER OF DAYS OFF	HOURS PER SHIFT(s)	NUMBER OF WEEKS IN CYCLE

▶ **Example:** 4 days on, 4 days off, 12 hours per shift, 8 weeks in cycle.

or,

- [ ] **(C.) Varied or Irregular Work Schedule** - Provide the total number of regular hours and shifts for each week for the 4 weeks prior to the accident/illness. (Do not include overtime hours or shifts here).

	Week 1	Week 2	Week 3	Week 4
From/To Dates (dd/mm/yy)				
Total Hours Worked				
Total Shifts Worked				

J. It is an offense to deliberately make false statements to the Workplace Safety and Insurance Board. I declare that all of the information provided on pages 1, 2, and 3 is true.

Name of person completing this report: (please print) _____   Official title: _____

Signature: _____   Telephone (____) ____   Ext. ____   Date: dd ___ mm ___ yy ___

THE WORKPLACE SAFETY AND INSURANCE ACT REQUIRES YOU GIVE A COPY OF THIS FORM TO YOUR WORKER

0007A (07/05)   Page 3 of 3

FIGURE **6.14**   Employer's Report of Injury/Disease, cont'd

WSIB
ONTARIO
CSPAAT

7 **Employer's Report**
of Injury/Disease (Form 7)

Claim Number

Please PRINT in black ink

| Worker Name | Social Insurance Number |

K. Additional Information

THE WORKPLACE SAFETY AND INSURANCE ACT REQUIRES YOU GIVE A COPY OF THIS FORM TO YOUR WORKER

0007A (07/05)

FIGURE **6.14**   **Employer's Report of Injury/Disease, cont'd**   *continued*

FIGURE **6.15**   **Health Professional's First Report**

Health Professional's Report (Form 8)

For

Chiropractors   Physicians   Physiotherapists   Registered Nurses (Extended Class)

Health Professionals, please use this form when:

- Your patient states that an injury/illness is related to his or her work.
- You believe that the cause of your patient's injury/illness is due to workplace factors.
- Your patient states that his or her current condition is a recurrence or re-injury of a previous work-related injury/illness. (Provide the patient's claim number from the previous injury/illness – if available).

Section 37 of the *Workplace Safety and Insurance Act, 1997* provides the legal authority for health professionals, hospitals and health facilities to submit, without consent, information relating to a worker claiming benefits to the Workplace Safety and Insurance Board (WSIB).

Your promptness in completing this form is key to our ability to process and adjudicate your patient's claim. Your patient, their employer and the WSIB depend on you.

When completing this report, please **print** using **black pen**.

Your patient should complete Section A of this report. If your patient needs assistance, please help. Please submit this report even if Section A is not fully completed.

Information for completing this report can be found on **Page 4**. For more details, refer to "Guidelines for Health Professionals – Completing WSIB Forms".

Please separate and send **Pages 2 and 3** to the Workplace Safety and Insurance Board:

By Fax to:

416 344 4684 or 1 888 313 7373

Or by Mail to:

Workplace Safety and Insurance Board
200 Front Street West
Toronto, ON M5V 3J1

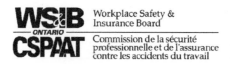

Workplace Safety &
Insurance Board

Commission de la sécurité
professionnelle et de l'assurance
contre les accidents du travail

Safety starts with you

www.wsib.on.ca

SOURCE: Reprinted with permission of The Workplace Safety and Insurance Board.

WSIB ONTARIO
CSPAAT

Health Professional's Report (Form 8)

Claim Number (If known)

A. Patient and Employer Information   (Patient to Complete this Section)

Last Name | First Name | Init.

Address (no. street, apt.)

City/Town | Prov. | Postal Code | Telephone No. ( )

Social Insurance No. | Job Title/Occupation | Health Card No. | Code

Date of Birth dd mm yy | Sex ☐ M ☐ F | Language ☐ Eng. ☐ Fr. | Does your employer have work duties that you can do while recovering? ☐ yes ☐ no ☐ don't know

Business or Company Name | Supervisor/Contact Name

Address (no. street, apt.)

City/Town | Prov. | Postal Code | Telephone No. ( )

Did you tell your employer about this injury/illness? ☐ yes ☐ no | Help us serve you better by telling us the size of your company: ☐ Small (1-19 workers), ☐ or Large (20 +)

The Workplace Safety and Insurance Board (WSIB) collects your information to administer and enforce the *Workplace Safety and Insurance Act*. The Social Insurance Number is used to register claims, identify workers and to issue income tax information statements as authorized by the *Income Tax Act*. The Health Card Number is collected under the authority of the *Health Card and Numbers Control Act* and is used for health administration and planning, research and studies. Questions? Contact the WSIB Privacy Officer at 1-800-387-5540 ext. 5323 or direct at 416 344-5323.

B. Health Professional Billing Information

☐ Chiropractor   ☐ Physician   ☐ Physiotherapist   ☐ Registered Nurse (Extended Class)

Service Code   **FORM8**

Health Professional Name   (please print)

WSIB Provider ID.

Address (no. street, apt.)

Your Invoice No.

City/Town | Prov. | Postal Code | FAX No. ( )

C. Incident Dates and Details Section

Date of Accident/ Recurrence   (dd/mm/yy)

1. What is your understanding as to how this injury/illness or re-injury occurred?

2. Have you previously treated this patient for this injury? ☐ yes ☐ no
If yes, please list dates of treatment since your last report:

3. Are you this patient's primary Health Professional? ☐ yes ☐ no | Location of this assessment ☐ Office ☐ Walk-in Clinic ☐ Emergency Dept. ☐ Other ☐ Workplace | Date of this assessment   (dd/mm/yy)

4. Did another Health Professional assess this patient before you? ☐ yes ☐ no | If yes, where and when did this take place? | Date (dd/mm/yy)

D. Clinical Information Section

1. Area of Injury (Body Part) - (Please check all that apply)

☐ Brain   ☐ Ears   ☐ Upper back
☐ Head   ☐ Teeth   ☐ Lower back
☐ Face   ☐ Neck   ☐ Abdomen
☐ Eyes   ☐ Chest   ☐ Pelvis
☐ Other:

Left / Right:
Shoulder ☐ ☐
Arm ☐ ☐
Elbow ☐ ☐
Forearm ☐

Left / Right:
Wrist ☐ ☐
Hand ☐ ☐
Fingers ☐ ☐

Left / Right:
Hip ☐ ☐
Thigh ☐ ☐
Knee ☐ ☐
Lower Leg ☐ ☐

Left / Right:
Ankle ☐ ☐
Foot ☐ ☐
Toes ☐ ☐

2. Type/Nature of Injury - (Please check all that apply)

☐ Abrasion
☐ Amputation
☐ Avulsion
☐ Bite
☐ Burn
☐ Contusion/Hematoma
☐ Crush Injury
☐ Degenerative Joint Disease

☐ Disc Herniation
☐ Dislocation
☐ Epicondylitis
☐ Fracture
☐ Ganglion
☐ Hernia
☐ Laceration
☐ Pain - Indeterminate Origin

☐ Puncture
☐ Repetitive Strain Injury
☐ Spinal Cord Injury
☐ Sprain/Strain
☐ Tendonitis/Tenosynovitis
☐ Other

☐ Asthma
☐ Dermatitis
☐ Fumes - Inhalation
☐ Hearing Loss

☐ Infectious Disease
☐ Needle Stick
☐ Poisoning/Toxic Effects
☐ Psychological

0008A (11/03)   Page 2

FIGURE **6.15**   **Health Professional's First Report, cont'd**   *continued*

WSIB ONTARIO
CSPAAT

Health Professional's Report
(Form 8)

Claim Number [| | | | | | |]

Patient's Last Name | Patient's First Name | Social Insurance No. [| | | | | | | |]

D. Clinical Information Section (continued)

3. Patient's Present Complaints (subjective complaints)

☐ Pain ☐ Paresthesia ☐ Stiffness ☐ Swelling ☐ Weakness ☐ Other _____

Description:

---

4. Physical Examination (objective findings)

☐ Bruising ☐ Crepitation ☐ Joint Effusion ☐ Lump/Swelling ☐ Tenderness ☐ Other _____
☐ Burns ☐ Deformity ☐ Laceration ☐ Scar ☐ Wasting

Description:

---

5. Are there abnormal signs for any of the following   If so please describe:
☐ Active ROM ☐ Passive ROM ☐ Gait
☐ Strength ☐ Reflexes ☐ Sensation ☐ Other

6. Are you aware of any pre-existing or other conditions/factors that may delay recovery? ☐ yes ☐ no

7. Diagnosis/Working Diagnosis

E. Treatment Plan and Return to Work Information

☐ **1. Treatment Plan**
Provide your proposed treatment plan for this patient (include goals, duration, frequency, etc..).

☐ **2. Medication(s) Prescribed**
Provide prescription details and anticipated medication adverse effects that could possibly impact ability to Return To Work.

☐ **3. Assistive Devices Prescribed**
Provide details (cane, crutches, orthotic, supports, etc..).

Treatment Plan/Medication details.

---

4. Investigations & Referrals:

☐ None ☐ Labs ☐ X-rays ☐ CT Scan ☐ MRI ☐ EMG/NCS ☐ Other

☐ Family Physician ☐ Specialist   Name

☐ Chiropractor ☐ Massage Therapist ☐ Occupational Health Centre

☐ Physiotherapist ☐ Occupational Therapist ☐ Other:

Name of Referral or Facility (if known) | Phone Number (| |) | | | | | | | | Appointment Date (dd/mm/yy)

---

5. Please indicate the patient's status and task limitations in relation to the diagnosis (please see Page 4 for details)

A. ☐ **No Limitations**
B. ☐ **Specified Limitations**
(Please Specify)
C. ☐ **No Return to Work**
(Rationale Required)

{ ☐ Standing
☐ Sitting
☐ Lifting
☐ Bending/Twisting

☐ Kneeling
☐ Climbing Stairs/Ladders
☐ Use of Upper Extremities
☐ Operating Heavy Equipment
☐ Limitations Due To Environmental Conditions

☐ Personal Protective Equipment
☐ Use of Public Transportation
☐ Operation of a Motor Vehicle
☐ Other _____

Explanation:

---

6. From the date of this assessment, the above status(es) will apply for approximately: ☐ 1 to 2 days; ☐ 3 to 7 days; ☐ 8 to 14 days; ☐ 14+ days

7. Have you discussed Return To Work and these task limitations as part of your treatment with your patient? ☐ yes ☐ no

8. Follow-up Appointment ☐ None Required ☐ next day; ☐ 2 to 3 days; ☐ 1 week; ☐ 2 weeks;

It is an offence to knowingly make a false or misleading statement or representation to the WSIB. I hereby declare that the information being submitted is true and complete.

Health Professional's Signature | Phone Number (| |) | | | | | | | | Date (dd/mm/yy)

0008A2 (11/03) | Page 3

FIGURE **6.15**   **Health Professional's First Report, cont'd**

Health Professional's Report (Form 8)
Guidelines for Completion

The following information provides some assistance in completing the Form 8. For additional details please see "Guidelines for Health Professionals – Completing WSIB Forms".

Section A - Patient and Employer Information (Patient to complete this section)

- The information in this section helps to register and administer the patient's claim. It also ensures that the Health Professional's report is sent to the correct claim file. If a patient is unable to complete this section, the Health Professional can assist.

- The patient's personal information is collected under the authority of *The Workplace Safety and Insurance Act* and is used to administer the claim. For more information contact the WSIB Privacy Office toll-free at 1-800-387-5540 ext. 5323 or (416) 344-5323.

- If the patient is unable to supply the SIN and OHIP numbers, or other information, the form should still be completed and submitted to the WSIB.

Sections B, C, D and E (to be completed by the Health Professional)

Section C – Incident Dates and Details Section

- *"Did another Health Professional assess this patient before you*?" Check (✓) Yes or No. "*If yes, where and when did it take place*?" Please provide this information, if you can. It will enable the WSIB to request a report from the other Health Professional.

Section D – Clinical Information Section

Please check (✓) all that apply. Include all relevant clinical and/or objective findings or symptoms. Space has been provided for any additional findings/symptoms not listed, or for any other details.

Section E – Treatment Plan & Return to Work Information

- "Please indicate the patient's status and task limitations in relation to the diagnosis." Always complete this question and check (✓) all that apply:

    A. "*No limitations*": Patient is able to return to work now; no task limitations needed.

    B. "*Specified Limitations (Please Specify)*": Please check all limitations that apply (e.g. standing, sitting, lifting). If you wish to provide further details, please use the space provided.

    C. "*No Return to Work (Rationale Required)*": If the patient is unable to return to work in <u>any</u> capacity, the WSIB needs to know why in order to make a determination on entitlement to benefits. Use the space provided to give us this information.

- Please note: You can check more than one status or time period if needed and give an explanation in the space provided e.g., - No return to work for 1 - 2 days, then a return to work with a lifting limitation for 3 - 7 days.

- "*From the date of this assessment, the above status(es) will apply for approximately:*" Check (✓) the time period. Please note that for anything beyond 14 days, the WSIB will request a Progress Report.

This Health Professionals Report (Form 8) is not intended to replace the

Functional Abilities Form for Timely Return To Work (FAF).

If your patient or the employer requests a FAF, please complete as usual.

0008A (11/03)   Page 4

FIGURE **6.15   Health Professional's First Report, cont'd**

Administrative Assistant's Responsibilities

1. Secure the Treatment Memorandum upon arrival of the injured worker at the doctor's office. This has already been completed by the employer confirming the accident or injury.
2. Ensure that the Health Professional's Report has been completed and send it to the WCB within 48 hours. This is done after the doctor has seen the patient, and has provided the necessary information. Complete the billing portion in the bottom right corner of the form to reimburse the physician for completing the report.
3. Place a copy of the Health Professional's Report, or both, in the patient's chart and document when it was submitted.
4. Keep a financial record of the charges for patients seen by the doctor on behalf of the WCB. Payment for services rendered is received from the MOH. Complete and submit a MOH claim using the same procedure as for regular health service claims. Enter "WCB" in the "Payment Program" block on the health claim card.
4. Keep a record of fees claimed for completing reports on behalf of the WCB.
5. Complete a Health Care Accounts Inquiry Form and send it to the WCB.
6. Forward a Physician's Progress Report. This will be done under certain circumstances only, and completed by the doctor. Be sure to complete the payment portion in the bottom right corner of the report form. Place a copy in the patient's chart and document when submitted.
7. If a physician is required to submit to the WCB a supporting document such as a consultation or operating report, complete a Form 0150 and affix it to the bottom right corner of the report. Form 0150 is referred to as a "payment label." You should ensure that all portions of the form contain the required information.

The medical administrative assistant is not required to have considerable knowledge concerning workers' compensation, because reporting work-related injuries is the responsibility of the employer and employee. The doctor is responsible for diagnosing the injuries, and the WCB makes the decision on compensation to the injured worker. The medical administrative assistant should, however, have a general knowledge of the system and be capable of completing all forms related to the doctor's involvement with the WCB.

The medical administrative assistant is responsible for submitting WCB claims. The additional information required is listed as follows:

- Identify as WCB (WSIB) claim
- Patient's Social Insurance Number (SIN)
- Date of original injury
- Claim number (if one has been assigned)

If you have questions or need clarification of information, call the Workers' Compensation Board's head office. The number is in the telephone directory in both the white pages and the blue pages "government services" section.

RELEASE OF WORKERS' COMPENSATION INFORMATION

Before releasing any WCB information to a third party you must obtain a release of information. This form is usually entitled "WCB Medical Waiver Form" and is signed by the injured patient and witnessed by a second party.

ASSIGNMENT **6.2**

Dr. Plunkett provides you with the necessary information, and you are responsible for the completion of all reports, the doctor's account forms, and the submission of this information to the WCB.

 Using the following information, complete the Health Professional's Report (on the accompanying CD) and the Ministry of Health health claim.

On February 16, 20__, Tim Peters was involved in an industrial accident. Dr. Plunkett was doing rounds at the hospital (no. 1220) and Tim was transported to the hospital for examination. On examination, it was discovered that he had a severe sprain in his left ankle. The doctor recommended bed rest for one week, after which time he felt Tim would be able to return to work. Dr. Plunkett feels that three weeks of physiotherapy (twice weekly) will be required to restore the muscles in the ankle.

Tim Peters's social insurance number is 416 274 963. He is employed at Smith and Smith Limited, 372 Parkview Drive, Ottawa. The claim number has not yet been issued. Dr. Plunkett first saw Tim at 1535.

THIRD-PARTY INSURANCE

In addition to healthcare plans and workers' compensation, the public may wish to carry additional healthcare insurance to cover expenses not reimbursed by their respective plans.

Many private insurance companies issue group and individual policies to cover these additional expenses. London Life Mutual, Blue Cross, Green Shield, and Manulife are examples of third-party private insurance companies.

Some Benefits Available through Third-Party Insurance

1. Semi-private or private hospital accommodation (available on an individual pay-direct or a group basis).
2. Extended healthcare plans (available on an individual pay-direct or a group basis) provide protection against the costs of health services not covered by basic government health plans. The plan can be tailored to the needs of any group.
3. Prescription drug plan (available on a group basis), to help protect group subscribers and their families against the costs of prescribed drugs and injectables.

4. Vision care plan (available on a group basis), to provide payment toward the purchase of eye glasses and contact lenses.
5. Dental plan (available on a group basis).
6. Nursing home plan (available on a group basis).
7. Health plan for visitors (on an individual or a family basis), designed to provide visitors to Canada with protection against unexpected costs of hospital care.
8. Health plan for Canadians while travelling outside Canada (on an individual or a family basis), designed to protect people from unexpected costs of medical bills incurred while on business or vacationing anywhere outside Canada.

A general knowledge of what is available through third-party insurance companies is an asset. Although each private company offers its own plan, most benefits offered are very similar.

HOW THE MINISTRY OF HEALTH COMMUNICATES WITH MEDICAL ADMINISTRATIVE ASSISTANTS

The MOH communicates with medical administrative assistants in various ways. The following is a list of some of these ways:

1. Provincial Fee Schedule—Sent to the provider whenever ministry fees are renegotiated.
2. Bulletins—Sent whenever updates in rules or fees are required.
3. Brochures/Posters/Forms—Available for a variety of subjects. Additional copies are available from your local ministry office. Also available are all forms mentioned earlier in this chapter.
4. Claim Submission Manual—Available to all providers' offices. This manual assists administrative assistants in completing claims.
5. Medical Administrative Assistant Seminars—The ministry periodically conducts seminars in various cities. You will be invited to attend whenever one is to be held in your vicinity. These seminars have proved to be very popular and informative.

CONCLUSION

All of the preceding information will prove helpful once you begin your work as a medical administrative assistant. However, it is intended as a basic outline only. As in all professions, additional on-the-job training must be gained before you are proficient in your field.

Remember that your local MOH office will be available for assistance whenever possible.

ASSIGNMENT 6.3

Your instructor will provide you with the material required to complete this assignment.

ASSIGNMENT **6.4**

If your class is interested in more detailed information about third-party insurance, appoint a group to arrange for representatives of private insurance companies to visit your class to expand on the benefits offered by their particular organizations.

TOPICS FOR DISCUSSION

1. A patient arrives in the office for a visit. He has travelled over 300 kilometres for this visit and is complaining to you of the cost to him. How would you handle this situation?

2. Your healthcare claims are sent by diskette. It is almost the end of your billing cycle and the computer system has crashed. You still have to submit your claims. What will you do?

3. Your physician has given you a billing to submit. He saw the patient on a Sunday at 1730 in the hospital. He has given you the service code and diagnosis. What do you need to complete this billing?

4. Mr. Thomas has been sent to your office with an injury that occurred at work. What do you need to complete this billing?

CHAPTER 7

Financial Records

CHAPTER OUTLINE

Managing Finances in the Medical Office
Banking

Payroll
Topics for Discussion

LEARNING OBJECTIVES

After reading this chapter, you will be able to outline

- How to record cash disbursements, cash receipts, and patient charges in journals.
- How to prepare and post information from journals.
- How to prepare patient statements of account.
- How to control petty cash.

- How to prepare cheques and cash for deposit.
- How to reconcile bank statements.
- How to interpret payroll deduction tables and prepare payroll sheets.
- How to complete Revenue Canada payroll remittance forms.

KEY TERMS

Disbursement: The money that is being paid out.

Invoice: An invoice provides an itemized list of charges and prices owed.

Remittance: The money that is being paid to you.

Schedule of Benefits: The physicians' book that outlines the services they can provide, the premiums they are entitled to, and the fee that they can bill the Ministry of Health.

Statement: A financial accounting sheet.

Transaction: An exchange or transfer of goods, services or funds.

FIGURE **7.1** **Manual Accounting System**

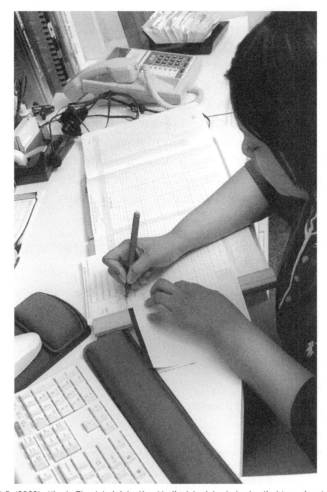

SOURCE: Young, A.P. (2003). *Kinn's The Administrative Medical Assistant: An Applied Learning Approach* (5th ed., p. 266: Figure 14.5). St. Louis: Elsevier/Saunders.

MANAGING FINANCES IN THE MEDICAL OFFICE

It is essential for any business to keep accurate and complete financial records. Large organizations such as hospitals, clinics, and health service organizations employ graduate accountants and have a separate finance department because their accounting systems are very complex. Generally, a small service organization maintains an adequate set of accounting records to enable a chartered accountant to complete the financial statements and process the proprietor's income tax returns.

A medical administrative assistant in a single-proprietorship practice should be knowledgeable about single-entry bookkeeping, writing cheques, bank deposits, petty cash records, completing patients' accounts and statements, and bank reconciliations (see Figure 7.1). Most medical administrative assistants take care of these accounting functions at a time when the doctor is not seeing patients or at other times when the office is not busy.

Since billing methods vary among the provinces, this chapter will follow Ontario procedures.

In many medical offices, all accounting procedures will be computerized, including medical plan billing, **remittance** advice reconciliation, cash receipts and **disbursements**, cheque writing, and so on. In a single-entry bookkeeping system, a multicolumn journal is used to record all daily receipts and expenditures. Look at Figure 7.2. This is a cash disbursements journal. You must record where the money is spent. Therefore, the payment entry is extended into a column that groups similar payouts. The accountant who sets up your doctor's accounting records will suggest basic column headings for disbursements. In order to fully understand the material necessary for computer input, it is first necessary to work with material using manual procedures.

Recording in the Cash Disbursements Journal

On a typical day in the doctor's office, you might record the following **transaction** in your cash disbursements journal.

January 2, 20__, purchased 2 gross (1 gross = 12 dozen) needles from AFAXEL Co. at $24.95 per gross. This transaction has been recorded in Figure 7.2 using the procedures outlined in the next paragraph:

FIGURE **7.2** **Cash Disbursements Journal**

| | | | CASH DISBURSEMENTS JOURNAL | | | | | | | | | | PAGE 1 | |
Date	Explanation	Ch. #	Amount	Office Supplies	Med. Supplies	Wages	U.I.C. C.P.P. In. Tax	Heat, Hydro, Tele.	Auto Maint. & Gas	Office Rent & Maint.	Draw'ng	Travel & Enter.	Misc.
20- JAN. 2	AFAXEL Co (2 gr. needles)	123	49 90		49 90								

At the top of the date column, the year is entered. On line one, the month and day are entered. Do not repeat the month again until it changes. The year appears only at the top of the date column on each page. Following along horizontally, enter the reason for payment—company name and 2 gross needles—in the "Explanation" column; the number of the cheque used to make payment in the "Ch.#" column—123; the amount of the purchase in the "Amount" column and also in the "Med. Supplies" column— $49.90.

ASSIGNMENT 7.1

(For the assignments in this chapter, record the transactions on the text figures or use the blank form provided on the accompanying CD.)

Following the same procedure described above, record these additional transactions (use consecutive cheque numbers, starting at no. 124):

January	2	Establish petty cash fund for $50
	2	The doctor entertained at a dinner party and spent $50 (Romeo's Cafe)
	2	Paid Purolator $7.62 for delivery of laboratory reports
	3	Purchased letterhead and envelopes $48.29 (ABC Supplies)
	3	Paid January rent $400 (Medical Services Inc.)
	4	Paid automobile credit card charges for gas and oil $71.65 (Jay's Gas Bar)
	5	Paid your wages $450, and janitor's wages $280 (Don James)
	5	The doctor withdrew $350 for personal use
	8	Sent cheque to Ontario Hydro for $147
	8	Made $100 contribution to the United Way
	9	Paid telephone bill of $56.50 (Bell Canada)
	11	Paid Campbell's Florist $25 for roses sent to the doctor's wife for anniversary
	12	Paid your wages $450, and janitor's wages $280 (Don James)
	12	The doctor withdrew $350
	13	Submitted cheque to the Receiver General of Canada for income tax $290; employment insurance, $15.18; Canada Pension $12.92
	13	Reimbursed petty cash $47.41

Examine your entry on January 2 for the dinner party. If a businessperson entertains for the purpose of promoting the business, the expense is tax deductible. However, a businessperson must not charge personal expenses against the business. You may have entered the $50 dinner expense under "Travel and Entertainment," assuming it was a business engagement. Or you may have assumed it was a personal engagement, in which case the entry would be made under "Drawings."

FIGURE **7.3** **Business Cheques**

BAL.	$ 3,912.10
DEP.	1,069.00
TOTAL	4,981.10
CHEQUE	7.62
BAL.	4,973.48

PAY TO *PuROLATOR*

FOR LAB REPORTS

SUM OF *7.62*

DATE *JAN. 2/--* NO. *126*

THE BANK OF NOVA SCOTIA

Scotiabank **S**

126   *JAN 2, 20--*
NO.   DATE

PAY TO THE ORDER OF — *PuROLATOR* $ *7.62*

SUM OF — *SEVEN* —   *62* DOLLARS
                                                    ⎯⎯
                                                    100

ACCOUNT NO. *00000*

J. C. Plunkett

BAL.	$
DEP.	
TOTAL	
CHEQUE	
BAL.	

PAY TO

SUM OF

DATE   NO.

THE BANK OF NOVA SCOTIA

Scotiabank **S**

NO.   DATE

PAY TO THE ORDER OF $

SUM OF   DOLLARS

ACCOUNT NO.

Writing Cheques

A safe and convenient way to handle the payment of accounts is to write cheques. Since you will not have large amounts of cash on hand, you can eliminate the possibility of theft and loss. Also, mailing a cheque rather than making a personal visit to pay cash is a more efficient business practice. Never put cash in the mail. Cheques used by business are similar to those shown in Figure 7.3. (The January 2 payment is recorded on the first cheque.)

A running balance is kept on the cheque stub. This allows you to double check your accounting accuracy. The cheque number, amount, name of person to whom the cheque is issued, and purpose of the cheque also appear on the stub. On the actual cheque, the amount of the cheque in figures, as well as in words, and the payer's signature must be recorded.

In a computerized system the cheque is written and automatically posted to the chosen account. The program then balances the account.

ASSIGNMENT **7.2**

Write cheques for the first four entries in your cash disbursements journal. The beginning balance on cheque no. 123 is $4062. Assume that on January 2 you deposited $1069. (An extra cheque form can be found on the accompanying CD.)

Patients' Charges (Uninsured Services)

Physicians bill for the services provided. The billing amount is outlined in the provincial **Schedule of Benefits (SOB)**. At one time, physicians could be "opted out," which meant that they could bill the patient an amount over and above the fee assigned in the Schedule of Benefits. It is now illegal for physicians to extra-bill, therefore, there is no longer a benefit to be "opted out." The physician does perform some services that are no longer covered by the Schedule of Benefits. At one time all infant circumcisions were covered, but as they are not deemed medically necessary, the parent is now required to pay the physician directly if this is the procedure of choice. Patients need to be aware of uninsured services. See Figure 7.4 for an example of how this information can be communicated to your patients.

You must keep a record of all charges and payments for all patients. You may choose to record charges on a family or individual basis. The computerized system keeps track of charges and outstanding balances for each patient. As seen in Figure 7.4, a patient can pay an annual fee for uninsured services or they can choose to pay on a fee for service basis. The College of Physicians and Surgeons provides guidelines to practitioners for this billing process. See Box 7.1 for a listing of uninsured services.

7.1 Uninsured Services

Telephone advice
Prescription renewal by telephone (at patient's request)
Tax disability
Long distance phone calls or fax (at patient's request)
Transfer of medical records
Private insurance forms
UIC or maternity certificate
Return to Work form
Third-party medical examinations (adult)
Drivers' medical exams
Employment physicals
University/college physicals
Camp physicals
Photocopies
Summary of records requested by a third party
Procedures that are not deemed medically necessary

Physician Billing (Insured Services)

The physician submits a fee for each patient to the Ministry of Health and is reimbursed for these charges when his or her monthly medical insurance payment is received. This amount is deposited directly into the physician's bank account.

FIGURE **7.4**   **Letter Explaining Uninsured Services**

JOHN E. PLUNKETT
PHM.B.,MD.,CM.,FRCPC.,FACP.
278 O'Connor Street Ottawa, ON Tel: 613-722-7176
J5Z 2X8

Dear Patient(s),

I am writing to you regarding the payment of services not covered by O.H.I.P. For years I have absorbed these costs but am no longer able to provide these services for which I am not paid. Firstly, the demand for uninsured services has increased dramatically. This required more time and more staff. Secondly, our expenses continue to rise like everyone else's and thirdly, my staff is dependable, well-trained and hard working. Accordingly they deserve wage increases that keep pace with inflation. Accordingly, I would ask each of you to review the following information and select a method of payment that you feel would suit your needs.

OPTION #1: COMPREHENSIVE ANNUAL FEE

The Comprehensive fee covered all uninsured services for 1 year **regardless of how often they are used.** The annual fee is $50.00 per adult (over 21) and $20.00 to cover all dependent children under 21. The maximum fee for a family with dependent children is $120.00.
This fee does NOT cover missed appointments.

OPTION #2: FEE FOR SERVICE

Should you choose not the pay the Comprehensive fee, each service rendered will be billed to you according to the following fees:

TELEPHONE ADVICE	$15.00 per call
TAX DISABILITY	$30.00
PRESCRIPTION RENEWAL BY PHONE (at your request)	$15.00
LONG DISTANCE PHONE CALLS or FAX (at your request)	$15.00
TRANSFER OF MEDICAL RECORDS	Adults-$25.00- $100.00
	Child -$15.00 - $30.00
PRIVATE INSURANCE FORMS	$20.00 -$75.00
UIC OR MATERNITY CERTIFICATE	$25.00 minimum
RETURN TO WORK FORM	$20.00
DISABILITY PARKING FORMS	$25.00
THIRD-PARTY MEDICAL EXAMINATIONS ADULT 16 YEARS AND OLDER	
DRIVERS MEDICAL EXAMS	$95.00
EMPLOYMENT PHYSICALS	
UNIVERSITY/COLLEGE PHYSICALS	
CHILDREN AND ADOLESCENT (i.e. CAMP PHYSICALS)	$40.00
RETURN TO WORK ASSESSEMENT	$25.00
PHOTOCOPIES	$ 2.00
SUMMARY OF RECORDS REQUESTED BY A THIRD PARTY	$50.00 and up

<u>Please note: payment for forms will be requested prior to pick up</u>

Please note the guidelines set out by the College of Physicians of Ontario regarding this issue:

1.   You cannot be charged an annual fee for less than one year.
2.   The services covered by this fee must be clearly written.
3.   You must be told the cost of each service.
4.   You do not have to pay an annual fee. You may pay for each service not covered by OHIP.

5.   The decision on whether or not to pay the annual fee is yours and will not be a condition of your being seen by the doctor.

6.   Before indicating your agreement to pay an annual fee you must be given a copy of these rules.

7.   Your doctor cannot charge for being available to render a "service" in advance.

Should you be interested in the Comprehensive Fee coverage for this year please complete and return the form below with your payment by June 01, 20__. This will be effective until May 31, 20__.

Please contact me if you have any questions.

Also, if you would like a flu shot this fall, please call us after October 1st to make an appointment.

Prescriptions will not be filled over the phone if there is an outstanding bill for previous renewals. You will have to come in to the office to receive your scripts until this bill is paid.

Please refrain from calling in for prescriptions before 10:00.

We only book after 5:00 pm if it is an emergency. Please do not walk into the office and expect to see the doctor. Please make an appointment.

Patients Name(s)   _____

Address   _____

Please check either A or B and enclose the appropriate payment.
Receipt will be provided upon request

☐   **Plan A: Payment enclosed for annual fee $50.00 per adult and $20.00 to include any number of dependent children (under 21) maximum $120.00.**

Signature: _____ **Date:** _____

☐   **Plan B: Bill me on a Fee for Service basis.**

Signature: _____ **Date:** _____

John E. Plunkett, M.D.

FIGURE **7.4**   **Letter Explaining Uninsured Services, cont'd**

Patient's Statement of Account

At the end of each month, the administrative assistant must review the patient's account of uninsured services and send a **statement** to those who show a balance owing. Examine the statement of account in Figure 7.5 (see also Figure 7.6). A statement of account form may vary in its format, but the information required is generally the same (see itemized list that follows):

1. Name of statement
2. Originator's name, address, and telephone number
3. The date the statement is issued
4. Name and address of the debtor
5. Date of each service
6. Explanation of the service
7. Amount of the charges
8. Amount of any payment received
9. Balance owed
10. Notification of service charge for overdue accounts

It may be helpful to keep copies of outstanding statements (or a list) near the telephone. When patients call about their accounts or come into the office to pay an outstanding balance, the information is readily available.

Petty Cash

Most doctors' offices maintain a small petty cash fund to purchase stamps, coffee supplies, and so on. It is essential that an accurate record be maintained for the petty cash. This record does not have to be elaborate, but simply a record of the amount received to replenish the fund and a record of what payments were made from the fund (see Figure 7.7).

7.2

Sometimes a doctor is faced with unpaid accounts. After several unsuccessful attempts to collect the overdue account, a decision must be made whether to put the account in the hands of a collection agency or write off the account as a bad debt. The doctor's accountant generally makes this decision and takes the necessary action.

Let us assume that on January 2, 20__, a cheque for $50 was issued to establish a petty cash fund. The entry would be: year at the top of the "Date" column; date, January 2; explanation—cheque no. 124 to establish petty cash; received, $50; balance, $50.

FIGURE **7.5**   **Statement of Account**

STATEMENT

JOHN E. PLUNKETT
PHM.B.,MD.,CM.,FRCPC.,FACP.
278 O'Connor Street Ottawa, ON Tel: 613-722-7176
J5Z 2X8

Statement Date
31-Aug-20__

PLEASE RETURN THIS PORTION
WITH YOUR PAYMENT

DOE, JANE
1234 CHERRY LANE
PTBO, ONT, CA K1K 1K1

Statement Date
31-Aug-20__

DOE, JANE

IF PAYING BY INVOICE, CHECK
INDIVIDUAL INVOICES PAID

AMOUNT REMITTED_____

Page   1

Transaction Date	Description	Amount	Balance	Invoice No.	Amount Due	✓
31-Aug-20__		15.00	15.00	473	15.00	

Age	Current	31 - 60	Over 60	Total	Balance Due	Total
Amount	$15.00	$0.00	$0.00	$15.00	‹ ›	$15.00

FIGURE **7.6** **Invoice**

INVOICE

JOHN E. PLUNKETT
PHM.B.,MD.,CM.,FRCPC.,FACP.
278 O'Connor Street Ottawa, ON Tel: 613-722-7176
J5Z 2X8

| Invoice No.: | 0000 |
| Date: | 8/31/04 |

Bill To:

DOE, JANE
1234 CHERRY LANE
PTBO, ONT K1K 1K1
CA

Business No.: 88930 4861

Description	Amount
Prescription Renewal - Aug 20, 20__	15.00
	15.00
Terms: 2%/10, Net 30 Due 30-Sep-20__	

Comments	0.00
Total Amount	$15.00

FIGURE **7.7**   **Petty Cash Record**

PETTY CASH RECORD								
Date		Explanation	Receipts		Payments		Balance	
20- Jan 2		ESTABLISH PETTY CASH	50	–			50	–

ASSIGNMENT **7.3**

Using the form in Figure 7.7 or one from the accompanying CD, record the following transactions for January:

January	2	Bought paper clips, $1.29
	4	Paid for collect telegram, $1.35
	8	Purchased sugar, cream, and coffee, $11.27
	10	Bought stamps, $30
	13	Doctor's lunch, $3.50

When the cash in your petty cash box gets low, it is time to replenish the fund. You should have $2.59 in your cash box to agree with the balance column in your petty cash record. In order to bring your petty cash up to $50, you would write a cheque made out to cash in the amount of $47.41, have the doctor sign it, and then cash it when you go to the bank.

The petty cash box is generally a small metal box approximately 20 cm × 15 cm × 8 cm (8 inches × 6 inches × 3 inches) and is kept in the administrative assistant's desk or a file cabinet. You should be able to lock the drawer containing the petty cash box. You should always ask for receipts when making payment from the petty cash box to verify the amount of cash paid out. Occasionally, fellow workers may ask to borrow money from the cash box. If you are responsible for petty cash, it is advisable to refrain from making such personal loans.

BANKING

The three main banking duties required of the administrative assistant follow:

1. Making deposits
2. Writing cheques
3. Reconciling the monthly bank statement

We discussed cheque writing earlier in this chapter. We will now examine depositing and reconciling the bank statement.

Making Deposits

The doctor's *main* source of revenue is the fee paid by the Ministry of Health for the doctor's services.

As explained previously, the doctor submits a service fee for each patient to the Ministry of Health. The ministry issues a cheque or makes a direct deposit to the provider's bank every month for the amount of fee submissions during the period covered by the cheque. Other deposits will mainly consist of the revenue generated by uninsured services. In a complementary care setting such as chiropractic, physiotherapy, or massage therapy, the *main* source of revenue is through direct billing to patients/clients or to individual insurance companies. When you receive a cheque, it is a good safety measure to use a "For Deposit Only" stamp on the back of the cheque (see Figure 7.8). This is a form of endorsement.

FIGURE **7.8** **"For Deposit Only" Stamp**

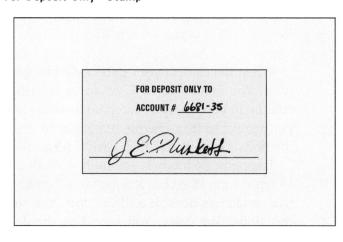

FIGURE **7.9**   **Deposit Slip**

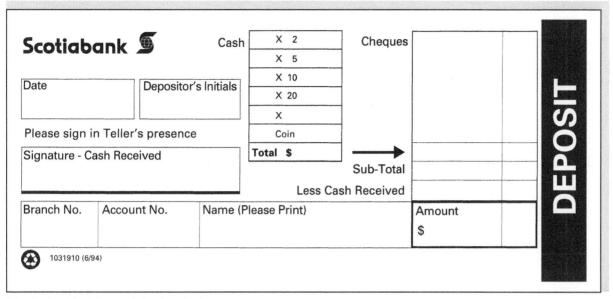

SOURCE: Reprinted with permission from Scotiabank.

If the cheque is lost or stolen but has this stamp on the back, it cannot be cashed. Each time you receive a cheque, you deposit it in the practitioner's business account.

A deposit slip may be used, similar to that in Figure 7.9, and is completed before presenting the deposit to the bank teller. Most offices use a deposit book (see Figure 7.10) rather than deposit slips, as the slips can be easily misplaced. The deposit information remains part of the book, therefore eliminating this risk.

It is never wise to accept a post-dated cheque. You cannot deposit a post-dated cheque until it is due, and collection on a post-dated cheque returned "not sufficient funds" (NSF) can sometimes cause problems.

ASSIGNMENT **7.4**

Enter the following information on a deposit slip (see accompanying CD) for Dr. Plunkett: date, January 13, 20__; cash $152.57 consisting of 9 ones, 4 twos, 3 fives, 6 tens, 3 twenties, and 57 cents in coin; cheques for $13.42 from E.C. Westran, $35 from C.S.A. Insurance Co. (for writing a patient history), $116.28 from W.C. Post, and $52.50 from R.A. James; account no. 6681-35; name of account, Dr. J.E. Plunkett (you made the deposit).

ASSIGNMENT **7.5**

Your instructor will provide you with the information required to complete this assignment.

FIGURE **7.10**   **Deposit Book**

DATE					CREDIT ACCOUNT OF:		

		DATE			INITIALS	
		DAY	MONTH	YEAR	DEPOSITOR'S	TELLER'S

Cheques	Amount
Total CAD $ Cheque Amount	
Total # CAD Cheques	

Wallet No. (if applicable)	
x 5	
x 10	
x 20	
x 50	
x 100	
Total CAD Cash	
Total Coin	
Total # Total CAD $ Cheques	
Total VISA	
Total Foreign Cash (do not include exchange)	
Total # Total Foreign $ Cheques	
Subtotal	
Bank Use Only	
Exchange	
Total ➡	
Deposited by	

If total cash exceeds $10,000, complete Declaration of Source of Funds on reverse.

Bank Copy

Bank Reconciliation

Each month, the bank sends a statement of account and all cancelled cheques to its current account customers. (A business bank account is called a current account.) The administrative assistant must check his or her figures with the bank's balance to make sure the two accounts agree.

The cancelled cheques received from the bank are checked off the chequebook and a small check mark (√) is placed beside the corresponding amount on the statement. After completing this procedure, you are ready to reconcile your statement. Divide a sheet of paper in two and write "Bank Balance" on one side and "Chequebook Balance" on the other (see Figure 7.11).

FIGURE **7.11** **Bank Reconciliation**

January 13, 20___				
Bank Balance		$2,769.20	**Chequebook Balance**	$1,326.50
Outstanding Cheques			1) Service Charge	−3.50
(a) S.O.S.	$ 732.60			1,323.00
(b) Jones	1,072.91		2) Interest earned	+127.50
(c) R.G. of				1,450.50
Canada	427.50	2,233.01	3) Loan interest paid	−200.00
		536.19		1,250.50
(d) Jan. 11			4) Safety deposit box	−5.70
Deposit		+543.21		1,244.80
			5) NSF Cheque Thomas Bell	−165.40
BANK BALANCE		$1,079.40	CHEQUEBOOK BALANCE	1,079.40

On your statement, you see five items that are not checked off. Item (1) is a service charge for $3.50; item (2) is a credit memo for $127.50 for interest you received on your term deposit; item (3) is a debit memo for $200 interest charged on a loan; item (4) is a $5.70 charge for safety deposit box rental; and item (5) is a debit memo for an NSF cheque from Thomas Bell for $165.40.

The procedure to record these items is as follows:

No. 1   The bank has charged you for service, but you have not recorded the charge on your books. Subtract $3.50 from the chequebook side.

No. 2   A savings deposit at the bank has earned $127.50 interest. The bank has recorded it in your account; now you have to enter the amount in your records. Add to the chequebook side.

No. 3   The bank has made a loan to the business. Two hundred dollars for interest on the loan is deducted from your bank account. You must make an equal deduction from your chequebook record.

No. 4   The bank charges $5.70 yearly for rental of a safety deposit box. The bank has charged your account; you must charge your records with the same amount.

No. 5   A patient, Thomas Bell, gave you a cheque for $165.40. You deposited the cheque in the bank and added the amount to your records. When you received your bank statements, you discovered that Mr. Bell did not have sufficient funds in his account to cover the cheque. It was, therefore, returned to you. The bank did not add $165.40 to its records. You must therefore subtract the amount from your records.

Items (1), (3), and (4) would be entered in your cash disbursements journal after your statement is reconciled. Although you would not write cheques for these items, you would have to subtract the amounts from your cheque-book stubs in order to keep your running balance accurate. For item (2) you would record it on your chequebook stub in the deposit space and label it "interested earned". Item (5) would require a notation in the patients' charges and payments journal beside the entry that recorded the receipt of Mr. Bell's payment, indicating that the cheque was returned NSF. The amount of the cheque would have to be deducted from the chequebook stub, and an adjustment to Mr. Bell's account would have to be made.

When you examine your chequebook stubs, you discover that three cheques you have written have not been cashed. The cheques are to Smith Office Supplies, $732.60; Jones Medical Service, $1072.91; and the Receiver General of Canada, $427.50.

You have deducted all these cheques from your chequebook. But since they have not been cashed, the amounts have not been deducted from your bank account. See items (a), (b), and (c) in Figure 7.11.

Your bank statement was mailed on January 12, and on January 11 you made a deposit of $543.21. You notice that the amount does not appear on your statement. You have added this deposit to your chequebook; you must now add it to your bank statement (d).

Your bank statement and your chequebook balance are now in agreement.

Many offices do not require the completion of a formal printed reconciliation statement. However, you should be aware of the correct format. Based on the information used in Figure 7.11, a formal keyed bank reconciliation statement would resemble that shown in Figure 7.12.

At the end of every month a computerized printout of the general ledger, balance sheet, income statement and bank reconciliation statement should be

FIGURE **7.12**   **Bank Reconciliation Statement**

J.E. PLUNKETT M.D.
Bank Reconciliation Statement
January 13, 20___

Balance as per bank statement, January 13		$2,769.20
Add: Deposit of January 11 not recorded by bank		543.21
		$3,312.41
Deduct Outstanding Cheques:		
#236 S.O.S.	$ 732.60	
#239 Jones Medical Services	1,072.91	
#244 Receiver General of Canada	427.50	2,233.01
Adjusted Bank Balance		$1,079.40
Balance as per Chequebook, January 13		$1,326.50
Add: Interest on term deposit		127.50
		$1,454.00
Deduct: Debit memo for safety deposit box rental	$ 5.70	
Bank interest on demand loan	200.00	
Monthly service charge	3.50	
NSF Cheque of Thomas Bell	165.40	374.60
Adjusted Chequebook balance		$1,079.40

available to the employer. Often, a comparative income statement and bank statement are completed to show the previous year versus the current year to date.

ASSIGNMENT **7.6**

Using the following information, prepare rough draft bank reconciliation statements for Dr. Plunkett.

a. The bank reported the balance of $2751.16. Your records show a balance of $2823.70. A cheque issued to us from J.P. Sands for $50.75 was returned NSF. Cheque no. 42 is still outstanding. The bank charged $2 for service. Cheque nos. 46 and 53 are outstanding. The account was debited $10 for interest on the demand loan. Cheque no. 55 for $127.50 is outstanding. Cheque stub no. 40 revealed an error: the cheque was recorded as $36 when it should have been $72. The amounts of cheque nos. 42, 46, and 53 are $19.75, $75.80, and $68.30, respectively. Bank deposit made but not recorded on bank statement $295.14. Bond interest paid by bank $37.50. Safety deposit charges $7.50. Date the statement November 30, 20__.

b. Final bank balance as shown on bank statement $3241.82. Cash account balance (agreeing with chequebook balance on February 29) $3544.22. Outstanding cheques: no. 140, $31.40; no. 144, $40.00; no. 147, $7.15. Deposit in night depository on last day of February, outstanding on bank statement, $234. Dishonoured cheque from W.J. Krestel, $144. Bank service charge $2.75. A cheque issued to Kraus Novelty Company (no. 141) was issued for $14.40, but incorrectly recorded in the cash journal and on the cheque stub as $14.20. Date the statement March 31, 20_.

ASSIGNMENT **7.7**

Prepare a bank reconciliation statement for Dr. Plunkett using the following information. Date the statement April 1, 20__. Students may use a computer software package.

Cash account $2140 and March 31 bank statement $2012. Deposit entered in books on March 30 was not taken to the bank until March 31 (amount $530). The bank sent a credit memo for $215 for interest earned on Canada Savings Bonds. The amount is shown on the account. However, the memo has not yet been received. Bank service charges $6. A patient's cheque for $50, included in the March 27 deposit, has been charged back by the bank on the statement as NSF. The patient is J. Wren. Cheque no. 502 was made out to cash for $35 to reimburse the petty cash; this cheque is recorded in the cash payments journal as $53. The following cheques were not returned by the bank with the March statement: no. 521 to R. Smith for $10; no. 523 to J. Jones Ltd. for $50; no. 524 to Metrics Limited for $100 (certified on March 27); no. 525 to P. Brown for $75; and no. 526 to J. Smith and Company for $90.

PAYROLL

In order to follow this section of the chapter, each student must have a copy of the Canada Pension Plan (CPP), Employment Insurance (EI), and Income Tax Deduction tables. These tables are now included with most accounting programs. If not, a diskette is available from the Receiver General. The software company or the Receiver General will provide updates semi-annually in January and July.

Before beginning the instructions for payroll, please read the preambles at the beginning of the CPP, EI, and income tax tables. It is essential that anyone working with payroll be familiar with the instructions given in these two manuals. Because you require the tables to compute any payroll, reprinting the guidelines in this text is unnecessary.

In a large organization, payroll is fairly complicated and requires several employees to process the employee paycheques each pay period. However, in a small organization, of say ten or less, the payroll procedure is fairly simple. You can purchase a payroll book from an office supply store to cover 52 pay periods (or one year). Each employee has a separate sheet similar to that in Figure 7.13. Many offices use a computerized payroll system. However, in order for you to understand a payroll process, we are providing information on the manual procedure.

Let us assume that in your office you are the only salaried employee. The doctor does not have a registered nurse. A part-time janitor looks after cleaning and maintenance duties and is paid on an hourly basis. The doctor is not on the payroll; he or she is the proprietor of the business. A proprietor cannot draw wages from his or her company. The money the doctor extracts for personal use is called "drawings," which you learned about earlier in the chapter.

The first step is to complete the personal data portion on the payroll page. In order to read the Income Tax Deduction table, you must establish the employee's code. This is done by completing a TD1 form, which lists your total exemptions and places you in one of fourteen categories in the Income Tax Deduction table. The CPP, EI, and tax are calculated according to the pay period, which can be weekly, bi-weekly, or monthly.

ASSIGNMENT 7.8

Let us assume that you are single with no dependents; your deductions would be read from column 1. The janitor's deductions are read from column 4. Using blank payroll forms from the CD, we will complete the payroll for the week of January 15, 20__.

You are paid $450 weekly and work 40 hours. The janitor, Mr. Don James, earns $8 an hour. Mr. James lives at 321 Jane Street, Manotick, K2E 7Z3. His phone number is 626-9731. He was formerly employed as a toolmaker at Tool and Die Co. Ltd. He was born September 25, 1939, and is a widower. He looks after his elderly mother and two teenage children. He began working in Dr. Plunkett's office two

FIGURE **7.13** **Payroll Journal**

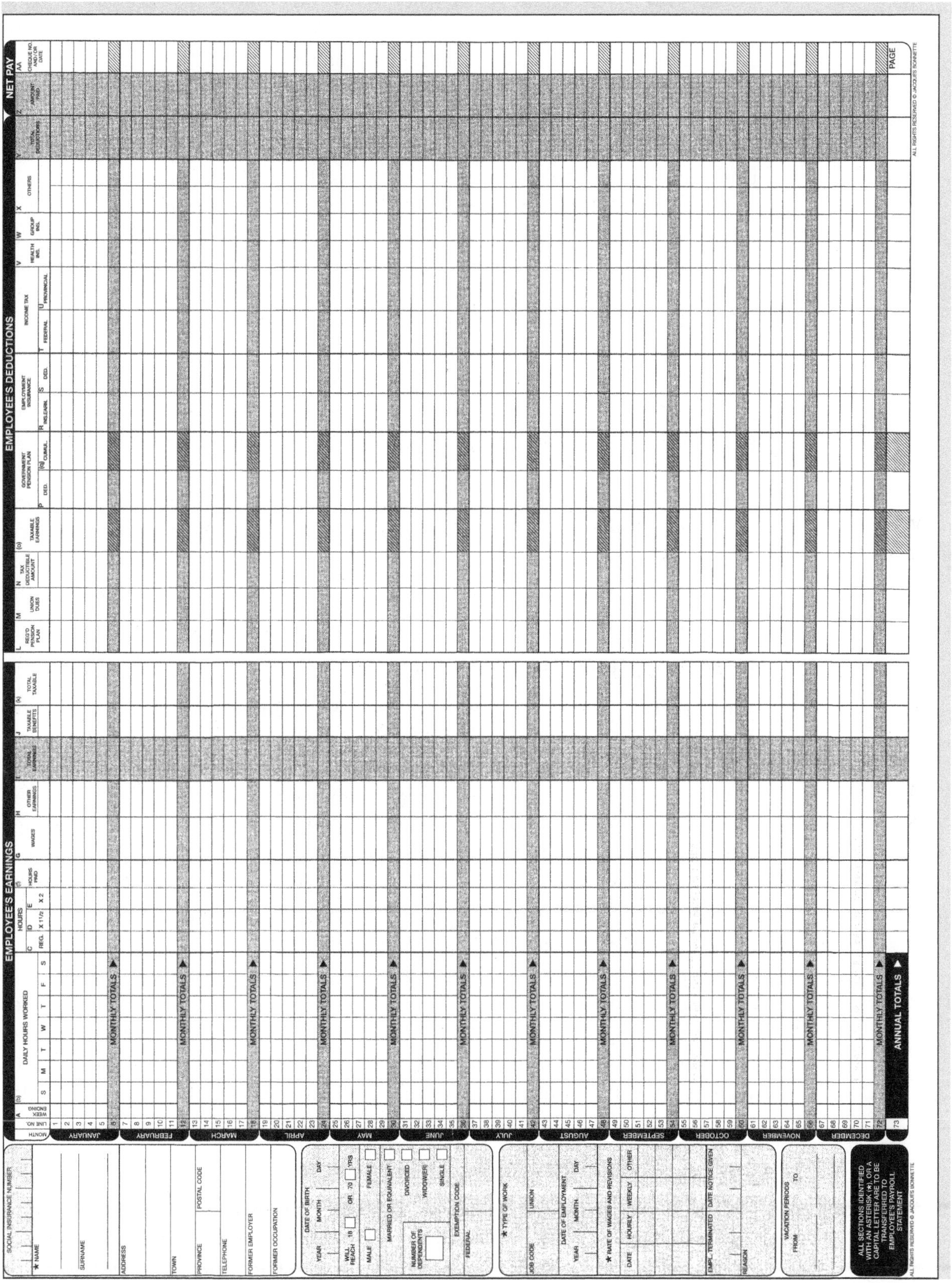

years ago on June 12 at a salary of $7 an hour. He receives a 50-cent-an-hour increase every year on the anniversary of his employment. His vacation period is negotiable. He is paid every two weeks. Complete Mr. James's data portion of the payroll sheet. Mr. James's social insurance number is 472 237 942.

Complete your portion of the personal data sheet on the payroll. You are paid every week, were not previously employed, were hired on the first day of June this year, and have not received an increase in your salary. Your vacation is negotiable. Use your regular street address and Ottawa as the city in which you live.

Now complete the earnings and deductions portion of the payroll. Mr. James has worked the following hours over the past two weeks. Week ending January 8: Sunday $4^{1}/_{2}$ hours, Tuesday 5 hours, Thursday 6 hours, Friday 4 hours. Week ending January 15: Sunday 8 hours, Monday 8 hours, Tuesday 10 hours, Wednesday 8 hours, Thursday 10 hours, Friday 8 hours. Mr. James is paid time-and-a-half for hours worked from 41 to 49 inclusive, and double time for hours above 49. In addition to deductions for CPP, EI, and income tax, Mr. James pays $28.35 each pay period for OHIP and $5 each pay period for group insurance. Mr. James also contributes $10 each week to his registered pension plan and $1 each pay period to the United Way.

Your $450 salary is paid every week. In addition to CPP, EI, and income tax, you pay $5 each week to a registered pension, $6.50 for OHIP, $2 for group insurance, and $1 to the United Way.

(Keep this payroll assignment for use in Assignment 7.10 at the end of the chapter.)

Employee Payroll Statement

An important part of any payroll system is the employee payroll statement. The statement may be attached to the employee's cheque, or it may be included as a separate statement in the employee's pay envelope. Figure 7.14 is an example of an employee payroll statement.

You will note that it gives a complete account of hours worked, earnings, each deduction, and the net amount of the paycheque. For practice, after you have completed Mr. James's payroll sheet for the two-week period ending January 15, fill in his employee payroll statement on Figure 7.14 or use a statement form from the accompanying CD.

A three-part employee cheque can be computer generated (see Figure 7.14) or a copy can be made for the employer by using a two-part NCR cheque-book. If you receive the tax tables on diskette from the government, copies of the employee payroll statement are included. These can be inserted into your printer. When using accounting software, the employee payroll statement is printed on the cheque stubs.

Payment of EI, CPP, and Income Tax Deductions

On the fifteenth day of each month, an employer must submit to the Receiver General of Canada the amount of money deducted from employees' cheques, combined with the employer's contribution to CPP and EI. A Statement of Account for Source Deductions form (see Figure 7.15) must be completed to

FIGURE **7.14** **Payroll Statement**

DEAN / LEFEBVRE EMPLOYEES' PAYROLL STATEMENTS No 81-200

SOURCE: All rights reserved © Jacques Bonnette, 1994. Reprinted with permission from Dean & Fils, Inc.

accompany the payment. The top half of the form is retained by the employer as a record of payment. The administrative assistant should calculate the total amount required for CPP, EI, and income tax and insert the figures in the proper areas of the form. If payment is made at the bank, the teller will stamp the receipt and return part one. If you remit by mail, submit part three in with your cheque and keep part two for your records. Let us assume that for the month of March, $47.52 has been deducted from your employees for EI, $57.64 for CPP, and $237.98 for income taxes. The calculations for your payment would be as follows:

EI	Employee contribution	$ 47.52	
	Employer contribution (47.52 x 1.4) =	$66.53	(for every $1.00 contributed by the employee, the employer contributes $1.40)
	Total EI submission	$114.05	

CPP	Employee contribution	$ 57.64
	Employer contribution	$ 57.64
	Total CPP submission	$115.28

Income Tax (amount deducted according to tax schedule) $237.98

You should write a cheque for the Receiver General of Canada in the amount of $114.05 + 115.28 + 237.98 = $467.31. The Statement of Account for Source Deductions form (see Figure 7.16) is completed as follows:

Part 1: Write amounts for CPP and EI premium contributions, tax deductions, current payment, gross monthly payroll, and number of employees in the appropriate boxes.

FIGURE **7.15** **Three-Part Employee Cheque**

THIS DOCUMENT CONTAINS SECURITY FEATURES · SEE REVERSE

2493

CITY BANK
399 SIMPSON STREET
WINNIPEG MB R3B 1X3

CHEQUE

PAY

TO THE
ORDER
OF

DATE

AMOUNT

DR. ROGER HOLMES

PER ______________________________

THIS DOCUMENT CONTAINS SECURITY FEATURES · SEE REVERSE

CHEQUE 2493

2493

FIGURE **7.16**   **Statement of Account for Current Source Deductions**

| Canada Customs and Revenue Agency | Agence des douanes et du revenu du Canada | STATEMENT OF ACCOUNT FOR CURRENT SOURCE DEDUCTIONS |

Statement of account as of
August 18 2004

Business number

Employer name

006579

Balances on last statement		Current balances	
Amount paid for 2004	Assessed amount owing	Amount paid for 2004	Assessed amount owing
4,520.87Cr	0.00	5,343.24Cr	0.00

EXPLANATION OF CHANGES

| Aug 17 | Payment July 2004 | Recd Aug 16 2004 | 822.37Cr |

Thank you for your payment.

Please use remittance voucher to make your next remittance or explain on the last page why you will not be remitting.

For general information about this notice, please call 1-800-959-5525.

Alan Nymark
Commissioner of Customs and Revenue

CPP contributions	EI premiums	Tax deductions	Current payment	Gross payroll	No. of employees in last pay period

PD7A E (03)   Tear off here and return lower portion with your payment.

| Canada Customs and Revenue Agency | Agence des douanes et du revenu du Canada | CURRENT SOURCE DEDUCTIONS REMITTANCE VOUCHER | PD7A E (03) |

ST. JOHN'S NL A1B 3Z1

Business number

6

Do not use this area

Gross payroll in remitting period (dollars only)

0,0

| Number of employees in last pay period | End of remitting period for which deductions were withheld | Year | Month |

Amount paid

⑆122204⑈1171⑈   96

The current payment is the sum of EI premiums, CPP, and income tax. Part 1 is kept by employers for their records.

Part 2:   This section is retained for communiqués from Revenue Canada.

Part 3:   Write proper amounts in the corresponding boxes.

After the first submission, the government will send a blank form for you to complete for the next remittance. The form will have the following information preprinted on it:

Part 1:   Date of last remittance, amount of remittance, any balance owed, and taxation centre contact

Part 2:   Employer account number and name, and address of business

Part 3:   Employer account number

ASSIGNMENT **7.9**

Dr. Plunkett has asked you to write a letter to Thomas Bell, informing him that his cheque for $32.50 was returned NSF and asking him to make arrangements to rectify the situation. (Use your imagination.)

Mr. Harris has not yet paid his account in full. It is now four months overdue. Dr. Plunkett sends a statement of account the first month, a reminder notice the second month, an inquiry the third month, and an appeal the fourth month. You have completed the statement of account. Compose the correspondence for the remainder of the collection series. (Use an appropriate reference book from the library and your imagination to assist you in completing the letters—*do not copy* letters from a textbook.) The balance outstanding on Mr. Harris's account is $37.50.

The cost of living has been increasing rapidly over the past year, and your employer and Mr. James have negotiated a 10 percent cost of living increase in the salary schedule. Complete the payroll book for the weeks of January 22 and January 29. Mr. James worked 8 hours each day Monday to Friday the week of January 22. For the week of January 29 he worked 12 hours Monday, 14 hours Tuesday, 10 hours Wednesday, he was off work Thursday, and he worked 8 hours Friday. During the week of January 22, you were granted two days off work to participate in a curling bonspiel. Of course, you were not paid for those two days. The salary increase became effective the week of January 22.

Calculate the CPP, EI, and income tax deduction figures for January to be submitted to the Receiver General of Canada, and insert them in the appropriate areas on the remittance form. (Include the figures from Assignment 7.8 for salaries paid January 8 and 15.)

ASSIGNMENT **7.10**

Complete an employee payroll statement for Mr. James's two-week pay period, January 22 and 29, and one for yourself for the week of January 29. Use the payroll sheets from Assignment 7.9.

TOPICS FOR DISCUSSION

1. Mr. Bell pays by cheque for his completed Medical Form. His cheque comes back NSF and he has another form that needs to be completed. How would you handle this situation?

2. Services such as circumcision, mole or tattoo removal, etc., that are not medically necessary have been removed from the Schedule of Benefits (SOB). Physician reimbursement for completion of medically necessary forms is also not available through the SOB. What are your feelings about this?

CHAPTER 8

Managing Office Supplies

CHAPTER OUTLINE

Ordering Supplies
Purchasing and Inventory Control

Cash Discounts
Sales Taxes

LEARNING OBJECTIVES

After reading this chapter, you will be familiar with

- Proper ordering procedures for billing supplies, medical supplies, drugs, cleaning products, and office supplies
- Safety when handling drugs and supplies

- Purchasing and inventory records
- Cash discounts
- Sales taxes

KEY TERMS

Controlled drugs: These are drugs that have been identified through the *Comprehensive Drug Abuse Prevention and Control Act* (1971), including all depressant and stimulant drugs, and other drugs of abuse or potential abuse. This act controls all distribution and use of these drugs.

Dispensing: Preparing or delivering medicines.

Workplace Hazardous Materials Information System (WHMIS): This system was created by federal, provincial, and territorial legislation to identify hazardous material, inform employees about the risks, and make sure that workers have the opportunity to use the material safely through education.

FIGURE **8.1** **It is the medical assistant's responsibility to ensure a steady stock of supplies.**

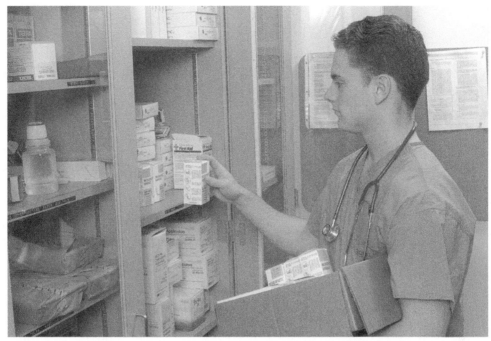

SOURCE: Hunt, S.A. (2002). *Saunders Fundamentals of Medical Assisting* (p. 185: opener). Philadelphia: Saunders.

An important responsibility of the medical administrative assistant is to ensure that adequate supplies for all facets of the practice are readily available (see Figure 8.1). When the physician arrives in the office he or she will expect that everything needed to provide patients with appropriate medical care is available.

It is the administrative assistant's duty to check through the stock of supplies to see how much is being used daily or weekly. You should ensure that you always have supplies available, and that reordering of stock is done before supplies are exhausted. It is advisable to produce a list of supplies contained in a specific area and post it in a readily visible place. This serves as a good reminder to check for depleted stock.

It is an easy task, when carefully monitored, to see how quickly supplies are used and to maintain a sufficient balance of stock.

ORDERING SUPPLIES

Billing Supplies

As you learned in Chapter 6, in order for providers to make a claim for their services, they must submit billing information for each patient seen. A busy doctor may see as many as 200 plus patients each week. Physicians submit their fee for service to the Ministry of Health via electronic media. It is essential that you maintain an adequate supply of diskettes to ensure that billing information can be submitted in a timely fashion.

Medical Supplies

Doctors use a large quantity of different medical supplies in their practice. Following is a list of the necessities. These will vary, of course, depending on the type of physician you are working with.

- Dressings
- Disposable needles
- Surgical gloves
- Sutures
- Tongue depressors
- Thermometers
- Disposable speculums
- Adhesive

A salesperson will usually contact the physician, who, in turn, will inform you of the companies with which to place medical supply orders.

Paper Supplies

Paper supplies will be ordered in the same way, with a preferable supplier identified by your physician.

- Examination paper (for the examination tables)
- Disposable gowns
- Drapes
- Paper towels

If you are the only employee in the office, you will be responsible for ordering and maintaining all medical and office supplies. If there are two or more employees, you may want to designate one person responsible for ordering supplies. On a busy day, it can be very disruptive to patient care if the supplies are not available.

Drugs

If you are responsible for ordering drugs, remember that drugs deteriorate over time. Keep in mind the drug's shelf life and your office usage when ordering, to avoid unnecessary waste and expense. Do not make quantity purchases without consulting your employer.

Most offices do not stock **controlled drugs.** These are drugs that are at high risk for addiction or abuse, such as painkillers, sleeping pills, and tranquilizers. Drugs that are kept in the office include vaccines for influenza and other common diseases, Adrenalin, various ointments and creams, antibiotics, aspirin, Novocaine, penicillin, and so on. Controlled drugs need to be kept in a securely locked cabinet with strict **dispensing** documentation witnessed by the physician and another health professional (usually a nurse). As most doctors' offices or clinics are not open 24 hours a day, this also eliminates the risk of someone breaking in.

All drugs should be stored as specified on the container—for example, in a dark dry place or in the refrigerator (check the temperature). When drugs are stored, the ones with the most recent expiry date should be located at the front. Keep all drugs for external use stored away from drugs to be used for internal use.

In the past, when a drug's shelf life expired, the drug was usually flushed down the toilet. It is no longer acceptable to dispose of drugs in this manner because of the harm it may cause to the environment. Outdated drugs must be incinerated. Many drug companies will collect outdated drugs and have a disposal company incinerate them. Private offices will empty the drugs from the smaller containers into one large disposal container. This container is then taken to a pharmacy for appropriate disposal. Larger medical clinics often have a pharmacy in the building. When disposing of drugs (solid or liquid), you should wear appropriate safety apparel (gloves, goggles, apron).

Used needles are placed in a "sharps container." When the container is full, the lid is snapped shut, and it is taken to the pharmacy for disposal. If you cannot arrange for this service, contact a local company or the pharmacy at your community hospital, to ensure that disposal is carried out in an environmentally safe manner.

Drug manufacturers employ salespersons who call on doctors to keep them informed of new drugs. Most doctors are aware of the services provided by these people and will give them a few minutes if possible. The preferred procedure to schedule drug representative appointments is discussed in Chapter 2.

Toiletries and Cleaning Products

Items such as soap, paper towels, toilet paper, disinfectants, cleansers, and cleaning cloths are necessary to maintain a clean, sanitary, and safe environment. A local cleaning and maintenance supplier can provide you with these items as well as with safety instructions.

The **Workplace Hazardous Materials Information System (WHMIS)** system is designed to identify hazardous materials, inform employees about their risks, and educate individuals on how to use certain materials safely in the work environment (see http://www.whmis.net for more details).

The bleach cleaner, toilet bowl cleaner, correction fluid, liquid hand wash soap, hairspray (for Pap smears), and fax and photos copier toner are some examples of materials that are identified as hazardous material under the WHMIS system. The type of hazard is identified by a symbol, as illustrated in Figure 8.2. Keep all cleaning supplies separate from drug supplies (see Box 8.1).

When disposing of or using such materials, the employee should have gloves, goggles, masks and aprons, or both, available, as well as appropriate disposal methods. There should also be an eyewash station available if needed. This station can be installed onto a faucet for quick access.

FIGURE **8.2**   **WHMIS Symbols, Health Canada**

	Class A Compressed gas	Contents under high pressure. Cylinder may explode or burst when heated, dropped or damaged.
	Class B Flammable and combustible material	May catch fire when exposed to heat, spark or flame. May burst into flames.
	Class C Oxidizing material	May cause fire or explosion when in contact with wood, fuels, or other combustible material.
	Class D, Division 1 Poisonous and infectious material: Immediate and serious toxic effects	Poisonous substance. A single exposure may be fatal or cause serious or permanent damage to health.
	Class D, Division 2 Poisonous and infectious material: Other toxic effects	Poisonous substance. May cause irritation. Repeated exposure may cause cancer, birth defects, or other permanent damage.
	Class D, Division 3 Poisonous and infectious material: Biohazardous infectious materials	May cause disease or serious illness. Drastic exposures may result in death.
	Class E Corrosive material	Can cause burns to eyes, skin or respiratory system.

SOURCE: Reproduced by permission of The Minister of Public Works and Government Services Canada, 2005.

> **8.1**
>
> CLEANING SUPPLIES AND DRUGS SHOULD *NEVER* BE KEPT
> IN THE SAME LOCATION.

Office Supplies

The medical administrative assistant requires a variety of items to perform daily office duties. The physician generally has preprinted stationery, such as letterhead, envelopes, statements, and prescription forms. In addition, a supply of pens, pencils, paper clips, staples, notepads, photocopier paper and toner, erasers, plain bond paper, file folders, and requisition and business forms should always be available. It may be helpful to flag supplies at a point where reordering should take place. This can be done easily by fastening a note indicating "Reorder now."

Arrangements should be made with equipment suppliers to have all equipment (i.e., computers, printers, fax machines, photocopiers, scales) serviced on a regular basis. In order to have an efficient office, equipment must be in good working order. Some office suppliers will fax you when your fax toner needs to be reordered. Bear in mind that toner is very expensive; do not order unnecessarily. Prescription pad forms are often obtainable free of charge through drug suppliers.

Contact your local hospital or other external diagnostic centre to secure their requisition forms. Provincial lab forms can be ordered in bulk with your physician's name, address, and billing number imprinted on them.

PURCHASING AND INVENTORY CONTROL

The administrative assistant should have an order book in which to keep a record of supplies ordered, the name and address of the supplier, the cost of the item, and the date on which the order was placed. This information can be used for reference when reordering, as well as for cost comparisons. It will also give you a general idea of how long a quantity of a certain item lasts and when it will be necessary to reorder. It is good practice to also identify the amount of time between when an order is placed and when it arrives in your office. You should make routine reference to your order book to ensure your supply room is always adequately stocked.

The Purchase Order

In most office environments, ordering will be done by telephone, by fax machine, or on-line. A copy of the order will serve as a record. In some organizations, it may be necessary to complete a purchase order (see Figure 8.3).

A copy of the purchase order should be kept in a pending file until the material is received. If quoted prices have been received prior to the order, the amount should appear on the purchase order. It is good practice to obtain

FIGURE **8.3** **Purchase Order**

PURCHASE ORDER

JOHN E. PLUNKETT
PHM.B., M.D., C.M., F.R.C.P., F.A.C.P.
INTERNAL MEDICINE
278 O'CONNOR ST.   OTTAWA, ONT.

TO: Readymade Office Equipment
225 Rideau Crescent
Ottawa, Ontario
J3X 7X6

DATE: Sept. 25, 20___
ORDER NO.: 3754
REQ'D BY: A.S.A.P.
SHIP VIA: Paxy Transport
TERMS: 2/10/n/30

ITEM NO.	QUANTITY	DESCRIPTION	UNIT	UNIT PRICE		TOTAL	
1	1	Pedestal Desk	1	$525	00	$525	00
2	500	Hanger Files	100	25	00	125	00
		Total				$650	00
		Add G.S.T. 7%				45	50
		Add P.S.T. 8%				52	00
		Total Invoice				$747	50

the name of the sales person you spoke with when placing the order, as well as a confirmation number or service number.

The Packing Slip

A packing slip (see Figure 8.4) will be enclosed with your shipment of supplies. The items and quantities listed on the packing slip should be compared with the contents of the package. After it has been confirmed that there are no discrepancies in the shipment you received, the packing slip should be

FIGURE **8.4** **Packing Slip**

PACKING SLIP

READYMADE OFFICE EQUIPMENT
225 Rideau Crescent
Ottawa, ON J3X 7X6
Telephone: (613) 387-5567
Fax: (613) 387-5568
Toll Free: 1-800-772-8893

INVOICE NO. 337815-33   DATE: ___/09/29

SOLD TO: SHIP TO:
Dr. John E. Plunkett   Dr. John E. Plunkett
278 O'Connor St.   278 O'Connor St.
Ottawa, ON J5Z 2X8   Ottawa, ON J5Z 2X8

CUSTOMER ORDER NO. 3754

ITEM NO.	QUANTITY ORDER	QUANTITY SHIP	DESCRIPTION
1	1		1 Pedestal Desk
2	500		400 Hanger Files
			100 Hanger Files on Backorder

_____
Customer Signature

---

compared with the order record to ensure that your supply requirements
have been met.

The Invoice

The invoice (see Figure 8.5) is a statement of the amount owed for goods
shipped by the supplier. The quantities on the invoice should match those
documented on the packing slip. If you were quoted prices prior to shipment,
the prices on the invoice should match your order record.

FIGURE **8.5** **Invoice**

INVOICE

READYMADE OFFICE EQUIPMENT
225 Rideau Crescent
Ottawa, ON J3X 7X6

INVOICE NO. 337815-33   DATE: ___/09/29

SOLD TO: SHIP TO:
Dr. John E. Plunkett   Dr. John E. Plunkett
278 O'Connor Street   278 O'Connor Street
Ottawa, ON J5Z 2X8   Ottawa, ON J5Z 2X8

CUSTOMER ORDER NO. 3754

ITEM NO.	QUANT. ORDER	QUANT. SHIP	DESCRIPTION	UNIT	UNIT PRICE		TOTAL	
1	1	1	Pedestal Desk	1	$525	00	$525	00
2	500	400	Hanger Files	100	25	00	100	00
			Sub Total				$625	00
			Add G.S.T. 7%				43	75
			Add P.S.T. 8%				50	00
			Total Invoice				$718	75

_____
Customer Signature

If there are any discrepancies in price and quantity, or both, the supplier should be contacted.

CASH DISCOUNTS

Suppliers often allow a cash discount on purchases to encourage prompt payment; the cash discount is referred to as the "credit terms." Consult with possible suppliers about their terms. The credit terms on a purchase may be

"2 percent 10 days, net 30 days," meaning that if payment is received within 10 days after purchase, 2 percent can be deducted from the total cost; otherwise, payment is due within 30 days of the purchase. The terms are written "2/10/n/30" and expressed as "2, 10, net, 30."

SALES TAXES

A 7 percent federal Goods and Services Tax will be added to many items that you will purchase. In some provinces, a provincial sales tax will also be added. The amount of the tax varies from province to province. For example, in Ontario, 8 percent is added to the invoice as a tax on the sale. There are also many variations in the types of goods that are taxed. The medical administrative assistant is not expected to know the federal and provincial sales tax laws, but should be aware of the types of medical supplies that are *not* taxable. Information can be obtained by calling your provincial government sales tax branch (usually through a toll-free line). Most suppliers are aware of sales tax implications on the goods they supply and will add tax where applicable. However, if you know which items are taxable, you may wish to add the tax onto your purchase order.

ASSIGNMENT **8.1A**

Prepare a purchase order (see accompanying CD) for 2 boxes of pencils, HB lead, at $2.50 a box; 2000 carbon packs at $10 per thousand; 4 ballpoint pens/blue at 59 cents each; 10 boxes of paper clips at $2.32 per box; 4 ballpoint pens/red at 69 cents each; and 250 $\frac{1}{5}$ cut file folders at $10.35 per 100.

The purchase order no. 423 is dated February 16, 20__, and is required by February 19, 20__. Ship via Purolator. Supply company is Ottawa Valley Office Supplies, 213 Bank Street, Ottawa. Their terms are 2 percent 10 days and net 30 days.

ASSIGNMENT **8.1B**

Your instructor will provide you with a copy of the packing slip that accompanied your order from Assignment 8.1A. Compare the slip and note discrepancies, if any.

ASSIGNMENT **8.1C**

Your instructor will provide you with the invoice for goods ordered in Assignment 8.1A. Compare the invoice with the order record and packing slip and note discrepancies, if any.

ASSIGNMENT **8.1D**

When you compared the order record, packing slip, and invoice, you noted some discrepancies. Document the discrepancies and the follow-up action you would take.

Select a classmate and role play your conversation with the supplier. Remember that it is important to maintain a good relationship with your suppliers. Diplomacy and tact should be used when dealing with this and every situation.

ASSIGNMENT **8.2**

Before completing this assignment, select two students in your class to contact your provincial sales tax branch (if sales tax is collected in your province) and inquire if sales tax is applicable to the items to be included in the following purchase order.

Medical supplies are ordered from Merke & Parker Medical Suppliers, 337 Main Street, Ottawa. Their terms on all purchases are 2 percent if paid in 20 days and net due in 60 days; they have their own delivery service. You require 200 disposable needles at $50 per 100; 500 disposable thermometers at $72.50 per 100; 12 dozen pairs of surgical gloves at $14.25 per pair; 20 dozen 5 cm × 10 cm gauze dressings at $8.75 per dozen; and 10 adhesive rolls (245 cm × 5 cm) at $7.50 per roll. A purchase order form can be found in the Working Papers (on the accompanying CD).

CHAPTER 9

The Procedures Manual

CHAPTER OUTLINE

Components and Style
Uses

Topics for Discussion

LEARNING OBJECTIVES

After reading this chapter, you will be able to

- Identify and recognize the components and style of a procedures manual
- Develop the knowledge to create a procedures manual for efficient office use

- Understand the uses of a procedures manual

KEY TERMS

Procedure manual: The procedure manual describes the necessary steps involved in completing any and all jobs relating to the business and position, or both.

All businesses, whether they are healthcare providers, manufacturers, wholesalers, retailers, or services, should have a procedures manual for easy reference by all employees.

COMPONENTS AND STYLE

A **procedures manual** describes the necessary steps involved in completing any and all jobs relating to the business. If you are the only person dealing with the administration, it is a simple task to describe in detail how you go about completing individual duties in specific areas. If you are one of many employees and you are responsible for producing a procedures manual, you will have to ask each employee to describe the procedures involved in completing his or her particular job. In large facilities, each department has its own procedures manual. This usually also outlines policies pertaining to the department as well as interdisciplinary guidelines.

The manual should adhere to the following criteria:

1. It should be printed on loose leaf sheets.
2. It should have a table of contents in alphabetical order.
3. It should be alphabetized by procedure description.
4. It should be organized to be used as a reference manual.
5. It should be separated with tabbed dividers to identify each section.

Figure 9.1 is a sample of how a page in a procedures manual might be formatted.

If you are employed in an office that does not have a procedures manual, or has a manual that needs updating, some topics you might consider covering are the following (listed alphabetically, not by order of importance):

Accounting Procedures
Appointments
Banking
Bill Collections (overdue)
Daily Activity Routine
Dress Code
Drug Disposal
Emergency and Referral Telephone Numbers
Employee Benefits
Equipment
Filing [colour-coding or order of filing (i.e., Mc's at end of "M" file)]
Health Card Billing
Hospital Requisition Forms
Insurance—Claim Forms and Policies Carried
Insurance Forms—Completion for Patients
Inventory

FIGURE **9.1**   **Procedures Manual**

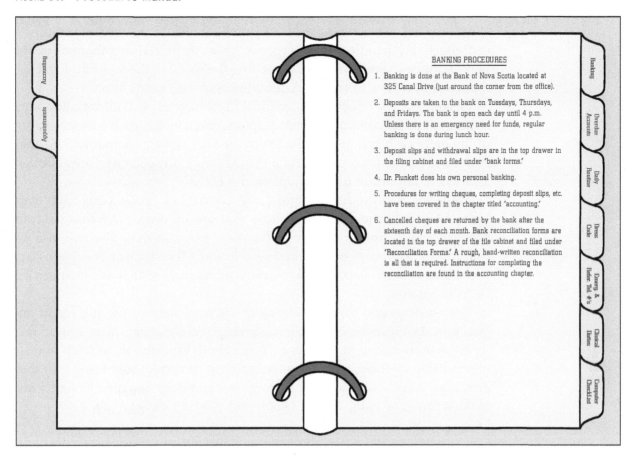

BANKING PROCEDURES

1. Banking is done at the Bank of Nova Scotia located at 325 Canal Drive (just around the corner from the office).

2. Deposits are taken to the bank on Tuesdays, Thursdays, and Fridays. The bank is open each day until 4 p.m. Unless there is an emergency need for funds, regular banking is done during lunch hour.

3. Deposit slips and withdrawal slips are in the top drawer in the filing cabinet and filed under "bank forms."

4. Dr. Plunkett does his own personal banking.

5. Procedures for writing cheques, completing deposit slips, etc. have been covered in the chapter titled "accounting."

6. Cancelled cheques are returned by the bank after the sixteenth day of each month. Bank reconciliation forms are located in the top drawer of the file cabinet and filed under "Reconciliation Forms." A rough, hand-written reconciliation is all that is required. Instructions for completing the reconciliation are found in the accounting chapter.

Job Description
Medical Transcription Formats and Guidelines
Office Policies
Payroll
Personnel
Petty Cash
Photocopier
Staff Replacement (for holidays and emergency staffing)
Supplies (ordering and storing)
Telephone
Travel Arrangements
Work Schedule

Specific procedures are unique to each organization. You would add to or delete from the above list as required.

The chronological order or time sequence (daily, weekly, or monthly) in which jobs should be completed should also be recorded in the manual, so that no job is left undone. By looking through the manual, the new administrative assistant can verify if any vital duties have been overlooked.

USES

When explicit instructions are documented for all jobs, a substitute employee can effectively handle any emergency tasks. A procedures manual is also helpful for new employees. After reading the manual, the new employee has a general overview of the job requirements of the organization.

Of course, to be effective, the manual must have explicit information, such as passwords for computers, photocopiers, and telephones; the exact location of the petty cash box; where the list of medical supply companies and their addresses can be found; what time the mail and lab specimens are collected; and where important phone numbers are listed.

Preparing a procedures manual can sometimes reveal poor time management in a particular job. Because you are involved in writing a comprehensive description of how to handle a job, you may discover you are duplicating a process or performing a facet of the job that is unnecessary. From time to time, you should review your manual so that any changes can be incorporated.

Cost savings and time management are important to the success of any business. As a responsible medical administrative assistant, you should take a personal interest in minimizing waste of both time and material. If you see others being inefficient, and you feel you can diplomatically bring it to their attention, you should do so. If the organization does not run efficiently and make a profit, or both, you will soon find yourself out of a job.

ASSIGNMENT **9.1**

When you begin your duties for Drs. Plunkett and Pelham, assume that the office does not have a procedures manual. Using your imagination, prepare a section for the manual describing appointment scheduling. The description should include such things as type of appointment scheduling used, what appointments are considered emergency bookings, amount of time to book for physicals, and so on.

ASSIGNMENT **9.2**

Following is an example of a patient billing from a medical office. Key the instructions, improving on format and information provided.

PATIENT HEALTH CLAIM BILLING
Physician sends out billing information on patient.
Enter information into computer billing screen.
Check off on day sheet that billing complete.
Save billing to diskette.
File patient chart.

Remember, the important thing to decide before completing this assignment is whether you would be able to perform the patient billing based on the preceding information. If not, you must improve the instructions so that *anyone* who may be involved in following the procedure would be able to do so without having to ask questions.

Assume this is an office where there is only one administrative assistant, and she is ill. You have been called to substitute during her illness. You have never been in the office before. The billing needs to be completed before you go home. The only instructions available for undertaking the task are found in the procedures manual as previously shown.

It will be necessary to use your imagination and previous knowledge to fill in missing information and clarify the information provided.

ASSIGNMENT **9.3**

Prepare a page for a medical office procedures manual entitled "Daily Activity Routine." You will have to imagine what duties you would perform and the order in which they would be done. Also, decide whether the doctor has office hours all day or just in the morning or afternoon. Choose the type of medical office (private practice, hospital admitting, clinic reception, or other) in which you hope to find employment when you graduate. Insert this assignment in your portfolio.

TOPICS FOR DISCUSSION

1. You have been asked on short notice to fill in at a general practitioner's office where you have never worked before. The only employee there is ill, and there is no one to show you what to do. What information would help you get through your first day?

2. Do you feel that procedures manuals are helpful, or not? If not, what would be more helpful to you?

CHAPTER 10

Meeting Organization

CHAPTER OUTLINE

Notice of Meeting
Meeting Agenda
Convention Agenda

Minutes
Topics for Discussion

LEARNING OBJECTIVES

After reading this chapter, you will be familiar with

- The steps required in the preparation of a notice of meeting

- The agenda format
- The minutes format

KEY TERMS

Proxy: When a vote is scheduled and a voting member cannot be present, he or she can give written permission to another member to vote for him or her on a specific issue.

Quorum: When a vote or action is recommended, the majority of members need to be present to approve or disapprove it. The number needed is referred to as a quorum.

A medical administrative assistant may be responsible for arranging meetings, as well as recording and producing minutes. A meeting can be very informal, involving a committee of three or four persons, or formal, involving a convention of several hundred participants.

The administrative assistant may also be responsible for sending out notices of the meeting, reserving an appropriate meeting place, deciding on and supervising suitable table placement, ordering beverages (coffee, tea, water, juice) for participants, compiling an agenda, recording the minutes, and producing and distributing printed copies of the minutes. For large convention-type meetings, public address systems and meals may also need to be arranged.

NOTICE OF MEETING

When the date and time of the meeting have been established, the first responsibility of the administrative assistant is to find an appropriate physical space in which to hold the meeting. The number of participants will determine the size of the room; if participants will be taking notes, tables, notebooks, and pencils should be available; if a number of people will be participating, a public address system may be necessary. These requirements, and any others necessary for a well-organized meeting, must be taken into consideration. Once an appropriate area has been reserved, the administrative assistant must inform the participants of the details in a notice of meeting (see Box 10.1).

> ### 10.1
>
> A meeting of the Medical Aid Association will be held at 5 p.m. on December 15, 20__ in the Blue Room at the Holiday Inn, 215 Front Street, Ottawa, Ontario. All committee heads are required to have their annual reports completed for presentation. Please confirm your attendance by (insert required date).

Notices can be simply stated as shown in Box 10.1, and sent to the attendees by e-mail. The notice can also be in a poster format and sent as an e-mail attachment to the attendees (see Box 10.2).

10.2 Notice of Meeting
DATE: December 15, 20__ *TIME:* 5 p.m. *PLACE:* Holiday Inn, Blue Room 215 Front Street Ottawa, Ontario *(All committee heads are required to have their annual reports completed for presentation.)* *Please confirm your attendance by (insert required date).*

Attendees should be requested to confirm their attendance when the notice has been received. Some meetings will require a vote to take place. It is important to know the number of attendees, as a **quorum** is required in order for the vote to pass. If the required number of members will not be present, the meeting may need to be moved to another date, the agenda item may have to be put on hold, or the vote may need to be achieved by **proxy**.

This notice should be distributed approximately ten days before the meeting. Timing of notices is crucial: if sent too early, they may be forgotten; if sent too late, members may have made other commitments for the date you have arranged.

MEETING AGENDA

Discuss with the chairperson of the meeting the topics to be covered. A planned order for the meeting will avoid confusion, wasted time, and missed items.

Some groups have an agenda committee as part of their executive. In this case, the administrative assistant would attend an agenda meeting approximately two weeks prior to the meeting; an appropriate agenda would be discussed and the administrative assistant would print and distribute the details. A computer template would be developed in a style that will suit the meeting and/or organization. Figure 10.1 is an example of an agenda.

ASSIGNMENT 10.1

Assume that your doctor/employer has just informed you that the meeting outlined in the previous boxes will be held. You are responsible for making all physical arrangements for this meeting. The doctor is also secretary of this society, and has asked you to take care of all the secretarial duties.

With your instructor's help, prepare a checklist of all items that you will have to attend to, including phone calls, paperwork, and so on. After you have completed your first list, determine the approximate date on which each task should be completed, and then prepare a chronological list of these tasks.

FIGURE **10.1**   **Meeting Agenda**

Agenda			
Meeting:	Medical Aid Association		
Date:	December 15, 20____		
Time:	17:00		
Place:	Blue Room, Holiday Inn, 215 Front Street, Ottawa, Ontario		

Type of meeting:		Facilitator/Chairperson:	
Note taker:		Timekeeper:	

Agenda topics		Presenter	Time
1.	Call to order	Chair	
2.	Review of ground rules	Members	
3.	Approval of the agenda	Members	
4.	Approval of the minutes	Members	
5.	Business arising		
	5.1 Correspondence	Secretary	
	5.2 Financial report	Treasurer	
	5.3 Purchase of resuscitating equipment	G. Farley	
	5.4 Revision of constitution	D. Moore	
6.	New business		
	6.1 Charity project for 20____	Nominating	
	6.2 Election of officers	Members	
	6.3 Guest speaker – 'Crib Death'	J.A. Coons, MD	
7.	Attachment – FYI		
	7.1		
8.	Round table/information sharing		
9.	Next meeting		
10.	Adjournment		
Parking lot items			
	1.		
	2.		
	3.		
	4.		

Members:				

FIGURE **10.2**   **Convention Agenda**

AGENDA

Friday, June 2, 20___

2:00 - 6:00	Registration
6:30	Barbecue
8:30	Travelling Theme Party

Saturday, June 3, 20___

7:30 - 9:00	Breakfast (8:00 President's Round Table)
9:00 - 9:30	Opening Ceremonies and Welcome
9:30 - 10:00	Annual Meeting
10:00 - 10:15	Coffee
10:15 - 11:00	"Rules My Grammar Never Taught Me" - Sylvia Smith
11:00 - 12:00	"M.O.R.E." (Multiple Organ and Retrieval Exchange) - L. Lars, Representative • Heart Transplant Recipient • Lung Transplant Recipient • Mother of a young donor
12:00 - 1:00	Lunch

1:00 - 2:00	"Emergency Medicine" - Dr. A. Vince Emergency Department Peterborough Civic Hospital
2:00 - 2:45	"What's Happening in Health Care ... What's Coming Up" - D. Jones Health Policies O.M.A.
2:45 - 3:00	Coffee
3:00 - 4:00	"Laughter is the Best Medicine" - Tom White, Humorist
5:30	President's and International Reception
6:30	Social Time (Cash Bar)
7:00 - 9:00	Banquet Awards/Presentations
9:30	Academy Awards

Sunday, June 4, 20___

8:00 - 9:00	Continental Breakfast (Delivered personally to your cottage)
9:30 - 11:30	Country Store & Craft Sale
11:30 - 1:00	Buffet Brunch Fashion Show

Visit the displays
on Saturday
in the Whistle Stop Room

Elmhirst Resort Total Convention Package is $242.94 per person

Includes: All Taxes and Gratuities
2 Nights Accommodation/
Fully Equipped Cottages
All Meals/Entertainment
Use of All Facilities/
Pool/Hot Tub/Sauna
Nature Trails

To reserve your accommodations or meal packages, please see enclosed flyer.

Convention Registration

Registration Fee:

Members	$30.00
Non-Members	$75.00
Retirees	$30.00

Please complete the reverse side, tear off this portion and return to OMSA by April 27, 20___.

To be eligible for an **Early Bird Draw**, registrations must be received at Head Office by May 1, 20___.

CONVENTION AGENDA

Preparation for a convention begins several months in advance. A planning committee is responsible for all facets of the event including engaging speakers, setting the agenda, and publicity. Once details are finalized, the administrative assistant produces the agenda (Figure 10.2) and ensures that all those registered to attend the convention receive a copy. The agenda may be sent out prior to the convention, or used as a handout on the day of the event.

ASSIGNMENT **10.2**

Assume you are employed as the administrative assistant of the doctor responsible for organizing a convention. Prepare a printed copy of the convention schedule (Figure 10.2) using an appropriate and attractive format (use your creativity). Computer programs have many formats, symbols, and pictures to choose from. A copy of the schedule would be mailed to each convention delegate. Insert a copy of the completed schedule in your portfolio.

The schedule for the convention is the same each day except for the registration beginning at 10 a.m. on May 14 and the dinner on May 18 at 6 p.m.

On May 14, the convention meetings begin at 1 p.m. and conclude at 4 p.m. On May 15, 16, and 17, morning sessions begin at 9 a.m. and conclude at 11:30 a.m.; afternoon sessions are from 2 p.m. to 4 p.m. On May 18, sessions conclude at 11:30 a.m., and the afternoon is free.

The afternoon sessions are lecture meetings and the morning sessions are workshops. The speakers are Dr. John McGilvray, anaesthetist, on "Advances in Administering Techniques"; Dr. Scott Hayes, pediatrician, on "Learning Disabilities"; Dr. Fraser McGee, heart specialist, on "The Killer Disease"; and Dr. Terry Fisher, neurologist, on "The Human Mind."

The workshops are discussions pertaining to the previous afternoon's lecture.

MINUTES

You may be required to attend the meeting and record the minutes, or your employer may record the minutes and ask you to prepare them from handwritten notes; alternatively, a recording device may be used, and you would produce the minutes from the transcription tape. Regardless of the method used to record the minutes, they must be printed and distributed to the participants in an acceptable format. A general guideline for producing minutes follows:

1. Identify the type, the location, and the time of the meeting.
2. Identify those in attendance, those who have sent regrets, and those who are absent.
3. Identify the chairperson and the recording secretary.
4. Use the prepared agenda as a guideline for recording the minutes. It should be noted if deviation from the agenda order occurs.
5. Place subject captions such that they can be easily located and that the number of the subject corresponds to the agenda number (see Figure 10.1).
6. Some minutes are produced with "motion" captions formatted in the same manner as the subject captions.
7. The words "motion carried" or "motion defeated" should be in all capitals, underlined, and should follow each motion. The recording secretary might also wish to note the number "for," "against," and "abstaining."
8. Do not record personal comments or opinions such as, "John Smith thought it would be wise if . . ." Only business matters are recorded.
9. Try to summarize discussions; motions should be recorded exactly as presented.
10. If a thank-you letter is requested, or if an expression of gratitude recommended, it should be in the form of a resolution.

11. Attach any pertinent reports to the minutes.
12. All motions must be seconded and voted on by the membership (a motion of adjournment is an exception). Be sure to include both the "mover" and "seconder" when recording the minutes.

For an example of completed minutes, refer to Figure 10.3.

ASSIGNMENT **10.3**

You are the administrative assistant to Dr. John Lawson, chairperson of the medical records committee. Using the following minutes as a guide, produce a notice of the meeting and the agenda that would be sent to the committee members prior to the meeting.

Reproduce the minutes and agenda using the format provided in the CD.

MINUTES

Minutes of a meeting of the Medical Records Committee held on May 20, 20__, at 1215 hours in Conference Room A, Peterborough Regional Health Centre (PRHC).

PRESENT: Dr. J. Lawson, Dr. T. Chromie, R. Smith, Dr. Trims, S. Adams, R. Sevich, L. Bazio, N. Taylor, A. Rawlins, P. Clark, Z. Copping, T. Kezia, R. Jacobs, Dr. Roberts, T. Dawson.

MINUTES: The minutes of the previous meeting were approved on a motion by Dr. M. Roberts, seconded by Mrs. S. Adams.

BUSINESS ARISING FROM THE MINUTES
1. New Medical Records Policy for Incomplete Charts

    Dr. Chromie noted that the policy recommended by this committee has now been passed by the Medical Advisory Committee and the Board of Governors. It is now up to the Medical Records Committee to decide when and how the new policy should be implemented. It was agreed that a notice should be sent to all medical staff members explaining the policy and including a copy of the policy. Mrs. R. Smith noted that the next count would be taken on Friday, May 21. It was agreed that overdue charts would be ignored for this one week. The notice to physicians would be sent out as quickly as possible and implementation of the new policy would begin the week of May 25.

2. Patient Profile Form

    There is nothing to report on this form at the present time. Dr. Chromie noted that she suggested to Miss Dawson that she obtain suggestions for the Patient Profile Form from all medical departments. Committee members agreed that medical staff input is necessary.

3. Obstetrical Form

    Mrs. Adams noted that the Obstetrical Form, which includes intrapartum risk factors, was used on a trial basis for several months. At the end of this

FIGURE **10.3** **Meeting Minutes**

Minutes

Meeting	Medical Aid Association Meeting	Date	December 15, 20___	Time	17:00	Location	Blue Room, Holiday Inn

Members present:

J. Hayes (President)	R. Mastrianni	T. Intersoll	A. Mosta	C. Fortran
M. Zincovich	T. Cavanagh	D. Moore	G. Farley	T. Fergus
D. Fergus	D. Dudley	J. Bluett	E. Chambers (Treasurer)	

Members absent:

Nil

Items for agenda	Presenter	Discussion/decision (Who do we need to consult prior to and inform after?)	Who is responsible for follow-up? Timeframe/deadline
1. Call to order	J. Hayes	The meeting was called to order at 17:15	
2. Review of ground rules			
3. Approval of agenda		The agenda was approved as distributed	
4. Approval of minutes (date)	T. Cavanagh	T. Cavanagh noted that Paragraph 2, section 5.2 of the November 14, 20___ minutes should read '...At a purchase price of $218.28.' Moved by D. Moore, seconded by T. Fergus that the minutes be accepted and amended. MOTION CARRIED	D. Moore/T. Fergus
5. Business arising			
5.1 Correspondence	Secretary	Letters were received from the Homecare Workers requesting a donation of baked goods for their Christmas Tea and Bazaar to be held on	

continued

5.2 Financial report	E. Chambers	Wednesday, December 3, 20____, and from the Heavenly Home for the Aged inviting our association to attend their Christmas party on December 10, 20____, tickets are $8.00. Treasurer Eleanor Chambers reviewed the financial statement (copy distributed) Moved by C. Fortran and seconded by M. Zincovich that the financial report be adopted as read and that all accounts be paid when properly vouched. MOTION CARRIED	C. Fortran/M. Zincovich
5.3 Resuscitating equipment	G. Farley	G. Farley reported on his investigation into the cost or purchasing resuscitating equipment for use by the fire department. The TX60 equipment discussed at the November meeting can be acquired for $4,926.50. Mr. Farley has discussed the purchase with the fire chief and he feels the TX60 would improve their efficiency 100 percent when dealing with cardiac and drowning victims. A. Mosta moved that we purchase the TX60 package at a cost of $4,926.50. D. Dudley seconded the motion. MOTION CARRIED D. Moore reported that the constitution committee is still meeting twice a month and they will be ready to present a draft revision at the January meeting.	A. Mosta/D. Dudley D. Moore
6. New business			
6.1 Charity project for 20____	T. Intersoll	T. Intersoll recommended that our charity project for 20____ be directed toward providing tables, chairs, cards, and trays for the Senior Citizens' Bridge Club. A brief discussion ensued. No other suggestions were brought forward. I. Bluett moved that we defer this topic to the next meeting and hopefully more suggestions will be made at that time. R. Mastrianni seconded the motion.	I. Bluett/R. Mastrianne
6.2 Election of officers	Nominating committee	The nominating committee presented a slate of officers for 20____ and an election was held. The new executives are: President: R. Mastrianni Vice-president: J. Bluett Secretary: T. Intersoll Treasurer: E. Chambers	
6.3 Guest speaker, 'Crib Death'	J.A. Coons, MD	Dr. J.A. Coons was introduced by A. Mosta. His presentation on crib deaths was both interesting and informative. G. Farley thanked Dr. Coons on behalf of the membership.	G. Farley
7. Attachment – FYI-Treasurers report			
8. Vision statement/committee effectiveness			

FIGURE 10.3 Meeting Minutes, cont'd

9. Round table/ information sharing		
10. Next meeting		
11. Adjournment	D. Moore	The meeting was adjourned at 19:15 p.m.
Parking lot items		Constitution committee
		Charity project

FIGURE **10.3** **Meeting Minutes, cont'd**

time, its use was reviewed by the department of obstetrics, which has recommended to discontinue use of the form.

Dr. Trims drew the attention of committee members to the vast amount of duplication from physicians completing medical records. He asked that the committee be aware of this when new forms are being considered, and that all possible attempts be made to avoid duplication wherever possible.

4. Diet Order Form

Mrs. Sevich reported that the new Diet Order Forms have been printed and are now in use throughout the health centre.

5. Dictating Line in Special Procedures Room

It was noted that this line has now been installed in the special procedures room and is in use.

6. Unit Number System

Mrs. Bazio reported that the conversion to a unit number system is complete and all patients' charts are now being handled in this fashion.

NEW BUSINESS

1. Letter from Wellesley Hospital re Transfer of Information

A letter was received from Wellesley Hospital asking precisely what information is sent with a patient being transferred from PRHC to another hospital. Wellesley Hospital is gathering this information from a number of hospitals in an effort to determine what is actually required when patients are transferred.

Mrs. Rawlins noted that what is sent with the patient depends on where the patient is being sent and what procedures are going to be done. She noted that it is one thing for a patient being transferred to Princess Margaret, and that it is quite a different situation if a patient is being transferred to Sunnybrook Medical Centre. Dr. Chromie noted that when a patient comes back from Toronto, we receive copies of almost the total chart, and he finds this very useful. She noted that it is difficult for one hospital to know what will be useful in another hospital and, therefore, sending the whole chart is often helpful. She stated that for patients being sent to Toronto for a CT scan, the whole chart (not copies) is sent with the patient and then returned when the patient comes back to Peterborough.

Mrs. Smith noted that nursing staff find it very helpful to receive the nursing notes with the patient and not at a later date. Dr. Trims noted that it can take up to six months for final notes to be received on patients being sent back to Peterborough from another facility.

Mrs. Sevich will respond to the Wellesley Hospital request, noting that it is very helpful to receive as much information as possible at the time of patient transfer.

2. Pre-op Histories

This item was included on the agenda because of an incident where one physician insisted on having a medical transcriptionist called back to the hospital at night to transcribe a pre-op history. This is an ongoing problem. On the day of surgery, transcriptionists frequently spend a great deal of time hunting for the pre-op history dictation. Mrs. N. Taylor noted that there are two outside priority lines that are cleared very early every morning. If pre-op histories are dictated on these lines, there should be no problem with histories being available for surgery that day.

Mr. Clark made the suggestion that for all elective surgery, pre-op histories be required before the patient is admitted; if no history is available, the patient is not admitted to the hospital.

Committee members agreed that the whole pre-op package should be reviewed once again, not just in light of difficulties in obtaining histories but also in light of laboratory work, and so on.

As an interim measure, Mr. Clark suggested that a cutoff time, after which pre-op histories will not be transcribed in the hospital, be set and if this deadline is not met, it then becomes the physician's responsibility to have the history transcribed elsewhere.

It was further suggested that doctors should be educated to dictate pre-op histories when they see the patient in their offices. If this were done, problems would be minimized.

Mr. Copping suggested that Mr. Jacobs and Mrs. Kezia be delegated to look at the whole problem and bring back suggestions to this committee. In the meantime, he noted, no transcriptionist should be called back after hours to transcribe pre-op histories.

3. Availability of Old Charts

Mrs. Kezia noted that the physicians like to have old charts added to their patients' current charts. The anaesthetists in particular find this most desirable, and it has been recommended that the old chart be added to the current chart in the ward. Mrs. Bazio outlined the procedure used for surgical patients. She is attempting to organize the logistical problems in order to reach the goal of having all old charts attached to current charts in the ward.

Mrs. Smith noted that she has received some complaints about physicians having to use microfilm charts. She noted, however, that space is an ongoing problem and in her department, there is little alternative to microfilming.

Mrs. Sevich noted that she is looking at ways in which to increase the storage potential in her department; however, she noted that those charts that have been microfilmed in the past cannot be restored to their previous form.

4. Chart Review

This item was tabled because of lack of time to deal with it adequately.

5. Problem Charts

Ms. Dawson noted that there were two charts for which she was unable to determine which physician should complete the record. Committee members looked at these charts and assigned them to physicians for completion.

ADJOURNMENT

Dr. Chromie moved the meeting be adjourned at 1530.

NEXT MEETING
June 21 20__, 1215, Conference Room A, PRHC.
John Lawson, M.D., Chairman
Medical Records Committee

ASSIGNMENT 10.4

Conduct a meeting as a class. Appoint one student as the chairperson. The chairperson will decide the topic for the meeting, draft an agenda, and chair the meeting. Appoint another student as the secretary/note-taker. The secretary will produce the agenda using an appropriate format and distribute it to the attending members (the rest of the students). The secretary will take the minutes, type the minutes, and distribute the finished product to the members. Have a class discussion about how the meeting ran. Was it on time? Was the discussion captured in the minutes? Your instructor will act as an observer.

TOPICS FOR DISCUSSION

1. You know that there is a major vote issue on the agenda for the upcoming meeting. You are not sure if there will be a quorum at the meeting. What will you do before you consult the chairperson?

2. You are coordinating a convention and you have several speakers coming. What information will you need from each speaker in order to arrange the convention?

CHAPTER 11

Hospital Records, Requisitions, and Reports

CHAPTER OUTLINE

Initiation of Hospital Records
Hospital Admission
Hospital Chart
Medical Chart
Surgical Charts

Hospital Notes
Processing Physician Orders
Confidentiality
Discharge of a Patient
Topics for Discussion

LEARNING OBJECTIVES

After reading this chapter, you will be familiar with

- Ways in which hospital records can be initiated
- Some of the medical administrative assistant's responsibilities in the hospital setting
- Proper procedures for completing hospital requisitions
- The responsibilities associated processing discharge records
- Recognized filing systems in health records departments

After reading this chapter, you will also be able to identify appropriate formats for

- History and physical reports
- Admission/consult notes
- Discharge summaries/final notes
- Operative records
- Delivery reports
- Patient admission forms
- Patient consent forms
- Request for accommodation forms
- The various types of investigative reports generated in a medical environment

KEY TERMS

Addressograph: This machine is used to imprint the patient's information from the admission card to the appropriate form or requisition. It is similar to a manual credit card machine in that it uses ink, pressure, and the raised letters on the card to transfer the information to a paper source.

Discharge: A discharge means that the patient is leaving the facility of admission or visit, either to go home or to be admitted to an

Elective: Elective means that the admission or procedure is not considered urgent or an emergency and can be pre-booked.

KEY TERMS—cont'd

Hospitalist: This physician works either full-time or part-time in the hospital to provide in-hospital medical services to patients who do not have a family physician or whose family physician has permanently or temporarily given up his or her admitting privileges. In some areas, these physicians provide short-term medical support for the patient on discharge.

PACU: This is the abbreviated form for Post-Anaesthetic Care Unit. It is also known as the Recovery Room.

Provisional Diagnosis: This is the original diagnosis made by the physician based on the patient's presenting symptoms.

Stat: In the medical environment, *stat* means "immediately." The action(s) should be completed right away.

In addition to discussing hospital records, this chapter will explain how to complete hospital requisitions, how to prepare notes, and the medical administrative assistant's responsibilities in a hospital setting.

INITIATION OF HOSPITAL RECORDS

Hospital records consist of out-patient visits and in-patient visits. Some examples of out-patient visits follow:

- Emergency
- Medical out-patient
- Cardiac catheterization
- Diagnostic imaging
- Physiotherapy
- Surgical out-patient

When out-patient visits such as medical out-patients and cardiac catheterization occur, a medical chart is assembled that may consist of the following:

- Physician's Orders (pre- and post-procedure)
- Consent
- Anaesthetic Questionnaire (pre- and post-procedure)
- Nursing Flow Sheet
- Multidisciplinary Notes

A hospital record can be as simple as an out-patient emergency visit consisting of one sheet or multiple pages on an in-patient admission.

The in-patient hospital record can be initiated in several ways:

1. The patient may be assessed in the Emergency Department and then admitted.
2. The patient may enter the hospital for an out-patient procedure and subsequently require admission.
3. The patient may be admitted for an **elective** medical or surgical procedure.

Admissions are processed in the admitting department. In some hospitals the Emergency Department or nursing units do their own admissions. The admitting physician will provide the **provisional diagnosis** (reason for admission), which is then recorded on the Admission/Discharge Record (see Figure 11.1). The provisional diagnosis cannot appear in abbreviated form. For example, U/A must appear as Unstable Angina. The original diagnosis stays the same on the Admission/Discharge Record even though the patient's diagnosis may change during the hospital stay.

When a patient is being admitted on a pre-arranged (elective) basis, the patient's sociological and medical information is provided to the admitting department prior to the admission date. As mentioned previously in Chapter 2, the physician's office will give the patient a Pre-Admission Form to complete and send to the hospital (see Figure 11.2). The office will also complete a Medical or Surgical Pre-Admission Card (see Figure 2.9) to be sent to the hospital prior to admission.

HOSPITAL ADMISSION

On admission, the sociological information, name, address, telephone number, and so on are checked for accuracy and the patient's health card is scanned or keyed in for verification. This information is very important for future reference, billing, and statistical purposes. The admitting facility is responsible for informing the patient how this information will be used by the hospital. This is usually done by information posters in admitting and on all floors. If the patient has concerns, the staff are aware of the appropriate steps to take to ensure the patient's requests are met. This is required under the provincial *Privacy Act*.

At this time, the patient will be asked to identify which accommodation he or she is requesting or which accommodation he or she is covered for by a third-party insurance. If the request is for private or semi-private and the patient has no additional insurance (most provincial healthcare insurances cover ward accommodation only—usually four beds per room), the patient will be responsible for paying the difference in cost.

At this time, a hospital card or **addressograph** plate (see Figure 11.3), or both, is prepared and used during the patient's stay. All forms and requisitions are imprinted with the patient's information from this card by using an addressograph machine. The addressograph machine is similar to a manual credit card machine. In some hospitals, the hospital card is given to the patient on **discharge** to use as identification for future visits. Some hospitals

FIGURE **11.1**   **Admission/Discharge Record**

PETERBOROUGH REGIONAL HEALTH CENTRE							
ADMISSION/DISCHARGE RECORD		Name				Unit #	
Hospital number		Acct.#		Admission Date 22 DEC	Time 1221	Health Card Number	MOH 50

Marital status M	Sex M	Age	Date of Birth:	Religion	ADM Clerk	
Address			Postal Code		Maiden Name	

ALERTS:	Next of Kin	WIFE	Person to Notify

	Req	Assign	Room number - bed	Insurance Info	2nd Insurance

Attending Physician	Family Physician	Admitting Physician	Transferred from

Admitting Diagnosis	LOS	Prev.Other	Prev.

Discharged Signed Out Death	Date and Time: dd mm yy / hours	Autopsy: Yes No	Coroner Yes No name	Transferred to:	LOS

(Do Not Use Abbreviations)

	Health Records
MOST RESPONSIBLE Dx: (Most significant/dx responsible for the most days of care)	
PRE-ADMIT COMORBIDITY: (Dx present on admission that significantly influences LOS and/or treatment)	
SECONDARY DIAGNOSIS: (Dx which may or may not have received treatment but did not contribute to LOS	
POST-ADMIT COMORBIDITY: (Dx arising after admission that significantly influences LOS and/or treatment)	
PROCEDURES:	

Discharge Summary

	ALC Days
	ICU Days
	Physio O.T.
	Speech Resp.
Note Dictated: Yes ☐ No ☐ Assembled by:_____ Checked by:_____ Coded by:_____	Other Other
	Social Serv. Disch. Plan.
The undersigned confirms all orders for treatment contained in the herein doctors' order sheets. whether signed or not and the discharge of the patient on the date shown above.	Blood Given Hosp.Acq.Inf.
A.C.R. ☐ _____ _____ (Signature of Most Responsible Physician) Date	VRE ☐ MRSA ☐ C.DIFF ☐

SOURCE: Reproduced by permission of Peterborough Regional Health Centre.

PETERBOROUGH REGIONAL HEALTH CENTRE

ADMISSION/DISCHARGE RECORD

Health Card Number

Name	Unit #
Acct.# Admission Date Time	Health Card Number MOH

Marital Status	Sex	Age	Date of Birth:	Religion	ADM Clerk

Address	Postal Code	Maiden Name

Next of Kin	Person to Notify

Req	Assign	Room number - bed	Insurance Info	2nd Insurance

Attending Physician	Family Physician	Admitting Physician	Transferred from

WARD ☐
(Max. 4 patients per room)

Cost per day

___ Covered by Health Card

___ WSIB

___ Non-Ohip $_____

_____

___ Out of Province $_____

___ Out of Country $_____

SEMI-PRIVATE ☐
(2 patients per room)

Cost Per day

$_____

___ Covered by Insurance

___ Self-Pay

PRIVATE ☐
(1 patient per room)
(Room may not have private bathroom)

Cost per day

$_____

___ Covered by Insurance

___ Self-Pay

DISCHARGE DATE

_____

THE HOSPITAL DOES NOT ASSUME ANY RESPONSIBILITY FOR THE KNOWLEDGE OF YOUR INSURANCE COVERAGE.

THE HOSPITAL DOES NOT ASSUME ANY RESPONSIBILITY FOR PATIENT VALUABLES.

ASSIGNMENT OF BENEFITS / RELEASE OF INFORMATION / RESPONSIBILITY FOR PAYMENT:
I hereby assign to the Hospital named herein all benefits payable from this claim or so much thereof as may serve to satisfy my indebtedness or that of my Dependent.

I hereby authorize the above-named Hospital to release any information which may be required for insurance claim purposes.

I acknowledge that if, for any reason, my insurance agency (if applicable) does not honour my claim, I agree to make full and immediate payment for these charges.

Signature: _____

Witness: _____   Date: _____

FIGURE **11.1   Admission/Discharge Record, cont'd**

FIGURE **11.2** **Patient Registration Sheet**

REGISTRATION SHEET — PLEASE COMPLETE & RETURN TO THE ADMITTING DEPT. OF THE APPROPRIATE HOSPITAL IMMEDIATELY.

DEAR PATIENT: YOU HAVE BEEN BOOKED FOR A PROCEDURE AT:

ST. JOSEPH'S HOSPITAL & HEALTH CENTRE
384 ROGERS ST.
PETERBOROUGH, ONT. K9H 7B6
ADMITTING: TEL. (705) 740-8000 FAX (705) 740-8001

PETERBOROUGH CIVIC HOSPITAL
ONE HOSPITAL DRIVE
PETERBOROUGH, ONT. K9J 7C6
ADMITTING: TEL. (705) 876-5068 FAX (705) 876-5107

☐ A.M. ADMIT
☐ IN–PATIENT
☐ SURGICAL OUT–PATIENT
☐ MEDICAL OUT–PATIENT

PATIENT'S NAME: _____ AGE _____

DATE OF ADMISSION: _____ _____ _____   DATE OF PROCEDURE: _____ _____ _____
Month   Day   Year   Month   Day   Year

ATTENDING DOCTOR: _____ ( ) _____ FAMILY DOCTOR: _____ ( ) _____
                                    INITIAL   INITIAL

PROCEDURE: _____

1. LAST NAME	ALL GIVEN NAMES (No Initials) (Underline Name Used)	ANY PREVIOUS LAST NAME

2. HOME ADDRESS (STREET, R.R., BOX, APT.)	CITY/TOWN	POSTAL CODE	TOWNSHIP

3. IF YOU ARE FROM: HOME FOR THE AGED_____ NURSING HOME_____ RESIDENTIAL FACILITY_____

NAME THE FACILITY _____

4. HOME TELEPHONE:	DATE OF BIRTH:	MONTH DAY YEAR	AGE	SEX	MARITAL STATUS (Please Circle)
AREA CODE_____ - _____		___ / ___ / ___	___	__ M__ F	S M D W SEP CL

5. RELIGION & _____

NAME OF CHURCH _____

IF YOUR "CLERGY PERSON" OR THE PASTORAL CARE DEPT. WERE TO INQUIRE, WOULD YOU LIKE THEM TO BE MADE AWARE OF YOUR HOSPITAL ADMISSION?

YES ☐   NO ☐

TO ENSURE THAT YOUR "CLERGY PERSON" IS AWARE OF YOUR ADMISSION, PLEASE CONTACT HIM/HER YOURSELF BEFORE COMING TO THE HOSPITAL.

6. NAME OF NEXT OF KIN OR FRIEND:

SPOUSE _____ TELEPHONE _____ ADDRESS _____

PARENT _____ TELEPHONE _____ ADDRESS _____

OTHER & _____ TELEPHONE _____ ADDRESS _____

RELATIONSHIP _____

7. IF WORKERS' COMPENSATION: MON.   DAY   YR.

YES _____ NO _____   SIN # ___ ___ ___   DATE OF ACCIDENT ___ / ___ / ___   CLAIM # _____

NAME OF EMPLOYER _____   ADDRESS OF EMPLOYER _____

8. IS THIS HOSPITAL VISIT DUE TO COSMETIC SURGERY? YES _____ NO _____   COVERED BY ONT. HEALTH INS.? _____

9. HEALTH CARE # :	VERSION CODE:	PLEASE BRING YOUR HEALTH CARD WITH YOU
⌊_⌋_⌋_⌋_⌋_⌋_⌋_⌋_⌋_⌋_⌋_⌋_⌋	⌊_⌋_⌋ 1 OR 2 LETTERS BOTTOM RIGHT OF CARD.	_____

10. PATIENT'S EMPLOYER: _____   ADDRESS: _____

(Please Circle)

11. IF YOU ARE ADMITTED DO YOU WISH A   STANDARD WARD   SEMI-PRIVATE   PRIVATE ROOM?
(YOU WILL BE RESPONSIBLE FOR SEMI OR PRIVATE ROOM CHARGES IF YOUR INSURANCE DOES NOT COVER THIS ACCOMMODATION REQUEST.)

12. ADDITIONAL INSURANCE FOR SEMI-PRIVATE:

NAME OF INSURANCE _____   NAME OF EMPLOYER _____
                                     (IF A GROUP PLAN)

IDENTIFICATION/POLICY # _____   GROUP # _____

INSURANCE HOLDER'S NAME _____   INSURANCE HOLDER'S SIN # ___ ___ ___

13. ADDITIONAL INSURANCE FOR PRIVATE:

NAME OF INSURANCE _____   NAME OF EMPLOYER _____
                                     (IF A GROUP PLAN)

IDENTIFICATION/POLICY # _____   GROUP # _____

INSURANCE HOLDER'S NAME _____   INSURANCE HOLDER'S SIN # ___ ___ ___

14. WHAT CONTACT HAVE YOU HAD WITH THE HOSPITALS?

PETERBOROUGH CIVIC   YEAR _____   PREVIOUS SURNAME _____   ST. JOSEPH'S   YEAR _____   PREVIOUS SURNAME _____

15. ALLERGIES: FOOD _____ DRUG _____ NONE _____ UNKNOWN _____

FORM # 0505021 JF   (PAGE 2 OF 5)

SOURCE: Reproduced by permission of Peterborough Regional Health Centre.

FIGURE **11.3** **Addressograph**

EXAMPLE A

Patient's Medical Record #	40442
Patient's Sex/Name	M Shultz, Erik
Patient's Address	17 Bond St., Ottawa, ON
Health Card #	7819749313

EXAMPLE B

Patient's Medical Record #/Visit Specific #	40442 95-03751
Patient's Sex/Age/Name	M55 yrs Shultz, Erik
Patient's Visit Date/Birth Date	16 Oct 20____ BD26 May 20____
Patient's Address	17 Bond St., Ottawa, ON
Health Card #/Doctor's Name	7819749313 Dr. Plunkett

do not use an addressograph at all. When the patient is admitted, a sheet of labels is printed off and sent to the unit with the admission information. The ward secretary then peels off a label when needed.

The patient's armband is created on admission and is placed on the patient's wrist. Each time the patient has lab work done or is having a treatment, the armband is checked to verify the patient's identity. Allergy bands are put on the patient on arrival on the nursing unit.

If the patient is not being admitted from out-patient or emergency status, the Admission/Discharge Record will be the first of several documents that will make up the patient's chart.

HOSPITAL CHART

The chart will follow the patient to the nursing unit, where the patient will be treated, and to any department within the hospital to which the patient needs to go (e.g., Diagnostic Imaging or Physiotherapy).

In some hospitals, all charting and ordering of tests (Order Entry) is done through a computer network. With this system, the patient's chart can be accessed from any department or unit when necessary. When the patient's name is entered, a list of names will appear on the screen. The staff must be sure to choose the correct patient. The most accurate way to verify a patient is by entering the Medical Record number for the search. If there is still some doubt, the health card number and date of birth should be checked with the patient name. There may be quite a few John Smiths in the system, but there will only be one John Smith with the same health card number and date of birth. Some hospitals still do manual charting on the units, but diagnostic imaging reports, lab reports, and transcription notes are accessible through the computer, therefore eliminating the amount of phone requests and paper delivery.

The Medical Record number is also known as the Health Record number, the Unique number, or the Patient ID number. This number is assigned to the patient on their first visit to that hospital and remains a unique number to that patient for any other visit. The health record chart, diagnostic imaging files, etc., are filed by this number. The account number or visit number will change with each separate visit, but the Medical Record number remains the same.

In some software, the patient status will be shown in different colours. For example, out-patient visits may be in red, current in-patient visits may be in bright green, and discharged patients may be in black. A deceased patient's name may be followed by a small "x."

MEDICAL CHART

A medical admission is facilitated by a physician who is not a surgeon. All physicians must have admitting privileges at the facility they want to admit patients to. If they do not, they must arrange for a physician to assume care for their patients while in hospital. The role of the **hospitalist** will be discussed later in this chapter.

The forms shown in Figures 11.4 to 11.14 are part of a medical admission chart.

NOTE: The Patient Care Plan is also referred to as a "Kardex" in a manual system. It is usually the same format for Surgical and Medical admissions but may be different for units such as Labour & Delivery. The Kardex is shown in Figure 11.4 as separate sheets; however, it is actually preprinted on 16 × 11 cardstock, folded, and 3-hole punched to fit in the chart binder.

SURGICAL CHARTS

When the patient is admitted for surgery or if surgery is required during the patient's hospital stay, additional records are required and added to the chart. For a surgical admission, the Most Responsible Physician (MRP) must be the surgeon. Figures 11.15 to 11.23 are examples of some of the additional records required.

Any changes that occur in the patient's condition are recorded on the progress notes and may be followed by a dictated Progress Note by the attending physician.

HOSPITAL NOTES

When a patient is admitted, the attending or admitting physician will dictate an Admission or Consult Note (it may read Admission/Consult note). This may also be entitled History & Physical/Admission note (see Figure 11.24). History of the present illness, past illnesses, family's health, and the patient's lifestyle must be reported because they may play a part in diagnosing the illness. The

Text continued on p. 253.

FIGURE 11.4   Patient Care Plan (Kardex)

RESUSCITATION STATUS		DIAGNOSIS	CONTACT PERSON:
DATE:			
ADVANCED DIRECTIVE: Yes ☐ No ☐		SPECIAL OBSERVATIONS/1:1 CARE REQUIRED: ☐	TRANSFER PLAN:
PERTINENT HISTORY		SURGERY & DATE DPO	DISCHARGE: INITIATED:
			DISCHARGE PLANS
			CARE PROGRAM
			HOME CARE REFERRAL: ☐ NEEDED ☐ COMPLETED ☐ SIGNED
HYGIENE			MOBILITY
BATHES SELF	☐		WALKING WITH ASSISTANCE/UP IN CHAIR ☐
BATHES SELF WITH HELP	☐		POST-OP MOBILITY ☐
Any Previous hospitalization in past 3 months Yes ☐ No ☐	☐	COMPLETE BATH	TWO PERSON TRANSFER ☐
ALLERGIES	☐	PM CARE/POST - OP BATH	BEDREST WITH ASSISTANCE ☐
	☐	MOUTH CARE Q1 - 2 HRS	BEDREST WITH TURNING ☐
			MECHANICAL LIFT ☐
DRUG		NUTRITION	TRANSFER TECHNIQUES ☐
		DIET	
FOOD	☐	FEEDS SELF/NPO/FAMILY FEEDS	
	☐	FEEDS WITH ASSISTANCE	VITAL SIGNS ROUTINE
	☐	TOTAL FEED	ROUTINE VS ☐
OTHER	☐	TUBE/GASTRIC FEED	V.S. UP TO Q 4 H/CLOSE OBS. ☐
PLANNED TEACHING EMOTIONAL SUPPORT		ELIMINATION	VASCULAR/NEURO V.S. ☐
	☐	TOILETS WITH HELP/BEDPAN/CATHETER/COMMODE/	OTHER
TIME: 15 MINUTES ☐ 20 MINUTES ☐ 30 MINUTES ☐	☐	OCCASIONAL INCONTENENCE	SAFETY
	☐	TOILETS WITH SUPERVISION	SPECIAL PRECAUTIONS
PATIENT CONFERENCE ☐		INCONTENENT CARE	
		CATHETER SIZE	
	☐	INSERTED REMOVED	
	☐	OSTOMY BAG CHANGE	
		OSTOMY CARE	
NAME:		ROOM:	MOST RESPONSIBLE PHYSICIAN:

continued

SOURCE: Reproduced by permission of Peterborough Regional Health Centre.

I.V. THERAPY		
DATE	☐ CV LINE	☐ P.I.V
☐	MAINTENANCE	
☐	TITRATED INFUSIONS	
☐	TPN	
☐	PAIN MANAGEMENT	
☐	IV PCA ☐ MORPHINE	
	☐ FENTANYL	
	☐ MEPERDINE	
☐	EPIDURAL	
	EPIMORPHINE _____ mg q _____ h prn	
	BUP/FENT@ _____ ml/hr	

DIAGNOSTIC TESTS		
DATE	FREQ	
		CBC, DIFF, PLTS, PTT, INR
		GLUC, LYTES, BUN, CR
		CK q 8H X3, AST, CK,ECG DAILY X3
		RESTART WITH ANY EPISODE > 20 MIN.
		ECG STAT WITH CHEST PAIN
		CHEST X-RAY
	DAILY	APTT

CULTURE COLLECTIONS		
DATE	SITE	RESULTS
	BLOOD	
	URINE	
	SPUTUM	
	WOUND	

TREATMENTS		
DATE		
		ECG ON DAY OF DISCHARGE - COPY TO F.P. & ATTENDING M.D.
		OXYGEN THERAPY

FIGURE 11.4   Patient Care Plan (Kardex), cont'd

MEDICATIONS

PERSONAL MEDICATIONS TO PHARMACY ☐ YES ☐ NO

DATE (mm/dd/yy)	MEDICATION	ROUTE	FREQ	07 - 19	19 - 07	STOP	DATE	PRN MEDICATION	STOP

REFERRALS & CONSULTS

DEPARTMENT/SERVICE	NOTIFIED	COMMENTS

LINE INSERTION & REMOVAL

LINE/DRAIN	INSERTION DATE (mm/dd/yy)	DRESSING CHANGE	SOLUTION CHANGE	TUBING CHANGE	REMOVAL DATE (mm/dd/yy)

PHYSIOTHERAPY ☐   OCCUPATIONAL THERAPY ☐

NUTRITION ☐   SPEECH THERAPY ☐

SOCIAL WORK ☐   RESPIRATORY ☐

ISOLATION ☐

VENTILATOR PHYSICIAN: _____

FAMILY PHYSICIAN: _____

CONSULTANT: _____

MOST RESPONSIBLE PHYSICIAN: _____

NAME: _____   ROOM: _____

FIGURE 11.4 Patient Care Plan (Kardex), cont'd

continued

PETERBOROUGH REGIONAL HEALTH CENTRE PATIENT CARE PLAN

DATE	NURSING ORDERS	NURSING ORDERS				DATE	EXPECTED OUTCOMES
		BP	HR	RR	NEURO V/S		
	ALTERATIONS IN CARDIOVASCULAR	CVP	PAPS	PAWP	CO		READY FOR TRANSFER WHEN:
	FUNCTION RELATED TO:	TEMP.	PULSES				1. VS & HEMODYNAMIC PARAMETERS WITHIN NORMAL RANGE FOR PATIENT
		PA CATCHER LENGTH AT INTRODUCER _____ CM					
		☐ TTVP MA _____ RATE _____					2. ABSENCE OF ARRHYTHMIAS
		☐ CHECK THRESHOLD _q_ SHIFT					
	ALTERATION IN RESPIRATORY	CHECK AUSCULATION _q_ _____ _h_					READY FOR TRANSFER WHEN:
	FUNCTION:	FlO2 _____ RATE _____					
	1. IMPAIRED GAS EXCHANGE	VENTILATOR MODE: SIMV AC PC CPAP					1. PATIENT'S RESPIRATORY FUNCTION IS ADEQUATE
	RELATED TO:	RATE _____ VT _____ CPAP/PEEP _____ PS _____					
		☐ BIPAP IPAP _____ EPAP _____					
	2. INEFFECTIVE BREATHING	ETT SIZE _____ @lip _____ cm					2. PATIENT IS MAINTAINING AN ADEQUATE AIRWAY
	PATTERNS RELATED TO:	☐ WEANING AS PER PROTOCOL					
		SUCTION PRN					
	3. INEFFECTIVE AIRWAY	CHEST PHYSIO _____ _q_ _____ _h_					
	CLEARANCE RELATED TO:	INCENTIVE SPIROMETRY _q_ _____ _h_					
		SPO2 MONITOR _____ _q_ _____ _h_					
		ETCO2 MONITOR _____ _q_ _____ _h_					
		TRACH CARE _____ _q_ _____ _h_					
	ALTERATION IN COMFORT/PAIN/						READY FOR TRANSFER WHEN:
	SLEEP						1. PATIENT'S PAIN IS CONTROLLED
	RELATED TO:						
							2. PATIENT'S NORMAL SLEEP PATTERN IS RE-ESTABLISHED

FIGURE 11.4   Patient Care Plan (Kardex), cont'd

FIGURE **11.5**   **Nursing Assessment**

Peterborough Regional Health Centre	BASELINE DATA:

Peterborough Regional Health Centre
Nursing Department
OREM
NURSING ASSESSMENT
DATE:_____
INITIATED
BY:_____

BASELINE DATA:

TPR _____

BP _____(R)

_____(L)

CHIEF COMPLAINTS:_____

SIGNIFICANT PREVIOUS ILLNESS:

APEX: _____

1. AGGRAVATES/ALLEVIATES:_____

WEIGHT:_____(kg)

2. DESCRIBE SYMPTOMS:_____

HEIGHT:_____(cm)

ALLERGIES:(MEDS & FOOD)

3. TIMING:_____

4. IF PAIN:
   a) REGION/RADIATION_____

   b) SEVERITY_____
      1   2   3   4   5   6   7   8   9   10

CURRENT MEDICATION:	DOSE	FREQUENCY	CURRENT MEDS.	DOSE	FREQUENCY

RISK FACTORS: [ ] FALLS   [ ] WANDERS   [ ] AGGRESSIVE

LEVEL OF AWARENESS: [ ] CO-OPERATIVE

[ ] ALERT   [ ] TIME   [ ] PLACE   [ ] PERSON

[ ] CONFUSED   [ ] DISORIENTATED   [ ] STUPOROUS
[ ] UNRESPONSIVE   [ ] UNCOOPERATIVE   [ ] ANXIOUS
[ ] DEPRESSED   [ ] RETICENT

DISCHARGE CONCERNS:_____

USUAL HEALTH PATTERNS

DIET:_____   ALCOHOL: _____

HEARING:_____   DRUGS:_____

VISION:_____   SMOKE:_____

SPEECH:_____   MOBILITY:_____

CURRENT COMMUNITY SUPPORTS

PHN _____

HOME CARE
_____

VON
_____

OTHER:
_____

FAMILY HISTORY
SPOUSE OR SIGNIFICANT OTHER:_____

FATHER:_____

MOTHER:_____

SIBS:_____

CHILDREN:_____

Form #1697 Rev. Feb./92

continued

USCR - ASSESSMENT OF SELF CARE AGENCY:

AIR (RESPIRATORY)	FOOD (GI)
ACTION DEMAND: TO MAINTAIN AIRWAY AND ADEQUATE RESPIRATION.	ACTION DEMAND: TO OBTAIN, PREPARE, INGEST AND DIGEST ADEQUATE QUANTITIES OF APPROPRIATE FOOD TYPES.
SELF [ ] SUPPORT [ ] ASSIST [ ] TOTAL [ ]	SELF [ ] SUPPORT [ ] ASSIST [ ] TOTAL [ ]
FLUID (CARDIOVASCULAR, GI)	ELIMINATION (GI, URINARY, REPRODUCTIVE)
ACTION DEMAND: TO MAINTAIN ADEQUATE INTAKE AND FLUID	ACTION DEMAND: TO REGULATE AND CONTROL EXCRETORY FUNCTIONS, INCLUDING SAFE AND SANITARY DISPOSAL OF WASTES.
SELF [ ] SUPPORT [ ] ASSIST [ ] TOTAL [ ]	SELF [ ] SUPPORT [ ] ASSIST [ ] TOTAL [ ]
ACTIVITY/REST (MUSCULOSKELETAL, SKIN)	SOLITUDE/SOCIAL INTERACTION (PSYCHOSOCIAL/SPIRITUAL)
ACTION DEMAND: TO MAINTAIN AN ADEQUATE BALANCE BETWEEN ACTIVITY AND REST.	ACTION DEMAND: TO MAINTAIN AN ADEQUATE BALANCE BETWEEN SOLITUDE AND SOCIAL INTERACTION
SELF [ ] SUPPORT [ ] ASSIST [ ] TOTAL [ ]	SELF [ ] SUPPORT [ ] ASSIST [ ] TOTAL [ ]
PREVENTION OF HAZARDS (NEURO, MUSCULOSKELETAL, PSYCHOSOCIAL)	NORMALCY (PSYCHOSOCIAL, NEURO)
ACTION DEMAND: TO MINIMIZE RISK FROM AND PROTECT SELF FROM INTERNAL, EXTERNAL AND ENVIRONMENTAL HAZARDS.	ACTION DEMAND: TO ACHIEVE AND MAINTAIN POSITIVE SELF ESTEEM
SELF [ ] SUPPORT [ ] ASSIST [ ] TOTAL [ ]	SELF [ ] SUPPORT [ ] ASSIST [ ] TOTAL [ ]

SUMMARY

IDENTIFIED S.C. DEFICITS IN:
AIR   [ ] ACTIVITY/REST [ ]
WATER   [ ] SOLITUDE/
FOOD   [ ] INTERACTION   [ ]
ELIMINATION [ ] PREV.OF HAZARDS[ ]
               NORMALCY   [ ]

NURSING SYSTEM
  WHOLLY COMPENSATORY   [ ]
  PARTLY COMPENSATORY   [ ]
  EDUCATIVE-SUPPORTIVE [ ]

DATE:
SIGNATURE:

ASSESSMENT: SEE NURSING DIAGNOSIS
              RECORD
PLAN:

Form #1697   Rev. Feb./92

FIGURE **11.5**   **Nursing Assessment, cont'd**

FIGURE **11.6**   **Nursing Diagnosis Record**

Peterborough Regional Health Centre

NURSING DIAGNOSIS RECORD

Nursing Diagnosis	Present Date	Potential Date	Resolved Date
1.			
2.			
3.			
4.			
5.			
6.			
7.			
8.			
9.			

SOURCE: Reproduced by permission of Peterborough Regional Health Centre.

FIGURE **11.7** **Physician's Order Sheet**

PETERBOROUGH REGIONAL HEALTH CENTRE

PHYSICIAN'S ORDER SHEET

M.R.P.: _____

Date (d/m/y) & Time	Sent to Pharmacy	Allergies: _____ ☐ No Known Allergies	S M O	K A R D E X	M A R	N O T I F I E D	Signature of Nurse Date & Time
		COMPLETE ALLERGY BOX (ABOVE) AT TIME OF INITIAL ORDERS					

Number Must Show Through Hole Before Physician Writes Orders

COPY **1**

STANDARD MEDICATION ADMINISTRATION TIMES (except psychiatry)
daily - 0800
hs - 2200
bid - 0800, 1800
q12h - 0800, 2000
tid - 0800, 1200, 1800
q8h - 0600, 1400, 2200
qid - 0800, 1200, 1800, 2200
q6h - 0600, 1200, 1800, 2400
q4hwa - 0600, 1000, 1400, 1800, 2200 (and 0200 if patient awake)
q4h - 0200, 0600, 1000, 1400, 1800, 2200
q3h - 0300, 0600, 0900, 1200, 1500, 1800, 2100, 2400

0505014JF-02/03

SOURCE: Reproduced by permission of Peterborough Regional Health Centre.

FIGURE 11.8 **Patient Assessment/Intervention Flow Sheet**

PETERBOROUGH REGIONAL HEALTH CENTRE

MEDICAL SERVICES

PATIENT ASSESSMENT / INTERVENTION FLOWSHEET

	Date (D/M/Y):								
	Time:								
Problem Name & #	Areas of Assessment								
Pain R/T	VAS (0 - 10)								
Impaired LOC / Orientation / Cognition R/T									
Other	RESTRAINT CARE / INCREASED OBSERVATION (Indicate Type)								
	TEACHING/ EMOTIONAL SUPPORT > 5 minutes - see note & min. count (Indicate Type / Topic)								
	ISOLATION PRECAUTIONS (Indicate Type)								
	SPECIMEN COLLECTION / TEST (Indicate Type)								
	ACCOMPANY/MONITOR PATIENT (Internal/External) MINUTES								

CLINICAL NOTE:

FORM 1693 // flowshee.med // Revised July 10, 2001

SOURCE: Reproduced by permission of Peterborough Regional Health Centre.

continued

PATIENT ASSESSMENT / INTERVENTION FLOWSHEET

LEGEND: √ Complete & Normal   * Abnormal Finding see clinical note   ➡ Abnormal Finding same as last time, therefore, no clinical note   / = Not Applicable

DATE: (D/M/Y)								
TOUR OF DUTY								
Nutrition F = Fluids R = Regular SD = Sp. Diet	Self							
	NPO							
	Feeds with Assist / Family							
	Total Feed							
	Feed w/ Constant Supervision							
	Enteral Feed: Solution:							
	Rate:							
	Time:							
	Water Flush (time & amount):							
	Gastric Residual:							
	Additional Dietary Needs / HS Snacks							
	N = Nausea V = Vomiting							
LEGEND: Mark 1-Adequate 2-50% 3-25%4-Refused								
Elimination	Toilets w/ Assist of 1 nurse (Count)							
	Toilets w/ Assist of 2 nurses (Count)							
	Incontinent/Involuntary Care (Count)							
	Ostomy Emptying (Count)							
	Number of Stools							
	Urine: Y - Yes N - No							
	Catheter Output							
LEGEND: Urinal; Bedpan; Commode; BR (bathroom)								
Hygiene	Bathes / Showers Self							
	Bathes / Showers Self w/ Help							
	Bath / Shower by Personnel							
	Dress / Undress: Street Clothes							
	HS Care							
	Emesis Care (Count)							
Activity	Chair / Ambulate							
	(Self w/ 1; w/ 2 or more) # of times:							
	Ambulate in hallway							
	(Self w/ 1; w/ 2 or more) # of times:							
	Mechanical Lift							
	Bed Rest							
	Turn q 2 - 4 hr							
	Reposition with Assistance							
	Side rails: 1 or 2 ☐ more than 2 ☐							
	Encourage Rest Periods / Sleep							
	Bed to Stretcher / Stretcher to Bed (Count)							
INITIALS ☞ ☞ ☞ ☞								

Nurse's Name & Status	INITIALS	Nurse's Name & Status	INITIALS	Nurse's Name & Status	INITIALS

FORM # 1693 // flowshee.med // Revised July 10, 2001

FIGURE **11.8**   **Patient Assessment/Intervention Flow Sheet, cont'd**

FIGURE 11.9   Vital Signs Record

PETERBOROUGH REGIONAL HEALTH CENTRE

VITAL SIGN RECORD

FORM #1519 Revised April 2000 - Forms disk 1B

SOURCE: Reproduced by permission of Peterborough Regional Health Centre.

FIGURE **11.10**   **Nursing Department Fluid Balance Sheet**

Peterborough Regional Health Centre
NURSING DEPARTMENT
FLUID BALANCE SHEET

NURSE'S SIGNATURE: _____ INITIAL _____
NURSE'S SIGNATURE: _____ INITIAL _____
NURSE'S SIGNATURE: _____ INITIAL _____
NURSE'S SIGNATURE: _____ INITIAL _____
NURSE'S SIGNATURE: _____ INITIAL _____
NURSE'S SIGNATURE: _____ INITIAL _____
NURSE'S SIGNATURE: _____ INITIAL _____

DATE: _____

MM/DD/YY

| | TBA | TBA | INTAKE | | | | OUTPUT | | | | |
	LV.	LV.	MEDS	ORAL	BLOOD	SITE	URINE	STOOL	GASTRIC	DRAIN	
0700											
0800											
0900											
1000											
1100											
1200											
1300											
1400											
1500											
1600											
1700											
1800											
12 HR TOTAL											
SIGNATURE											

| | TBA | TBA | INTAKE | | | | OUTPUT | | | | |
	LV.	LV.	MEDS	ORAL	BLOOD	SITE	URINE	STOOL	GASTRIC	DRAIN	
1900											
2000											
2100											
2200											
2300											
2400											
0100											
0200											
0300											
0400											
0500											
0600											
12 HR TOTAL											
SIGNATURE											

| 24 HOUR INTAKE ( ) | 24 HOUR OUPUT ( ) | 24 HOUR BALANCE ( ) |

FORM #1577, REV. NOV. 1994

.....OVER

FIGURE 11.11 **Routine Medication Administration Record (MAR)**

Peterborough Regional Health Centre
ROUTINE MEDICATION ADMINISTRATION RECORD

Allergies	Nurse's Signature	I	Nurse's Signature	I	Nurse's Signature	I
Diagnosis						

I = Ineffective E = Effective

ROUTINE MEDICATIONS YEAR ______	Date: Time
Order Date (d/m/y): ______________ Reorder: ______________ po IV IM Sub cu sl pr aerochamber nebulizer TOP Eye Ear Nose Checked by: _____/_____ Stop Date (d/m/y): ______________ Reordered by: _____/_____	
Order Date (d/m/y): ______________ Reorder: ______________ po IV IM Sub cu sl pr aerochamber nebulizer TOP Eye Ear Nose Checked by: _____/_____ Stop Date (d/m/y): ______________ Reordered by: _____/_____	
Order Date (d/m/y): ______________ Reorder: ______________ po IV IM Sub cu sl pr aerochamber nebulizer TOP Eye Ear Nose Checked by: _____/_____ Stop Date (d/m/y): ______________ Reordered by: _____/_____	

FORM # 1609 Revised 30 July 2004 G:\Clinical\ProfessionalPractice\14 Linda's Forms Folder - Not Ctee\General Use Forms\1609 Blank MAR-Routine.doc Side 1 of 2

SOURCE: Reproduced by permission of Peterborough Regional Health Centre.

FIGURE 11.12   PRN Medication Administration Record (MAR)

Peterborough Regional Health Centre
PRN MEDICATION ADMINISTRATION RECORD

Side 1 of 2

FORM # 1615   Revised 30 July 2004   F:\FORMS\1615 Blank MAR-PRN.doc

SOURCE: Reproduced by permission of Peterborough Regional Health Centre.

FIGURE **11.13**   **Stat Medication Administration Record (MAR)**

ALLERGIES	NURSE'S SIGNATURE	I	NURSE'S SIGNATURE	I	NURSE'S SIGNATURE	I
DIAGNOSIS						

STAT MEDICATIONS _____ **YEAR** _____

1. Order Date _____ Date to Give _____

Route: PO   IV   IM   SC   SL   RECTAL | Date Given _____ Time Given _____
Single Dose _____ Checked By _____ | Given By _____

2. Order Date _____ Date to Give _____

Route: PO   IV   IM   SC   SL   RECTAL | Date Given _____ Time Given _____
Single Dose _____ Checked By _____ | Given By _____

3. Order Date _____ Date to Give _____

Route: PO   IV   IM   SC   SL   RECTAL | Date Given _____ Time Given _____
Single Dose _____ Checked By _____ | Given By _____

4. Order Date _____ Date to Give _____

Route: PO   IV   IM   SC   SL   RECTAL | Date Given _____ Time Given _____
By _____ | Given By _____

5. Order Date _____ Date to Give _____

Route: PO   IV   IM   SC   SL   RECTAL | Date Given _____ Time Given _____
Single Dose _____ Checked By _____ | Given By _____

6. Order Date _____ Date to Give _____

Route: PO   IV   IM   SC   SL   RECTAL | Date Given _____ Time Given _____
Single Dose _____ Checked By _____ | Given By _____

7. Order Date _____ Date to Give _____

Route: PO   IV   IM   SC   SL   RECTAL | Date Given _____ Time Given _____
Single Dose _____ Checked By _____ | Given By _____

8. Order Date _____ Date to Give _____

Route: PO   IV   IM   SC   SL   RECTAL | Date Given _____ Time Given _____
Single Dose _____ Checked By _____ | Given By _____

9. Order Date _____ Date to Give _____

Route: PO   IV   IM   SC   SL   RECTAL | Date Given _____ Time Given _____
Single Dose _____ Checked By _____ | Given By _____

10. Order Date _____ Date to Give _____

Route: PO   IV   IM   SC   SL   RECTAL | Date Given _____ Time Given _____
Single Dose _____ Checked By _____ | Given By _____

11. Order Date _____ Date to Give _____

Route: PO   IV   IM   SC   SL   RECTAL | Date Given _____ Time Given _____
Dose _____ By _____ | Given By _____

12. Order Date _____ Date to Give _____

Route: PO   IV   IM   SC   SL   RECTAL | Date Given _____ Time Given _____
Single Dose _____ | Given By _____

SOURCE: Reproduced by permission of Peterborough Regional Health Centre.

FIGURE **11.14** **Multidisciplinary Note**

PETERBOROUGH REGIONAL HEALTH CENTRE

- ☐ Hospital Drive Site
- ☐ Rogers Street Site
- ☐ Haliburton Hospital
- ☐ Minden Hospital

Date d/m/y	Discipline	Time	Multidisciplinary Notes Signature/Status

FORM # 3514 Rev. 14. August.2002 g:\clinical\profpractice\forms\general use forms\3514

SOURCE: Reproduced by permission of Peterborough Regional Health Centre.

FIGURE **11.15** **Flowsheet**

Peterborough Regional Health Centre

Flowsheet

Tea/Coffee/Hot Water	200 mL
Styrofoam cup	150 mL
Soup (cup)	150 mL
Juice (pre-pkg)	125 mL
Jello/Ice Cream/Sherbert	100 mL

Date(d/m/y): _____________ Transfer INTO ☐ Transfer OUT OF ☐ SCC TIME: ______

	TBA I.V.	TBA I.V.	TBA I.V.	TBA I.V.	INTAKE			OUTPUT				
					MEDS	ORAL	BLOOD	URINE	COL	GASTRIC	DRAIN	C.T.
0700												
0800												
0900												
1000												
1100												
1200												
1300												
1400												
1500												
1600												
1700												
1800												
12 Hr												

12 HOUR INTAKE [ ] 12 HOUR OUTPUT [ ] 12 HOUR BALANCE [ ]

SIGNATURE & STATUS: SIGNATURE & STATUS:

1900												
2000												
2100												
2200												
2300												
2400												
0100												
0200												
0300												
0400												
0500												
0600												
12 Hr												

12 HOUR INTAKE [ ] 12 HOUR OUTPUT [ ] 12 HOUR BALANC [ ]

24 HOUR INTAKE [ ] 24 HOUR OUTPUT [ ] 24 HOUR BALANCE [ ]

SIGNATURE & STATUS: Prev Cumulative Balance _____________ New Cumulative Balance _____________

SIGNATURE & STATUS:

TUBING CHANGES: Arterial ☐ CVP / TPN ☐ CVAD ☐ PIV ☐

0700 - 1900 Hours		1900 - 0700 Hours	
Initial PCA Prescription Check:		Initial PCA Prescription Check:	
Drug / Concentration:		Drug / Concentration:	
Dose:	Delay:	Dose:	Delay:
Basal:		Basal:	
12 Hour Totals:		12 Hour Totals:	
Successes / Attempts:		Successes / Attempts:	
Total Amount Used:		Total Amount Used:	
Pump Cleared:	Initials:	Pump Cleared:	Initials:

FORM # 1674// 05.Feb.01// g:\flowsheet\flowshee.srg

SOURCE: Reproduced by permission of Peterborough Regional Health Centre.

continued

		0700	0800	0900	1000	1100	1200	1300	1400	1500	1600	1700	1800
C N S	Orientation Status												
	VAS (0 - 10) / Sedation Score	/	/	/	/	/	/	/	/	/	/	/	/
	Side Effects												
	Chair/Activity: Assist of 1 or 2 (Count)												
	Reposition w/Assist/Turn w/skincare												
	Bed-Stretcher/Stretcher-Bed (Count)												
	Rest and Sleep												
C V S	DP Pulses (R, L) Palpable / Doppler												
	PT Pulses (R, L) Palpable / Doppler												
	CMS / Edema												
	IV / CVP Site												
	IV Initiate / Restart												
	Arterial Line / Blood Draws (Count)												
R e s p i r a t o r y	Chest Tube Maintenance												
	O_2 / SpO_2												
	Incentive Spirometry / DB & C												
	Chest Sounds												
G I	Diet: NPO / Ice Chips / Self / Assist												
	Total Feed / Enteral												
	Additional Dietary Needs/HS Snack												
	Abdomen												
	Bowel Function												
	Ostomy Care / Changes (Count)												
	Toilets w/ Assist of 1 or 2 (Count)												
	Urinal/Hat/Catheter Emptying (Count)												
	Incontinence/Involuntary Care (Count)												
G U	Oral Hygiene/Emesis Care (Count)												
	Bathes Self / Assist / Total												
	Suprapubic catheter clamp/unclamp w/ residuals												
	Peri / Catheter Care (Count)												
	CBI Colour / # Bags												
Signature(s) / Status:													

FIGURE **11.15   Flowsheet, cont'd**

CLINICAL NOTES	0700 - 1900 HOURS	1900 - 0700 HOURS
Dressings (Simple, Moderate, Complex) Suture / Staple / Drain Removal		
Diagnostic Procedures Tests / Specimens		
Nursing Procedures (Insertion or irrigation of tubes, bladder scanner, IV (re) starts, removal vag packing, sitz baths, enema other than fleet, CBI setup, manual irrigation, strain urine, apply traction to catheter, hooking up drainage devices, d/c catheter or IV, application of anti-embolic stockings, chest physio by nurse)		
Emotional Support (type) (> 5 mins. indicate time)		
Teaching (Type) (> 5 mins. indicate time)		
Barriers to Care (Type) (additional note prn)	Isolation Precautions ☐	
Other (assist w/procedure, increased observation, restraints, constant observation (minutes), accompany & monitor patient (minutes), prepare patient for OR)		
Problem List		
SIGNATURE(S):		

FIGURE **11.15** **Flowsheet, cont'd**

FIGURE **11.16** **Consent for Treatment/Procedure/Operation**

Peterborough Regional Health Centre
Consent for Treatment/Procedure/Operation
Date of Procedure: _____

I, _____ , hereby consent to the treatment/
procedure/operation of _____

ordered by/to be performed by————————————————————upon
                              (Name of physician or health practitioner)
myself or _____ .

_____ has explained to me the nature of the treatment/
(Name of physician or health practitioner)

procedure/operation, the material risks of the treatment/procedure/operation and the alternative
courses of action, including the likely consequences of not having the treatment/ procedure/
operation.

I am satisfied with these explanations and I have understood them. I have received responses to
my requests for additional information.

I also consent to such additional or alternative treatments/procedures/operations as may be
immediately necessary or medically advisable during the course of such procedures. In addition, I
consent to the administration of such anaesthetics as are necessary. I further consent that other
physicians or health practitioners of the Health Centre may assist in the treatment/procedure/
operation as required and directed by the supervision of _____
                                                        (Name of physician or health practitioner)

Dated this _____ day of _____ Year_____ at _____ hours

_____   _____
Signature of Witness   Signature of Patient and/or Substitute Decision-Maker

                                _____
                                Relationship - Substitute Decision-Maker

                                _____
                                Address - Substitute Decision-Maker

                                _____
                                Telephone Number - Substitute Decision-Maker

Note: Consent to be signed by patient, if capable, or by the Substitute Decision Maker
in the case of an incapable patient.

Form #1605 - Oct. /99

FIGURE **11.17** Informed Consent for/Refusal of Blood and/or Blood Products

> ### INFORMED CONSENT FOR OR REFUSAL OF BLOOD AND/OR BLOOD PRODUCTS
>
> Patient Name _____ Date(d/m/y) _____ Time _____
>
> 1. I have been informed by Dr. _____ or his/her designate,
>   that in the course of my medical/surgical treatment I may need a transfusion of blood or blood products.
>   (Red Blood Cells, Platelet Concentrates, Frozen Plasma and/or Cryoprecipitate).
>
> 2. I understand that blood transfusions are usually provided from blood donated by volunteer donors that has been collected by Canadian Blood Services (CBS), which has been responsible for selecting blood donors, collecting, testing and storing blood and blood products. **Peterborough Regional Health Centre** and its staff have stored the blood products since receipt from the CBS and will prepare the product for transfusion.
>
> 3. I have been informed of and understand the benefits and risks associated with this therapy. All blood donors are volunteers and are carefully screened by medical history, physical assessment and laboratory tests in order to minimize the risk of infectious disease transmission. These include viral hepatitis, Acquired Immune Deficiency Syndrome (AIDS) and other possible viral diseases (known and unknown). A test to detect West Nile Virus will be in place in July 2003. Although in most cases the risks and consequences are very small, in some cases serious injury and/or death may result. I understand that these measures cannot completely eliminate these risks or the risks of other adverse reactions. Other possible reactions may include allergic reactions, fever, chills, and rarely, haemolytic reactions, which may cause kidney damage.
>
> 4. In some cases, my own blood (autologous) may be used for transfusion. I have been made aware that there are risks even with donating or receiving my own blood and I have discussed this with my doctor. I have been told that even if my own blood is used, it may sometimes be necessary to give me additional blood or blood products donated by others.
>
> 5. My doctor and I have discussed the possibility of using treatment other than a blood transfusion. I understand the benefits and risks of these alternative treatments.
>
> 6. I also understand the risk(s) of not receiving a blood transfusion.
>
> 7. I have read the information on the back of this form, "Risks, Benefits and Alternatives for Blood Transfusion" and have had the opportunity to ask questions about my treatment. All my questions have been answered to my satisfaction.
>
>   ☐ **I DO consent to the transfusion of blood and/or blood products if it becomes necessary during the course of my treatment.**
>
>   ☐ **I DO NOT consent to the transfusion of blood and/or blood products if it becomes necessary during the course of my treatment.**
>
> _____
> Signature of Witness
>
> _____
> Signature of Patient or Substitute Decision Maker (SDM)
>
> _____
> Relationship – Substitute Decision Maker (SDM)
>
> _____
> Address – Substitute Decision Maker (SDM)
>
> _____
> Telephone Number – Substitute Decision Maker (SDM)
>
> **OR, Physician Statement:** I certify that, due to the urgent need for a transfusion, I am unable to obtain informed consent prior to therapy and that I have no advanced directive indicating that transfusion in reasonable circumstances is rejected.
>
> _____   _____
> Physician Signature   Date (d/m/y)
>
> _____
> Physician Name - Printed
>
> ORIGINAL (WHITE) – PATIENT'S HEALTH RECORD   YELLOW COPY – GIVEN TO PATIENT OR SDM
>
> FORM # 1630   New : 11.Dec.2002; Rev. 22 May 2003   Approved by: MAC November 12, 2002; Nursing Practice November 19, 2002

SOURCE: Reproduced by permission of Peterborough Regional Health Centre.

FIGURE **11.18**   **Pre-Anaesthetic Questionnaire**

Peterborough Regional Health Centre

PRE-ANAESTHETIC QUESTIONNAIRE

Hospital Drive Site   ☐
Rogers Street Site   ☐

Patient's Name:-_____
Operation to be performed:_____
Date of Surgery: _____
Surgeon's Name: _____

PLEASE COMPLETE BOTH SIDES

ALLERGIES YES...... NO...... NOT SURE......	SKIN RASH/HIVES	BREATHING DIFFICULTY	OTHER
MEDICATIONS- *PLEASE LIST* (E.G. PENICILLIN, SULPHA)			
LATEX (E.G. RUBBER GLOVES)			
FOOD (E.G. SHELLFISH, NUTS, BANANAS)			
ENVIRONMENTAL (E.G. POLLEN, GRASS, PETS)			

HAVE YOU OR A BLOOD RELATIVE EVER HAD A PROBLEM WITH GENERAL OR LOCAL ANAESTHESIA?
☐ YES   ☐ NO   IF YES, WHO? ☐ YOURSELF ☐ RELATIVE (SPECIFY RELATION)
REACTION: ☐ NAUSEA/VOMITING   ☐ TROUBLE WAKING UP   ☐ TROUBLE BREATHING ☐ FEVER _____
COMMENTS

HAVE YOU EVER HAD A BLOOD TRANSFUSION?   ☐ YES   ☐ NO   DATE (IF RECENT) _____

HAVE YOU DONATED YOUR OWN BLOOD FOR THIS PROCEDURE? (ie is autologous blood available)   ☐ YES   ☐ NO
DO YOU HAVE ANY CULTURAL OR SPIRITUAL BELIEFS AGAINST RECEIVING BLOOD PRODUCTS?   ☐ YES   ☐ NO
COMMENTS _____

ARE YOU PREGNANT?   ☐ N/A   ☐ YES   ☐ NO
LIST THE MEDICATIONS/INHALERS THAT YOU ARE NOW TAKING (including over-the-counter medications, e.g. Tylenol, laxatives, vitamins, antacids, herbal medications):

NAME OF MEDICATION	HOW MUCH DO YOU TAKE?	HOW OFTEN DO YOU TAKE IT?

QUESTION	YES	NO	
DO YOU SMOKE?			# OF CIGARETTES PER DAY..... # OF YEARS.........
DID YOU EVER SMOKE?			STOPPED WHEN?....................
DO OTHER PEOPLE SMOKE IN YOUR HOME?			
DO YOU DRINK ALCOHOL/BEER/WINE?			QUANTITY......................

FORM # 3504 - Oct. 1999

PLEASE COMPLETE BOTH SIDES OF THIS FORM

SOURCE: Reproduced by permission of Peterborough Regional Health Centre.

PLEASE CHECK (✓) "YES" OR "NO" TO THE FOLLOWING QUESTIONS

QUESTION	YES	NO	COMMENTS
HAVE YOU HAD A HEART ATTACK?			WHEN?
HAVE YOU HAD CHEST PAIN OR ANGINA?			HOW OFTEN?
HAVE YOU BEEN TOLD THAT YOU HAVE A HEART MURMUR?			
HAVE YOU BEEN TOLD THAT YOU HAVE HIGH BLOOD PRESSURE?			
DO YOU HAVE A PACEMAKER?			
HAVE YOU EVER HAD HEART FAILURE?			WHEN?
HAVE YOU EVER HAD OR BEEN TREATED FOR TUBERCULOSIS?			
HAVE YOU EVER BEEN TREATED FOR BREATHING DIFFICULTIES? (i.e. asthma)			

HAVE YOU EVER EXPERIENCED OR BEEN TREATED FOR ANY OF THE FOLLOWING?

PROBLEM	YES	NO	COMMENTS
SEIZURES OR CONVULSIONS			
STROKE/TIA'S			
DO YOU HAVE DIFFICULTY WITH SEVERE HEARTBURN OR SWALLOWING?			
DIZZINESS, BLACKOUTS			
HEAD INJURY			
THYROID PROBLEMS			
KIDNEY PROBLEMS			
HEPATITIS			TYPE? ❏ A ❏ B ❏ OTHER.............
HIV/AIDS			
BREATHING PROBLEMS/BRUISING			
CANCER			WHERE?
DIABETES			
EMOTIONAL DISTRESS (E.G. STRESS, DEATH IN FAMILY, DEPRESSION, TROUBLE COPING, OTHER)			
OTHER			

HAVE YOU EVER BEEN TREATED OR HOSPITALIZED FOR ANY MAJOR ILLNESS OR HAD SURGERY IN THE PAST? ❏ YES   ❏ NO
IF SO, WHEN, WHERE, WHAT?

1. _____
2. _____
3. _____
4. _____

Form #3504 - Reverse

FIGURE **11.18   Pre-Anaesthetic Questionnaire, cont'd**

FIGURE **11.19**   **Anaesthetic Record**

ANAESTHETIC RECORD
PRE ANAESTHETIC EVALUATION   Peterborough Regional Health Centre

PRE MEDICATION

PROCEDURE

SIGNED CONSENT ☐

HISTORY	PHYSICAL	LAB
— GENERAL	— GENERAL	— HGB — URINE
— CVS	— CVS	— OTHER
— RESPIRATORY	— RESPIRATORY	
— CNS	— AIRWAY ASSESSMENT	ECG
— RENAL/HEPATIC	— CNS	X-RAY
— ALLERGIES	— DENTITION	
— ANAESTHETIC HX	— OTHER	MEDICATIONS
— FAMILY Hx	— WEIGHT	

POTENTIAL PROBLEMS AND COMMENTS	BLOOD CXT
	NPO from:
	FLUIDS
	SOLIDS

| ASA CLASS | 1 | 2 | 3 | 4 | 5 | E | EVALUATING PHYSICIAN   DATE |

IMMEDIATE POST-OP ANAESTHETIC EVALUATION

COMMENTS

POST-OPERATIVE CONDITION

SIGNATURE OF ATTENDING ANAESTHETIST

3505
Medical Staff
Jan 85

Page 2

NAME:	SURGEON (PRINT)	ANAESTHETIC RECORD
		DATE
PROCEDURE:	ANAESTHETIST (PRINT)	ANAESTHETIC TIME

TIME

| O2 | L/MIN |
| N₂O | L/MIN |

FIO₂

VOLATILE   AGENTS   %

SYMBOLS

BP

PULSE

START ANAES

START OPER'N

END ANAES.

RESP

220 200 180 160 140 120 100 90 80 70 60 50 40 30 20 10

CVP
TEMP
URINE

IV AGENTS AND FLUIDS

IV GAUGE		MONITORS			GENERAL ANAESTHESIA		REGIONAL
SITE		STETH	OES □ PRECORD □		TECHNIQUE		TYPE
		BP	CUFF □ ART LINE □		AIRWAY □	MASK □	
FLUIDS		SITE	#		TUBE & TYPE	SIZE	LOCATION
IN—		PULSE □	ECG □		ORAL □	NASAL R□ L□	
		CVP □	TEMP □		CUFF □	PACK □	AGENT
		LOW PRESS □	O2 □		POSITION CHECK □		
		OTHER			SYSTEM		DOSE
TOTAL					CO-AXIAL □	T PIECE □	
OUT—BLOOD—SUCTION		PRE-ANAESTHETIC CHECK LIST □			CIRCLE □		REMARKS
—SPONGES					OTHER		
—DRAPES		POSITION			VENTILATION		
—TOTAL					SPONT □	ASSIST □	
—URINE		PROTECTION:	EYES □		CONTROL □	VENTILATOR □	
—OTHER		ELBOWS □	OTHER □		VT	RATE	

FIGURE **11.19**   Anaesthetic Record, cont'd

FIGURE **11.20** **Surgical Checklist**

SURGICAL CHECKLIST		

PRE-OPERATIVE VITAL SIGNS		TIME: _____ HRS.		NSG. UNIT	O.R.
T:	P:	R:	ID Band On		
B/P:		WT: _____ Kg	Surgical Permit Signed		
ALLERGIES	NSG. UNIT	O.R.	History & Physical		
			Pre-Anaesthetic Questionnaire		
			Consultation		
Rubber / Latex			Anaesthetic & Order Sheet		
Bananas / Chestnuts			Operative Area Prepared		
Corn			Pre-op Enema (if ordered)		
Type of Reaction			Fasting as Ordered		
Medic Alert			Blood Work Done		
			Urinalysis		
			Results Known		
PRE-OPERATIVE MEDICATIONS	TIME	DATE	Voided or Catheterization		
Antibiotics			Jewellery Removed & Secured		
			Hair Pieces, Hair Pins, Make-up Nail Polish Removed		
			Contacts/Glasses Removed		
			Hearing Aid		
Other			Dentures Removed		
			Name Plate		
			Sacrament of the Sick		
			ECG Done		
			X-Ray Done - Location		
Patient on Low Molecular Weight Heparin? YES ☐ NO ☐			Nursing History		
			Old Charts		
			Operative Sites Verified		
			Surgeon		
DATE:			Family Waiting YES ☐ NO ☐		
NURSING UNIT NURSE:			Contact at:		
O.R. NURSE:					
			Patient has ride home:		

FORM # 1681 Revised November 23, 1999

FIGURE **11.21**   **Nurse's Operative Record**

Erik Shultz
17 Bond Street
Ottawa, Ontario   May 26, 20___
7819749313

NURSE'S OPERATIVE RECORD   ☐ SJH & HC
                                ☐ PCH

Date_____ Theatre_____ Room Ready_____

Patient Entry_____

Anaesthetic Start_____ Total_____

Anaesthetic Stop_____

Surgeon Start_____

Surgeon Stop_____ Total_____

Patient Left_____ Overall Total_____

Wound Classification: ☐ Clean   ☐ Contaminated   ☐ Clean/Contaminated   ☐ Dirty
☐ Session   ☐ Non-Session   ☐ Elective   ☐ Non-Elective

Operation: _____

Surgeon: Dr. _____ Assistants: Dr. _____ Dr. _____

Anaesthetist: Dr. _____ Anaesthetic: ☐ General ☐ Local ☐ Neuro ☐ Spinal ☐ Epidural
☐ Other ☐ Bear Hugger ☐ Fluid Warmer   S.N. _____

Circ. Nurse 1. _____ R.N.   2. _____ R.N.   ESU Pad Position

Scrub Nurse 1. _____   2. _____   ESU S/N _____   Skin Condition Post-Op _____

Relief Circ. Nurse 1. _____ R.N.   2. _____ R.N.   Relief Scrub Nurse 1. _____   2. _____

POSITION: LITHOTOMY   SUPINE   PRONE   KIDNEY   JACKNIFE   REV. TREND   TREND   RT./LT. SIDE

Counts	Nil	Correct	Incorrect	If incorrect see action taken below
Sponge				
Instruments				
Needle				

In _____ R.N.   In _____

Out _____ R.N.   Out _____
Circ. Nurse Signature(s)   Scrub Nurse Signature(s)

Pathology _____ Cytology _____ Culture _____

TOURNIQUET TIME   S.N.

Location	Pressure	Up	Down	Location	Pressure	Up	Down
R. Arm				R. Leg			
L. Arm				L. Leg			

PROTECTION DEVICES

		Padding: Elbow	L ☐ R ☐
Safety Strap	☐	Hand/Wrist	L ☐ R ☐
Induction Only	☐	Knee	L ☐ R ☐
Wrist Ties	L ☐ R ☐	Heel	L ☐ R ☐
Skids: Wrist	L ☐ R ☐	Other	L ☐ R ☐
Elbow	L ☐ R ☐		☐
Bolsters	☐		
Donut	☐	Armboard	L ☐ R ☐
Head rest	☐	Stirrups	L ☐ R ☐
Kidney rest	☐	Sandbags _____	
Other	☐	Pillows _____	

CODES

PRIORITY CODE	DELAY	COMPLICATION	CANCELLATION

Penrose	Catheter	Other	Packing	Hyster. Drain	Hemovac

REMARKS

GRASP_____   _____ R.N.
                         Circulating Nurse Signature

PATIENT TO PACU _____   I.C.U. _____   DISCHARGE PACU _____   FLOOR _____
1566JF 11/93   Time   Time   Time

FIGURE **11.22**   **Post-anaesthetic Record (PACU)**

Erik Shultz
17 Bond Street
Ottawa, Ontario   May 26, 20___
7819749313

POST-ANAESTHETIC RECORD   DATE: _____

PROCEDURE:	POST-ANAESTHETIC RECORD SCORE		ADM.	15 min.	30 min.	D/C
	RESPIR-ATIONS:	BREATHING DEEPLY) ADEQUATE COUGH) 2 AIRWAY REQ.ATTENT- 1 APNEA - 0				
ADMISSION TIME: _____	MOVE-MENTS:	PURPOSEFUL - 2 SOME PURPOSEFUL - 1 ATHETOID - NONE - 0				
AIRWAY NIL ORAL NASAL E.N.T. AIRWAY REMOVED @ ANAESTHETIC_____ **OXYGEN** NIL MASK CATHETER T-PIECE AEROSOL RESPIRATOR	COLOUR:	NORMAL - 2 PALE, DUSKY - 1 CYANOTIC - 0				
POSITION ON ARRIVAL _____ _____ DRAINS _____	CONSCIOUS-NESS:	FULLY AWARE - 2 AROUSABLE ON CALL) DROWSY) 1 NOT RESPONDING - 0				
PACKING _____ CATHETER _____	CIRCU-LATION:	B/P P- $\pm$ 10 of PRE-OP-2 B/P P- $\pm$ 20 of PRE-OP-1 B/P P- $\pm$ 30 of PRE-OP-0				
DRESSING DRAINAGE_____ NAUSEA AND/OR VOMITING	PRE-OP B/P _____ P._____	CODE FOR D/C POOR 6 GOOD 8-10 FAIR 6 - 8				
_____ MONITOR _____ BLOOD WORK_____ & RESULTS _____ X-RAY _____ OUTPUT: URINE _____ OTHER _____	COMMENTS:					

I.V. THERAPY				M 15 30 45 15 30 45 15 30 45 15 30 45
I.V. SOLUTION	ABS. IN OR	ABS. IN RR	TOTAL	240 220 200 180 160 140 120 100 80 60 40 20 0
3.3% D.-0.3% SAL.				
5% GL/.2% SAL.				
Ringers Lact.				
5% D/Plas. 56				
Normal saline				
_____				
_____				

Resp.
Temp.

  MEDICATIONS

TIME	DRUG	ROUTE	REASON GIVEN & EFFECT	SIGNATURE

DISCHARGE TIME: _____   CONDITION   GOOD   FAIR   POOR

SIGNATURE _____R.N.

Revised 6/86

Form #142

REPORT GIVEN TO _____R.N.

TIME	FEET TEMP. COLOUR	DSG.	C.V.P.	PEDAL R.	L.	POST TIB. R.	L.	HAND GRIPS R.	L.	MEASUREMENTS PUPIL R.	L.			URINE	BLOOD PARAMETERS	TIME	RESULT
															Hgb.		
															Hct.		
															Cl.		
															Na.		
															K.		
															B.U.N.		
															P.H.		
															CO2con		
															PCO2		
															H2CO3		
															HCO3		
															PO2		
															H-HRat		
															B.Exc.		
															% Sat.		

```
CODE   D. & I.   –   Dry & Intact        R.B.   –   React Briskly
       C.O.      –   Cold                R.S.   –   React Slowly
       C.        –   Cool                F.     –   Fixed
       M.        –   Mottled
```

NURSE'S COMMENTS

FIGURE 11.22   Post-anaesthetic Record (PACU), cont'd

FIGURE **11.23**   **PACU Record**

PETERBOROUGH REGIONAL HEALTH CENTRE

PACU RECORD

Page 1 (A)

I.V. SOLUTIONS	ABS. IN O.R.	ABS. IN PACU	TOTAL	TBA ON TRANSFER

TIME	MEDICATION	Route	REASON GIVEN	EFFECT/VAS	Signature or Initials

Form # 0505039//Apr.99/Form # 1582//Disk 1b - Reprinted January 2001

SOURCE: Reproduced by permission of Peterborough Regional Health Centre.

NURSES' NOTES: **PAGE 2 A**

Discharge Time:

Dressing Drainage on Transfer:

Must have score   = 8   (D/C = Discharge)
Resp. score must be   = 2
☐ Does Not Meet Criteria   ☐ Physician's Order

NIL_____ Type	Discharged by Signature:	R.N.
Codes for Discharge	Transferred by Signature/Initials	RN/SNG
GOOD 8 - 10 FAIR 6 - 7 POOR Below 6	Report Given To:	RN/RPN/NS6

FIGURE **11.23**   PACU Record, cont'd   *continued*

PACU RECORD   PAGE 2B

Time	NIPB	IBP	Pulse	Resp	SA0^2	CVP	PAP	Urine	Temp	Initial	PEDAL		POST TIB		TEMP FEET COLOUR
											Left	Right	Left	Right	

PAP - Pulmonary Artery Pressure

NIBP - Non-Invasive BP

IBP - Invasive BP

Temperature:
C - Cool
Wa - Warm

Pulses: P - Palpable
D - Doppler

Colour: G - Good
Cy - Cyanosed
W - White
M - Mottled

BLOOD PARAMETERS

	RESULT	TIME	TIME		RESULT	TIME	TIME
NA				Hb			
K				Hct			
CL				WBC			
Glucose				Platelets			
Urea				APTT			
Creat				I.N.R.			
CPK							
PH							
PCO^2							
PO^2				Reported			
HCO^2							
Base				Xray			

NURSE'S SIGNATURE	INITIAL

FIGURE **11.23**   **PACU Record, cont'd**

Date:_____ (m/d/y) Time of Arrival:_____

ANAESTHETIC:
General ▢   Epidural ▢   Spinal ▢   Regional ▢
Neuro ▢   I.V. Block ▢   Local ▢

AIRWAY:
Nil ▢   Oral ▢ ETT ▢ Nasal ▢ Laryngeal Mask ▢
Time of Removal:_____ Initials:_____

Conscious Time:_____
Report from Anaesthetist: Yes ▢   No ▢
Receiving Registered Nurse: Initials:_____
Position on Arrival:_____

OXYGEN:
Nil ▢   Nasal Prongs ▢   Mask ▢ · Croupette ▢
Isolette▢   Aerosol ▢ Tandem ▢ T. Piece▢ Vent ▢

TIME:
On:_____ Off:_____ Continuous ▢ Initials:_____

VENTILATOR:
Mode: Mode_____ Tidal Volume_____Peep_____
    FIO2_____ Rate_____

RESPIRATIONS		ADM	15	30	45	D/C
Coughs freely or deep breathes or crying or breathes easily	2					
Ventilator	1A					
Obstructed, snoring, dyspneic or limited breathing	1					
Apnea, total or periodic obstruction requiring maintenance	0					

MOVEMENT		ADM	15	30	45	D/C
Moves 4 extremeties volunatrily or on command	2					
Moves 2 extremeties voluntarily or on command	1					
Unable to move any extremeties, OR head, voluntarily or on command	0					

COLOUR		ADM	15	30	45	D/C
Pink, maintains SAO₂ .92% on room air OR colour comparable to pre-op status	2					
Pale, dusky, blotchy & needs 0₂ to maintain SAO₂ > 92%	1					
Cyanotic, SAO₂ < 92%	0					

CONSCIOUSNESS		ADM	15	30	45	D/C
Fully awake OR comparable to pre-op status	2					
Rouses to stimuli or calling	1					
Unresponsive	0					

CIRCULATION		ADM	15	30	45	D/C
BP(OR)pulse +/- 20% pre-anaesthestic level	2					
BP OR pulse +/- 20%-49% pre-anaesthetic level	1					
BP OR pulse< 50% OR > 50% of pre-anaesthetic level	0					
TOTAL						
INITIALS						

DRESSING:
No Dressing ▢ Dry ▢ Drainage:_____

DRAINS Hemovac ▢   Jackson Pratt ▢   Penrose ▢
    Chest Tube ▢ Urinary Catheter ▢ Naso Gastric Tube ▢
Packing   ▢ _____ Other_____

OUTPUT	O.R.	P.A.C.U.	TOTAL
URINE			
OTHER			
EMESIS			

MONITORING:
NIBP ▢   Oximeter ▢   Arterial Line ▢   Swan Ganz ▢
C.V.P. ▢   Temp ▢   ECG ▢
Epidural ▢   P.C.A. ▢
PRE-OP BP _____   PULSE_____
BP Codes: V Systolic   ∧ Diastolic   • Pulse

SIGNATURE	STATUS	INITIALS

FIGURE **11.23** PACU Record, cont'd

FIGURE **11.24** **History and Physical**

HISTORY & PHYSICAL

NAME: Peters, Timothy   **MR#:**

DOB: **HC#:**

DATE OF ADMISSION: **ROOM #:**

DICTATING PHYSICIAN: **COPIES TO:**

HISTORY

CHIEF COMPLAINT:

Acute onset, severe chest pain, and indigestion.

PRESENT ILLNESS:

This patient has had several bouts of prolonged heaviness and pressure across his chest, which were eventually relieved by nitroglycerin. He has also complained of increasing shortness of breath and sputum production with no fevers, chills, or pleuritic chest pain. He is also complaining of decreased urine output and bilateral low back diffuse pain. His energy seems to be stable. He has had no syncopal episodes, nausea, or vomiting. He has had no burning, frequency, or urgency. His bowels seem to be working all right.

PAST HISTORY:

He has had osteomyelitis of the right leg. Appendectomy. He had a lymph node removed from his right groin in his early 30s, which was possibly thought to be Hodgkin's and he received radiotherapy for this.

PHYSICAL

GENERAL:

The patient is an alert, co-operative male, clutching at the chest at times during the interview. He says that this is still uncomfortable. Pulse: 93 and irregular. Temperature 98.6.

HEENT:

React to L & A, no AV nicking. Ears are normal. Pharynx is normal. No thyroid enlargement or bruit noted.

CHEST:

Barrel-shaped with a decreased air entry, but no crackles or wheezes appreciated. Normal S1 S2 with faint heart sounds.

ABDOMEN:

Soft with no hepatosplenomegaly or tenderness.

RECTAL:

Deferred

ANALYSIS AND PLAN:

It would appear that this man is having bouts of prolonged angina. He may have an acute exacerbation of his C.O.P.D. and he may have anuria secondary to his renal failure. He will be admitted to hospital, some basic tests will be done, and he will be observed over the next two to three days. If all is well, he will be sent back home to his apartment.

S. Lawren, MD., FRCPC

/emc

D:
T:

physician will then proceed with a physical examination, and subsequently prepare a report on his or her findings. The information contained is generally documented in a specific order as follows:

Sociological Information—The patient's name, address, date of birth, and so on are recorded. If the patient is seen in the hospital, information such as date of admission, hospital records number, and room number is required.

Chief Complaint—This refers to the reason the patient has engaged the physician.

Present Illness—The patient is asked to give a detailed outline of the chief complaint, for example, when the discomfort first began and the severity of the discomfort. If the patient has been referred by another physician, the patient may be asked for details of previous tests and treatments. (The Present Illness section is sometimes referred to as History of Present Illness or History of Chief Complaint.)

Past History—The patient is asked about such things as previous surgery, illnesses, and diseases. This section may be broken down into specific areas with appropriate subheadings such as Surgeries and Diseases.

Family History—This section comprises documentation of the medical history of the patient's parents, brothers and sisters, grandparents, and so on. Other details such as age and cause of death of any of the individuals mentioned previously may be significant.

Personal History—This includes such things as hobbies, alcohol or drug use or abuse, use of tobacco, socio-economic and marital status, and type of employment. (This section may be included with Past History and entitled Past and Personal History.)

After the above details are recorded, the physician will undertake the physical examination. This section of the report may be entitled Physical Examination, or it may be referred to as a Systemic Review, Functional Inquiry, or Inventory of Systems.

The examination usually begins with the head area, and contains the following subheadings:

Skin—An examination of the appearance of the skin including rashes, discolouration, and so on.

Hair—Including thickness and texture.

HEENT—Pertains to the head, eyes, ears, nose, and throat and includes such things as use of glasses, blurred vision, loss of hearing, dizziness, pain, discharges, ability to smell, colds, condition of teeth, taste, dentures, gums, swallowing, neck movement, and so on.

Cardiorespiratory (CR)—Refers to the patient's heart and respiratory system.

Gastrointestinal (GI)—This is an examination of the digestive system and may include questions about appetite, indigestion, change in weight, and diet or bowel habits.

Genitourinary (GU)—Refers to the urinary organs and genitals and may include urgency, frequency, sexually transmitted infection, incontinence, hesitancy, and pain.

Neuropsychiatric (NP)—Refers to headaches, pains, paralysis, emotional state, convulsions, and so on.

Musculoskeletal (MS)—Discusses such things as pain, stiffness, movement ability, and fractures.

The physician does not necessarily cover all of the previous details. If the patient's history or any other aspect of the examination has been covered previously, the report will state, for example, "Past Illness: as outlined on previous charts." A physician's personal preference of terms will also determine the subheading titles; for example, "Gastrointestinal" may be broken down into "Abdominal" and "Rectal."

If the examination of a system does not reveal any problems, the physician may record "unremarkable" or "nothing of note" beside the subheading. If an examination of a system is not performed, the record may state "deferred" or "not done."

Usually, the report will conclude with a diagnosis of the complaint or the dictating physician's recommendations, and plan, or both, for the patient. The subheading may be "Impression," "Admission Diagnosis," "Clinical Impression," or perhaps "Analysis and Plan."

In most hospital settings, the dictated notes are transcribed internally by the Health Records Stenography (transcription) Department. Once completed, the reports will print out in the unit where the patient is admitted. A copy will be sent to the dictating physician and copies will be distributed to identified providers. All hospital reports require more than one copy.

The format for these reports will vary depending on which software the facility is using. The basic information, however, is as follows:

- Patient's name
- Medical record number
- Patient's date of birth
- Patient's Health Card number
- Patient location (i.e., room number, Medical Out-Patient, Surgical Out-Patient, Emergency)
- Admission date or date of visit
- Dictating physician
- Where copies are to be sent
- Date of dictation
- Date of transcription
- Transcriptionist's initials

The format for an Operative Record (see Figure 11.25) and a Delivery Record (See Figure 11.26) is different than that for the other hospital notes. A

FIGURE **11.25**   **Operative Record**

OPERATIVE RECORD

Patient: Smith, Heather

Date:
Room: Ward 457C
DOB:

PREOPERATIVE DIAGNOSIS:

Epigastric pain with
Egurgitation and heartburn

POST-OPERATIVE DIAGNOSIS:

Eesophagitis, 1 to 2+, patulous
oesophagogastric junction

OPERATION:

Oesophagogastroduodenoscopy

PROCEDURE:

The patient was sedated before coming to the operating room and this was further supplemented with demerol 80 mg and valium 10 mg I.V.
The throat was sprayed with Xylocaine. Satisfactory sedation was obtained. An 18 Levin tube was inserted into the stomach and 10 cc of
mucus with brownish curds was aspirated. The scope was introduced without difficulty down to the lower end of the esophagus. At the
esophagogastric junction there was some superficial erosion. Some reddening came up into the esophagus, particularly in the lower half.
No fissures or superficial ulceration above the esophagogastric junction. The antrum and body of the stomach appeared normal. I was able
to get into the duodenum with ease and into the second part of the duodenum; it was difficult to get good visualization. There was a rather
sharp turn between the first and second parts of the duodenum. I did not see any abnormality and in the duodenal cap it looked quite
normal. The scope was withdrawn and a U-turn was done in the body of the stomach. The fundus, esophagogastric area, and lesser
curvature were quite normal.   he scope was withdrawn and the patient was taken to the recovery room in good condition.

On talking to the patient, I understand she has been on Tagamet for about three years. She is having rather persistent difficulty. I'll have to find
out when she had her last cholecystogram or ultrasound of the gallbladder. If the symptoms continue, I think the patient would benefit from
an antireflux procedure.

Surgeon: Dr. W.B. Bell

Assistant: Dr. J.E. Plunkett

Anaesthetist: Dr. E.J. Pelham

Date: 08 12 __

_____
W.B. Bell, M.D.

/lbp
cc: J.E. Plunkett, M.D.
    E.J. Pelham, M.D.

D: 10 12 __
T: 11 12 __

FIGURE **11.26**   **Delivery Report**

DELIVERY REPORT

Name: Davis, Hazel   **No.:**   8765233
Address: **Date:**
                                                                   Doctor: R. Smock, M.D.
Date of Birth: **Ward No:**   557

1500:   Patient admitted to labour ward section with severe contractions q.10 minutes and slight red bloody show. Patient is a gravida 2, eight days past term. Head not engaged on admission.

1550:   Seconal 100 mg.

1800:   Continuous epidural established by doctor. Cervix 8 cm but presenting part still spines minus 2.

2035:   Membranes ruptured spontaneously. Some meconium staining but fetal monitor good. Head still above ischial spines.

2335:   Fully dilated.

0120:   Difficult mid forceps rotation from R.O.P. to L.O.A., L.M.L. episiotomy with left vaginal vault tear. A female child approximate weight 7 pounds, Apgar 8/9. Stiff traction for delivery.

0124:   Placenta removed manually. Cervix inspected and intact. Left sulcus tear repaired with continuous interlocking oo plain catgut and routine episiotomy repair.

Estimated blood loss 200 cc.

_____
R. Smock, M.D.

/lbp
cc: J.E. Plunkett

Delivery Record is produced with dates and times in chronological order each time the patient is examined. Each date and time appears as a heading at the left margin.

In a hospital environment, all investigations must be documented.

The physician will then fill out a Physician's Order Form (see Figure 11.7). This form outlines the medications (dosage and times to administer), tests to be done, appropriate diet, physical activity, and general instructions for the patient's initial admission.

The MRP will update the physician's orders as needed during the patient's hospital stay. At times, a consultant may be requested to see the patient. The consultant's orders will be added to the physician's order sheet. The consultant will also dictate a note with regards to his or her findings on this patient.

Many locations in Canada have a shortage of family physicians and many family physicians have given up their admitting privileges, which leaves patients without a primary healthcare provider. Some hospitals have physicians called "hospitalists" who care for patients who require hospitalization but do not have a physician able to look after them while they are in hospital for a medical admission. Patients admitted for surgery have the surgeon as the MRP. The hospitalists care for the patient while in hospital and, in some areas, also provide short-term support when the patient is discharged.

WARD SECRETARY/UNIT CLERK

In the hospital setting, the medical administrative assistant is referred to as a ward secretary or unit clerk. As in a physician's office, a large amount of time is spent working with patient charts.

11.1   Ward Secretary/Unit Clerk Responsibilities

Processing physician orders
Assembling/disassembling charts
Reception
Liaison with patients, families, and hospital departments
Ordering supplies
Maintaining confidentiality
Working as part of a multidisciplinary team

This can be a very fast-paced and ever-changing environment. The same skills that were discussed in Chapter 1 also apply to this position. The responsibilities of the ward secretary differ from those of a position in a physician's office. The ward secretary does not do health card or third-party insurance billing, perform medical transcription, or have much phone contact with patients. The many phone calls that are received are usually internal calls, physicians, or occasionally, a patient's family. The position requires awareness of appropriate communication throughout the hospital, for example, when to use overhead paging as opposed to pagers or direct phone extensions. Requisitions, etc., can be faxed to other departments, delivered through a portering service or entered into the computer if the facility has order entry.

Hospitals also have codes for emergency response and an extension to call to expedite awareness throughout the facility. See the Box 11.2 for a list of common codes.

11.2 For All Codes Dial 3333	
CODE BLUE	Cardiac arrest
CODE RED	Fire
CODE GREEN	Evacuation
CODE ORANGE	External disaster
CODE YELLOW	Missing patient
CODE WHITE	Violent patient
CODE BLACK	Bomb threat
CODE BROWN	Internal chemical spill
CODE PINK	Pediatric cardiac arrest

Many hospitals have specialty clinics such as a diabetic clinic, foot clinic, cast clinic, blood pressure clinic, pulmonary function clinic, etc. Even though these clinics are in a hospital setting, the clinic secretary's responsibilities can mirror those of a medical administrative assistant in a physician's office. The responsibilities could include scheduling appointments, maintaining charts, contacting patients, ordering supplies, and possibly transcription and health card billing.

In the Admissions/Registration department, clerks are responsible for entering patient data for *all* in-patient visits as well as *all* out-patient visits. This information is entered into the hospital database. As some hospitals are linked to other facilities, it is extremely important that this information is accurate and up to date. Departments and physicians depend on this information to access patients and patient records. Hospital billing to the provincial health insurances is also generated from this patient information.

As mentioned earlier, a sound knowledge of terminology and anatomy is needed for any of these positions. In the admission/registration position, the use of abbreviations is not permitted.

PROCESSING PHYSICIAN'S ORDERS

The physician's orders must be processed as soon as possible after a patient is admitted (see Figure 11.27). The orders are transferred to the appropriate requisitions line by line. Ward secretaries generally have the responsibility for transferring information from the physician's orders. The ward secretary should check for any **Stat** (urgent) orders and process them first. She will then assess the Stat order and notify the appropriate personnel or department (e.g., the nurse, lab, or diagnostic imaging department). When an order is completed, the ward secretary should date and initial beside the line. Short forms are used to identify what has been done, as exemplified in Box 11.3.

FIGURE **11.27** **Physician's Orders Form**

		PHYSICIAN'S ORDERS
Erik Shultz		START NEW SECTION FOR EACH NEW ORDER. MORE THAN ONE SECTION MAY BE USED FOR A LONG ORDER. DO NOT USE SECTION IF COPY IS MISSING.
17 Bond Street		
Ottawa, Ontario May 26, 20___		
7819749313		

D.M. Obese   ALLERGIES:

DATE/TIME	ORDERS	1	EXECUTED
	1) CBC c̄ ESR		
	2) Weigh please		
	3) Dietician to see		
	4) 1200 cal. D.D. NAS		
	5) Urine bid ac c̄ hs for sugar		
	6) Daily FBS		
	7) 2 hour ac lunch BS		
	8) Tylenol #2 tabs i q8h prn.		
	9) Halcion 0.25 mgs. hs. prn.		
	10) BRP		
	11) LES prn		
	12) CXR		
	13) ECG		
	14) BUN		
	15) Lytes		
	16) Proteins		

PHYSICIAN'S ORDERS   WRITE FIRMLY!

11.3

SMO = Slip Made Out
MS = Copied to Medication Sheet (MAR)
K = Copied to Kardex

In a computerized order-entry environment, a short form may be order entered (OE) to identify "order has been entered and directed to the appropriate department."

As the nursing units are extremely busy, it is unreasonable to expect the ward secretary to process *all* of the orders. The Registered Nurses, and Registered Practical Nurses, or both, will often share this task. It is good practice to have the charge RN check the orders to ensure that they are completed correctly. If some orders are unclear or illegible, it may be necessary to clarify them with the ordering physician.

As shown in Figures 11.11, 11.12 and 11.13, medication orders are identified by three divisions. These divisions are explained in Box 11.4.

11.4

ROUTINE medications: Must be taken at a specific time, either daily or on a regular basis (i.e., every other day or once a week).
PRN medications: Must be administered as needed. The frequency will be identified so the patient does not receive too much (e.g., Tylenol No. 2 tabs 1 q8h prn).
STAT medications: Must be administered immediately. These medications are ordered by the physician to get results in the patient's condition as soon as possible. These medications are usually single-dose medications, meaning they are only given one time.

It is imperative that an accurate record of all medication orders be kept for each patient.

The following is an example of a physician's order for Erik Shultz. Mr. Shultz has been admitted to the hospital by Dr. Plunkett after complaining of severe thirst, headaches, and dizziness. The provisional diagnosis is diabetes mellitus/obesity as indicated at the top of the order sheet. Steps 1-16 will explain the process line by line. Examples of the appropriate requisitions will follow.

1. CBC and ESR mean that a complete blood count and sedimentation rate are required. On the Blood Testing Requisition (Hematology and Biochemistry combined) (see Figure 11.28) or a separate Biochemistry Form, the boxes beside "CBC" and "ESR" would be checked. The term *CBC* and the term *Hemogram* are interchangeable.

2. Weight please: the patient's weight would be recorded by the nurse on the Nursing History Chart (see Figure 11.29).

3. Dietician to see: the dietician would be telephoned, and an appointment time arranged. This would be noted on the Kardex.

4. 1200 Cal. DD, NAS means a diabetic diet of 1200 calories with no added salt. The information would be recorded on the Kardex under "Nutrition: diet" as well as on the Nursing History Chart (Figure 11.29). The nutrition department would also need to be notified to ensure the proper meals are prepared. This would also be noted on the Kardex.

5. Urine bid ac & hs for sugar: the ward nurse is required to check the patient's urine twice a day, before breakfast and at night, to determine if there is sugar in the urine. This would be done by using keto sticks, and recording the results of the tests on the Nursing History Chart under section reminders. The box beside urine S & A would also be checked.

6. Daily FBS means that a fasting blood sugar test is to be done daily. The request for this test would be recorded on the Biochemistry Form (Figure 11.28) by placing a check mark beside "glucose fasting."

7. Two hours ac lunch BS means a blood sugar to be done two hours before lunch, requiring another Blood Testing Requisition to be completed, but this time placing a check beside "glucose random." A separate requisition is completed as this test is to be done at a different time.

8. Tylenol No. 2 tabs 1 q8h prn gives permission to administer one Tylenol No. 2 tablet every 8 hours as needed. This would be charted on the Kardex as well as the PRN Medication Administration Record (Figure 11.30).

9. Halcion 0.25 mg hs prn gives permission to administer 0.25 mg of Halcion at night as needed (see Figure 11.30).

10. BRP means that the patient is allowed bathroom privileges and would be so recorded on the Nursing History Chart beside "BRP."

11. LES prn gives permission to administer, when necessary, a laxative, enema, or suppository (Figure 11.30). Laxatives and suppositories are treated as prn medications. The enema order would be recorded on the Nursing History Chart (Figure 11.29) under "Treatments."

12. CXR is a request for a routine chest X-ray. This would include a PA (posterior/anterior) and lateral view. The information would be recorded on the Diagnostic Imaging Requisition (see Figure 11.31).

13. ECG means that an electrocardiogram is to be taken and the appropriate requisition (see Figure 11.32) would be completed.

14. BUN stands for blood, urea, and nitrogen, and a check mark would be placed beside "urea" on the Biochemistry Form (Figure 11.28) to order the test.

15. Lytes means a testing of sodium, potassium, and chloride is requested. This test would also be ordered on the Blood Testing or Biochemistry

Text continued on p. 268.

FIGURE **11.28** **Biochemistry Form**

PETERBOROUGH REGIONAL HEALTH CENTRE
LABORATORY MEDICINE - /BLOOD TESTING REQUISITION

□ PCH □ SJHC □ Haliburton □ Minden □ Other________ **□ Emergent**
□ In-patient □ Out-patient □ Referred-In
Collection Date:m\d\yr______________Time:________ **□ Urgent**
O.R. Date:______________________Time:________
Relevant Clinical Information/Special Instructions: **☑ Routine**
____
Ordering Physician:. DR. J. PLUNKETT **□ Timed ____**
Nurse:________________________________

✓	HAEMATOLOGY
✓	CBC 2000
	DIFF 2010
	CELL MORPH. 2030
	RETIC 2040
	MONO SCREEN 2060
✓	ESR 2050
✓	**COAGULATION**
	INR 2500
	A.P.T.T. 2510
	BLEEDING TIME 2520
	D-DIMER 2540
	FIBRINOGEN SCREEN 2560

✓	CHEMISTRY
	CBG 3503
✓	(NaKCl) LYTS 3052
✓	GLUCOSE FASTING 3003
	GLUCOSE RANDOM 3010
	GLUCOSE AC 3003
	GLUCOSE PC 3014
	CREATININE 3030
	TOTAL BILIRUBIN 3220
	MICRO-BILIRUBIN 3120
	CALCIUM 3100
	PHOSPHATE 3200
	MAGNESIUM 3110
	URATE 3210
	TOTAL PROTEIN 3240
	ALBUMIN 3250
	AST 3160
	LDH 3170
	CK 3070
	CK-2 3080
	ALK 3180 PHOSPHATASE
	ACID 3260 PHOSPHATASE
	AMYLASE 3090

✓	CHEMISTRY
	GGTP 3190
	UREA 3020
	TSH 3600
	FREE T4 3610
	VITAMIN B12 3625
	RBC FOLATE 3630
	FERRITIN 3340
	IRON 3310
	TIBC 3320
	IRON 3315 SATURATION
	CORTISOL AM 9350
	CORTISOL PM 9355
	BLOOD GASES ART 3489
	BLOOD GASES CAP 3519
	BLOOD GASES VEN 3504
	CHOLESTEROL 3270
	TRIGLYCERIDES 3280
	HDL-C 3290
	LDL (CALC)
	HbA1C GLYCATED PROTIEN 3350
	SPE 3580
	IMMUNO- 3540 GLOBULINS
	C3 3545
	C4 3550

✓	SEROLOGY
	ANA 5200
	ANTI-DNA 5220
✓	**DRUGS / MISC**
	ACETAMINO-PHEN 3380
	BARBITURATE SCREEN 3390
	SALICYLATE 3470
	ETHANOL 3430
	DIGOXIN 3410
	PHENYTOIN 3420
	PHENOBARB 3460
	CARBA- 3400 MAZEPINE
	THEOPHYLLINE 3480
	GENTAMICIN PRE 3440
	GENTAMICIN POST 3445
	LITHIUM 3450
✓	**MISC**
	HAPTOGLOBIN 360

orm # JF 5046
uly/96

SOURCE: Reproduced by permission of Peterborough Regional Health Centre.

FIGURE **11.29** **Nursing History Chart**

NURSING HISTORY

ADMISSION: Date: _____ Time: _____ From: _____ How: _____ Age: _55___

Dr. Notified: YES NO _____ Admission Bld. Work Drawn: YES NO

DIAGNOSIS: _____ Pt's Expected Length of Stay _____

Pt's Own Words re Reason Admitted: _____

Other Health Problems: _____

Erik Shultz
17 Bond Street
Ottawa, Ontario   May 26, 20___
7819749313

MEDICATIONS: Taking At Home: _____   Taken Today: _____   Brought to Hospital: (list) _____

OBSERVATIONS: T_____ p.o./rectal P_____ reg/irreg R_____ easy/difficult B/P_____ Wt._____ Ht._____ Denture: Upper Lower

Prosthesis (explain) _____ Glasses _____ Hearing Aid _____ False Fingernails _____   Partial

_____ Contacts _____ Hospital I.D. Band _____ Ostomy: YES NO Selfcare/with help

General Appearance, Skin Condition & Physical Limitations: _____

Emotional & Mental Status: _____

Other Comments: _____

Allergies: _____ Bladder Habits: _____

Diet: _____ Bowel Habits: _____ Sleep Habits: _____

Valuables Record Understood & Signed by Pt. and/or Family? YES NO Has Pt. ever had a Blood Transfusion? YES NO

SOCIAL PROFILE: Marital Status: M S W D R   Religion: _____ Anointed: _____ Smoker - Nonsmoker: _____

Ethnic Origins: _____ Languages Spoken: _____ Previous Hospitalization: _____

Occupation (or retired from) _____ Employed/Unemployed: _____ _____

Hobbies & Normal Activities: _____

Social Problems: _____

Discharge Plans: _____

Significant Others: _____

Persons to Notify in Case of Emergency: (1) _____ Phone Number _____

(2) _____ Phone Number _____

Signature of Nurse_____

continued

OBSERVATION & SUPERVISION		AGE: 55 DATE OF ADMISSION		
☐ Isolation	☐ Urine S & A	Family Physician:		Erik Shultz
		Diagnosis:		17 Bond Street
☐ Vital Signs	☐ Weight			Ottawa, Ontario May 26, 20__
B/P	Due:	Surgery:		7819749313
TPR	☐ Measurements:			
☐ Pedal Pulses	☐ Head Injury Routine	Surgeon:		Other Health Problems:
R/L		Consultant(s):		
	☐ Other Supervision			
☐ CVP		Allergy:		Transfers:
Swan Ganz				
Art Lines			PC Level:	Revised:
Hygiene	Comfort/Activity	Nutrition	Elimination	Respiration
Bath	Up ad Lib.	Diet:	Self Care	☐ O$_2$
☐ Self	☐ Up in Chair		☐ Bathroom with Help	LPM
☐ Partial	☐ Walking			☐ Humidifier
☐ Complete	Devices	☐ Self	Urinal	
		☐ With Help	☐ Bedpan	☐ Cough & Deep Breath
☐ Tub/Shower	Total Bedrest	☐ Complete Feed	Commode	
	BRP	☐ Fluids	☐ Incontinence	☐ Trach Care
S M T W T F S	☐ Skin Care & Position		Condom	☐ Aerosol
		☐ Bottle Fdg/Baby Food	☐ Diapers	
☐ Oral Hygiene			☐ Catheter	☐ Suction
☐ Beard Shave	☐ Active/Passive Exercises	☐ Gavage (eg. Barron's)	☐ Change:	OTHER
				☐ Teach
☐ Hair Wash	Restraints Siderails			☐ Communication
S M T W T F S	☐ Traction, Stockings		☐ Ostomy	
	Bandage, Prosthesis	☐ Intake – Output		

FIGURE **11.29** **Nursing History Chart, cont'd**

		ERIK SHULTZ					INTRAVENOUS	I.V. TUBING	
Date	MEDICATIONS ☐		0700	1500	2300	Renew	☐ THERAPY	☐ CHANGE DATE:	

☐ REMINDERS   ☐ Diagnostic Workup

Date

Date	PRN MEDICATIONS	Renew

Other Disciplines   ☐ Treatments

PATIENT'S NAME: ROOM:

FIGURE **11.29** **Nursing History Chart, cont'd**

FIGURE **11.30**   **Medication Administration Record Sheet**

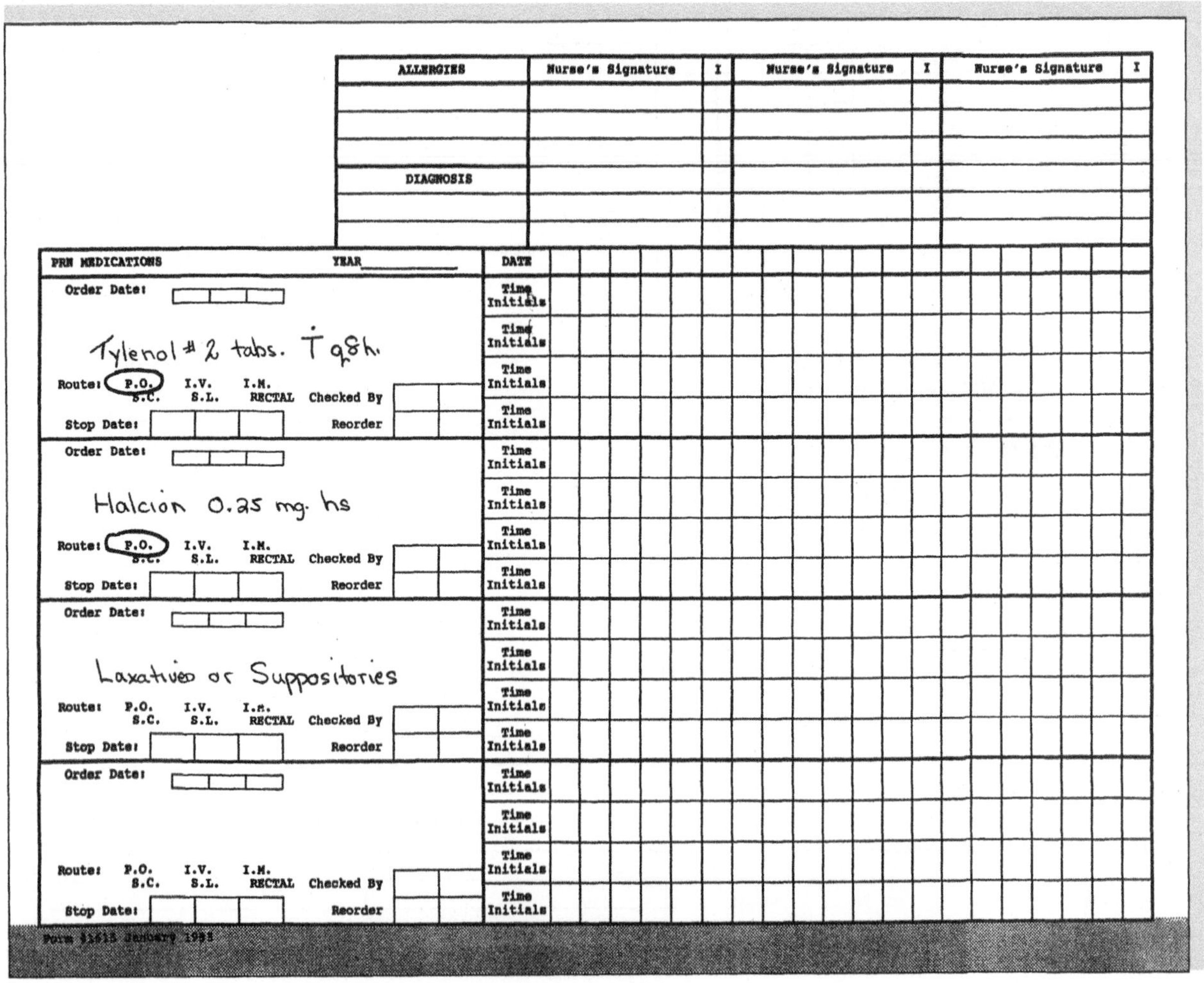

FIGURE **11.31** **Diagnostic Imaging Requisition**

Peterborough Regional Health Centre
Diagnostic Imaging Requisition

Patient Data (print or place imprint upper left corner)

Last Name ____________

First Name ____________

Address ____________

City ____________ Code ____________

Phone ____________ DOB [ ] d [ ] m [ ] y

HC no. [ ][ ][ ][ ] [ ][ ][ ] [ ][ ][ ] [ ][ ]

WCB/Adm. no. ____________

⇧ Place patient imprint in the above space only ⇧

Transportation (circle)

ambulatory — wheelchair (circled) — stretcher — ambulance

portable — isolation — I.V. — Oxygen CBI

Radiography ☑ Ultrasound ☐ Nuclear Medicine ☐

Examination(s) Requested:

chest (PA + lat)

History relevant to this request

Diabetes Mellitus

Physician Data (print or imprint below)

Name Dr. J. Plunkett

Phone

Billing no.

Copies to:

Diabetes	yes	☑	no	☐
Kidney Disease	yes	☐	no	☐
Serum creatine Level	____________			
Consent form completed?	yes	☐	no	☐
Previous IV contrast?	yes	☐	no	☐
Adverse Reaction?	yes	☐	no	☐
If yes, describe				

____________ Date ordered ____________ Physician's Signature

All of the above must be completed in full and signed by the physician

Form JF2209 Rev 08/99 Peterborough Regional Health Centrel (clipart by Corel)

To the Out Patient

Appointment location: ____________

time: ____________

date: ____________

You must bring this requisition with you!

If you think you might be pregnant, please inform the technologist
Please see over for instructions. Your doctor will check the appropriate box.

Peterborough Regional Health Centre
Hospital Drive Site
Phone 876-5039
Fax 743-1713

Peterborough Regional Health Centre
Rogers Street Site
Phone 740-8084
Fax 740-8089

SOURCE: Reproduced by permission of Peterborough Regional Health Centre.

FIGURE **11.32**   **Electrocardiogram Requisition**

```
                                                      5025/70
                                    ELECTROCARDIOGRAM
                                            REQUISITION
                                    DATE
                                    REQUEST
                                    SENT       ,  D  |  Mo.  |  Yr.
                                    DATE
                                    TO BE
                                    TAKEN      ,  D  |  Mo.  |  Yr.
                                    ADMISSION  DIAGNOSIS

                                    Diabetes mellitus

HISTORY

CHIEF  COMPLAINT
                                    Previous  E.C.G.   Yes ☐     No ☐
BLOOD  PRESSURE

                     Yes ☐                        Yes ☐
DRUGS - DIGITALIS                     Diuretic
                     No ☐                          No ☐

DRUGS - Other (Excluding Sedatives and Antibiotics)

BODY  BUILD    Short ☐        Medium ☐        Tall ☐
               Thin ☐         Medium ☐        Obese ☐
          Peterborough Regional Health Centre
```

SOURCE: Reproduced by permission of Peterborough Regional Health Centre.

Form by placing a check mark beside "Lytes." Some requisitions will require "sodium," "potassium," and "chloride" be checked individually. This can be included on the requisition ordering CBC, ESR, and glucose fasting.

16. Proteins are checked through urinalysis, and the order would be processed by completing a Urinalysis Requisition (Figure 11.33) and placing a check mark beside "protein."

NOTE: The same requisition can be used for numerous tests if they are to be completed at the same time.

All requisitions and forms have a blank space to addressograph stamp the patient information or attach the patient label. There is also space provided to write the patient information if needed.

During the patient's stay, new orders will be written in the patient's chart. Most hospitals use a "flag" system to identify that a new order has been written. It may be a coloured insert or tag for the chart that contains new orders. Physicians are asked to "flag" that they have written new orders that need to be processed. It is understandable that in a busy environment this can be forgotten or overlooked. The ward secretary should check the charts at the beginning of the shift and then periodically during the shift.

FIGURE 11.33   Urinalysis Requisition

Peterborough Regional Health Centre **LABORATORY MEDICINE**
URINALYSIS/OTHER BODY FLUIDS

☑ PCH   ☐ SJHC   ☐ Haliburton   ☐ Minden   ☐ Other_____

☑ In-patient   ☐ Out-patient   ☐ Referred-In

Date Ordered:m\d\yr_____

Ordering Physician:. _DR. J. PLUNKETT_

Nurse:_____

Specimen collected by:_____

Collection Date:m\d\yr_____Time:_____

☐ Random Urine   ☐ 24 Hour Urine

☐ **Emergent**   ☐ **Urgent**   ☑ **Routine**   ☐ **Timed**

O.R. Date: m\d\yr_____O.R.Time:_____

Clinical Information:_____

Special Instructions:_____

NOTE: USE MICROBIOLOGY TEST REQUISITION FOR ALL CULTURE REQUESTS

TESTS ON URINE	
ROUTINE URINALYSIS 3655	‖‖‖‖‖‖
MICROSCOPIC URINALYSIS 3660	‖‖‖‖‖‖
✓ PROTEIN 3241	‖‖‖‖‖‖
SODIUM 3045	‖‖‖‖‖‖
POTASSIUM 3055	‖‖‖‖‖‖
AMYLASE 3092	‖‖‖‖‖‖
URATE 3215	‖‖‖‖‖‖
CALCIUM 3105	‖‖‖‖‖‖
OSMOLALITY 3142	‖‖‖‖‖‖
PREGNANCY TEST 3640	‖‖‖‖‖‖
CREATININE 3035	‖‖‖‖‖‖
CREATININE 3038 CLEARANCE (NOTE:SERUM CREATININE ALSO REQUIRED)	‖‖‖‖‖‖
PATIENT - HT.	
WT.	
OTHER	

TESTS ON URINE	
CHLORIDE 3065	‖‖‖‖‖‖
PO4 3205	‖‖‖‖‖‖
URINE 3595 ELEXTROPHORESIS	‖‖‖‖‖‖

OTHER TESTS	
SWEAT CHLORIDES 3670	‖‖‖‖‖‖

STOOL	
OCCULT BLOOD 3635	‖‖‖‖‖‖
OTHER	
OTHER	

STONES	
STONE ANALYSIS 9525	‖‖‖‖‖‖
OTHER	

BODY FLUID TESTING

☐ CSF   ☐ JOINT   ☐ PLEURAL
☐ OTHER _____

GLUCOSE 3013	‖‖‖‖‖‖
CSF PROTEIN 3243	‖‖‖‖‖‖
PROTEIN OTHER FLUIDS 3242	‖‖‖‖‖‖
CSF CELLS 2070	‖‖‖‖‖‖
CELLS OTHER FLUIDS 2090	‖‖‖‖‖‖
CRYSTALS (JOINT FLUID) 2105	‖‖‖‖‖‖
PHOSPHATE	
ELECTROPHORESIS CSF 3590	‖‖‖‖‖‖
LD 3172	‖‖‖‖‖‖
URATE 3212	‖‖‖‖‖‖
AMYLASE 3092	‖‖‖‖‖‖
ALK PHOS. 3182	‖‖‖‖‖‖
SPECIFIC GRAVITY (OTHER FLUIDS) 3662	‖‖‖‖‖‖
OTHER	

*FOR LAB USE ONLY   Specimen Volume:_____mL   Surface Area:_____"

☑ **PETERBOROUGH CIVIC HOSPITAL**   ☐ **ST. JOSEPH'S HEALTH CENTRE**
One Hospital Drive, Peterborough, Ont., K9J 7C6   384 Rogers St., Peterborough, Ont., K9H 7B

Form # JF 5047   June/96

SOURCE: Reproduced by permission of Peterborough Regional Health Centre.

As in a physician's office, charts are taken away from their designated area. Physicians may take the chart with them to the patient's room, the ward secretary may need to photocopy information for a patient transfer, or the chart may need to go with the patient for a diagnostic test. The unit should have a system to track these charts. This can be accomplished with "out cards" or a "sign-out book."

CONFIDENTIALITY

As mentioned throughout this text, all areas of health care give personnel access to highly confidential information. In the hospital setting, personnel who are not involved in the direct care of a patient should not access charts or look up reports or notes on the computer. Even checking the computer to see if someone is in the hospital or coming into the hospital is a breach of confidentiality if the information it is not required for the job. This also applies to physicians.

If the ward secretary has concerns that confidentiality is being breached and is not comfortable confronting the individual, concerns should be reported to the unit charge nurse or unit director.

ASSIGNMENT 11.1

Your instructor will provide you with a Physician's Orders Form (Assignment 11.1A) for Erik Shultz. Mr. Shultz was admitted to the hospital last July 1. Requisitions were completed on July 2, 20__, hospital no. 56762, Room 2. You were the ward secretary responsible for transferring the doctor's orders onto the appropriate requisitions. (You will find the necessary forms on the accompanying CD.) After completing the requisitions, transcribe the orders on a sheet of plain white paper (for example, FBS would be fasting blood sugar; tid, three times in a day, and so on). Insert the completed assignment in your portfolio.

For Assignments 11.1B and 11.1C, use plain paper or write directly on the form and translate the physician's orders; indicate the appropriate requisition that would be used to document the order. Some orders have not been covered in the text. These assignments are intended to assess your ability to determine what requisitions would be needed to initiate the necessary action. Use Appendix B as a reference source.

ASSIGNMENT 11.1B

	PHYSICIAN'S ORDERS		
	START NEW SECTION FOR EACH NEW ORDER. MORE THAN ONE SECTION MAY BE USED FOR A LONG ORDER. DO NOT USE SECTION IF COPY IS MISSING.		
	EXPECTED DATE OF DISCHARGE		

ALLERGIES:

nl

DATE/TIME	ORDERS	1	EXECUTED
	DAT		
	AAT		
	Must sign on + off floor		
	Prozac 20 mg Po q prn	2	
	Psych consult		
	Social work consult		
	Tylenol E.S. ī-īī Po q4h prn.		
		3	
		4	

SEND TO PHARMACY   ADDRESSOGRAPH BACK - SEND TO PHARMACY   ADDRESSOGRAPH BACK - SEND TO PHARMACY   ADDRESSOGRAPH BACK - SEND TO PHARMACY

0505014 JF   **PHYSICIAN'S ORDERS**   WRITE FIRMLY!

ASSIGNMENT **11.1C**

PHYSICIAN'S ORDERS

START NEW SECTION FOR EACH NEW ORDER. MORE THAN ONE SECTION MAY BE USED FOR A LONG ORDER. DO NOT USE SECTION IF COPY IS MISSING.

EXPECTED DATE OF DISCHARGE

ALLERGIES:

DATE/TIME	ORDERS	1	EXECUTED
	Dx - acute (L) sciatica		
	DAT		
	bedrest c̄ BRP		
	Vitals - routine	2	
	CT scan - Lumbar spine		
	CBC, lytes, BUN, creatinine, B.S.		
	Demerol 50 mg. ī q 4-6 h. prn		
	Tyl. pl ī - īī q4h prn		
	Strax 15 mg qhs prn		

SEND TO PHARMACY

ADDRESSOGRAPH BACK - SEND TO PHARMACY

ADDRESSOGRAPH BACK - SEND TO PHARMACY

ADDRESSOGRAPH BACK - SEND TO PHARMACY

0505014 JF **PHYSICIAN'S ORDERS** **WRITE FIRMLY!**

DISCHARGE OF A PATIENT

The ward secretary is responsible for disassembling the chart when a patient is discharged from the unit. An out-patient chart is usually kept on a clipboard; an in-patient chart is kept in an individual binder for each patient. In both cases, the chart needs to be in a specific order on return to the Health Records Department. This order is dictated by hospital protocol.

The ward secretary will check the chart to ensure that all necessary signatures and initials are there (i.e., all orders must be signed by the ordering physician). The medication sheets will be taken from the MAR binder and inserted into the patient's chart. Once the process is complete, the chart is ready to be sent to Health Records. Any previous charts that have been sent to the unit for the discharged patient are to be returned at this time also.

NOTE: Only the current chart for the patient's admission is kept in the binder. If the patient has been in the hospital before (either as an out-patient or an in-patient), the previous chart is sent to the unit by Health Records for reference if needed on this admission.

The Admission/Discharge Record (see Figure 11.1) will identify the discharge date and the discharge diagnosis. The discharge diagnosis may be different from the provisional diagnosis. The signature of the MRP is required on this form.

A Discharge Summary or Final Note (see Figure 11.34) will be dictated regarding the patient.

If the patient has been to the hospital for an out-patient procedure, there will be a Clinical Note or an Out-Patient Operative Note dictated by the attending physician.

In the Health Records department, the record is analyzed by health records technicians for missing information and signatures. Hospitals have bylaws, rules and regulations, accreditation standards, and legislation that govern the content as well as the completion of records. If physicians do not comply with the regulations, various penalties may result, including loss of admitting privileges and a request to appear before the Medical Advisory Committee (Administrative Committee of Medical Staff); sometimes a report on the infraction may be sent to the College of Physicians and Surgeons.

Upon completion of the chart by the physicians involved, the Health Records staff assigns diagnosis and procedure codes. These are coded from the International Classification of Diagnoses and Procedures.

The chart is then filed according to a recognized filing system. The system generally used in Health Records departments is called *unit* numbering. The chart is filed by the patient's medical record number.

The key to the filing system used is the master patient index. This index is computerized so that in the case of a readmission, the patient's information can be readily accessed on the terminal and can easily be updated if necessary.

FIGURE **11.34**   Discharge Summary/Final Note

FINAL NOTE

Patient Number: 987654-32 _____   DOB: _____

Patient Name: Shultz, Erik _____   Admitted: _____

Address: _____   Discharged: _____

This ____-year-old man was admitted to hospital on the eighth day of August, 20__ with chest pain. The patient has a past history of possible pulmonary embolus and had surgery for carcinoma of the right ilium in 1999.

He was admitted to hospital with pain in the chest, and in the right foot. He had E.C.G. done which showed no abnormality.

SUMMARY

Serum enzymes were done and there was some elevation of the SGOT, but the CPK was normal.

BUN was normal. Alkaline phosphates was elevated to 204. Lung scan was done which showed a low to moderate possibility of embolism. Chest X-ray showed no significant abnormality.

The patient has now been up and around and has no further pain. He developed a bout of gout while in hospital, which was treated with indocid. He is to be allowed home and his condition followed with office visits.

A liver scan has been ordered but is not yet reported.

FINAL DIAGNOSIS

Acute gout, and chest pain with elevated liver enzymes, possible metastatic disease following carcinoma of the right ilium.

_____
R.M. Mann, M.D.

lbp
copies to: Dr. C.H. Hamblin
             Dr. R.M. McLeod

Each patient file is kept for many years in the Health Records department. The length of time is governed by provincial legislation. Records may be kept in the original file order or placed on microfilm for compact storage. Some hospitals are moving toward optical disk storage. The volumes of information produced in a hospital often necessitate off-site storage. This costly process has made optical disk storage much more attractive. If a patient is readmitted to the hospital, records are readily available for the attending physician's perusal.

The position in the Health Records department that would most likely be of interest to the graduate medical administrative assistant would be that of medical transcriptionist. The medical transcriptionist transcribes all medical reports dictated by the physicians. This position requires fast, accurate keyboarding skills and an excellent knowledge of medical terminology and anatomy.

ASSIGNMENT 11.2

Complete the following History and Physical Report using the format in Figure 11.24. Send appropriate copies.

Patient: Peter J. Scott—Admit today. The dictating physician is Paul T. Scole, M.D. The family doctor is Dr. Plunkett. The tape was dictated two days ago. Hospital no. 357914. His chief complaint is diarrhea and vomiting over the past 24 hours. Present Illness: This 10-year-old was perfectly well yesterday but awoke during the night with diarrhea and vomiting. There is severe cramping in the lower abdomen. Patient's last normal bowel movement was yesterday morning. His mother reports that he was at the movies yesterday and ate a large box of popcorn. Past History: Patient was born at Ottawa General Hospital—delivery uncomplicated. All childhood immunizations have been administered. He had a tonsillectomy at age 4 years and broke his right middle finger at age 7. Family History: Mother is 37 years old and is presently undergoing treatment for breast cancer. She reports that she had surgery and is on chemotherapy at the present time. Father is age 42 and well. They both had appendectomies, one for a ruptured appendix. A maternal great niece, uncle, and grandmother have had diabetes. No diabetes in the immediate family and no other history of familial disorders. Personal History: Allergic to morphine, is not on any medication at the present, is attending school, an excellent student. His hobbies include stamp collecting, hockey, water skiing, and cross-country skiing. Systemic Review: HEENT: There has been a muscle in one eye that has been off for years; his vision is good, hearing normal; CR: No known murmurs. No chronic cough, no recent cough, no dyspnea. N.P.: No history of head injury, no history of polio, paralysis, meningitis. Analysis and Plan: The patient will be admitted to hospital and examined further for possible appendicitis.

ASSIGNMENT 11.3

 This assignment is for additional practice and familiarity with using different formats to complete medical notes. Figure 11.35 is an example of a Pathologist's Report to be used as a reference. The forms and instructions can be found on the accompanying CD.

ASSIGNMENT 11.4

An Autopsy Report will be given to you by your instructor as a production assignment. You will be informed of the time allowed to produce the report. The patient's

FIGURE **11.35** **Pathologist's Report**

PATHOLOGIST'S REPORT

Department of Pathology   **Ottawa General Hospital**

Laboratory No: 6578-DP 56789   Date: **Adm. No:** 3546

Name: Steed, Robert   **Age:** 75   **Sex:** Male

Surgeon: Dr. Roger Jamieson   **Room No:** 304B

Material: Needle biopsy prostate. Prostatic tissue   **Date Rec'd:** 04/10/84

GROSS:

The specimen is received in formalin in two containers. The first is labelled needle biopsy of prostate. The specimen consists of six needle cores of white to tan prostatic tissue. A total length is approximately 7 cm. The biopsies are quite slim and are submitted in block A.

The second is labelled prostatic tissue. The specimen consists of 12 g of prostatic curettings with a somewhat nodular outline. The tissue is pink to tan in colour, a small amount of clot is received with the curettings. The tissue is submitted in toto in blocks B, C, and D.

MQ/hmb

MICROSCOPIC:

Multiple step sections of needle biopsy of prostate demonstrate in two fragments an adenocarcinoma of moderately well differentiated type associated with a marked chronic inflammatory cell infiltrate, lymphocytes being so numerous as to almost completely obliterate in some areas the markedly atypical glands. The remaining tissue shows predominantly fibromuscular bands in which large nerve fibres are identified.

Blocks B, C, and D. Multiple sections of curettage biopsy and prostate demonstrate a nodular outline in which hyperplastic gland elements are noted. A prominent feature is a marked granulomatous inflammation with central caseation. GMS, PAS, and ZN stains have been done but all are negative for identification of pathogenic organisms. It is, therefore, likely that these are the result of rupture of large ducts. In the fibromuscular stroma and areas away from the caseation there is moderate chronic inflammation. A single area in block D shows gland crowding. However, the glands are lined by a double layer of glandular epithelium and are AB PAS negative.

DIAGNOSIS:
1. Adenocarcinoma in needle biopsy of prostate.
2. Granulomatous inflammation in prostatic curettings.

Martin Quigg, M.D.

---

name is Mrs. Janet Bell. The student is responsible for making all necessary corrections in order to produce an acceptable document.

ASSIGNMENT **11.5**

This is a production assignment. Your instructor will provide you with the assignment material. Marks will be assessed for appearance, style, patient information, and ability to complete work in the allotted time. The patient's personal information can be obtained from the patient information forms in Chapter 3. Reports must

FIGURE **11.36A** Handwritten Physician's Orders

PETERBOROUGH REGIONAL HEALTH CENTRE

PHYSICIAN'S ORDER SHEET

M.R.P.: _____

Date (d/m/y) & Time	Sent to Pharmacy	Allergies:	S M O	K A R D E X	M A R	Signature of Nurse Date & Time
		☐ No Known Allergies _____				
		COMPLETE ALLERGY BOX (ABOVE) AT TIME OF INITIAL ORDERS				
May 11/20		Admit - Severe Epistaxis CBC, 'lytes, creatinine, BUN, INR in am ___ at 100 cc/hr Biaxin 250 b.i.d Fluids only _____ 0.5 mg tid po Metoprolol 25 mg bid po Zantac 150 mg bid po Tylenol c codeine elixir 2 tsp q4h prn Morphine 2 mg IV q2h prn Gravol 25 mg ____ IV q4h prn				
May 12/20		x match 2 units of packed cells - give both units				

Number Must Show Through Hole Before Physician Writes Orders	COPY 1	

0505014JF-5/01

continued

FIGURE **11.36B**   **Handwritten Physician's Orders**

PETERBOROUGH REGIONAL HEALTH CENTRE

PHYSICIAN'S ORDER SHEET

M.R.P.: _____

Date (d/m/y) & Time	Sent to Pharmacy	No Known Allergies	Allergies:	S M O	K A R D E X	M A R	Signature of Nurse Date & Time
			COMPLETE ALLERGY BOX (ABOVE) AT TIME OF INITIAL ORDERS				
08/05/20			Admit — Medical Bed				
			1550 KCal. Diabetic Diet				
			AAT				
			Vitals q shift				
			CBC / lytes / Creatinine				
			BS . fast + 1600h				
			ECASA 325 mg po OD				
			Glyburide 10 mg po BID				
			Lasix 40mg po BID.				
			Metoprolol. 25mg po BID				
			Altace 5 mg po OD				
			Humulin N 10 u sc ac				
			NTG spray sublingual prn				
			Colace 200mg po BID				
			MOM 30 cc's / Cascara 5cc po				
			— today and OD prn				
			Dulcolax suppositories ī OD prn				
			Serax. 7.5 ī 15mg po q HS prn				

Number Must Show Through Hole Before Physician Writes Orders	COPY	

0505014JF-5/01

be correlated with the patient list. Complete a preadmission form and a consent form for Jean Belliveau, inserting only information that you have available, and items 1 and 2 on day 1; items 3, 4, and 5 on day 2; items 6, 7, and 8 on day 3; items 9, 10, and 11 on day 4; and items 12, 13, 14, and 15 on day 5. Insert the completed assignment in your portfolio.

As the admitting doctor, Dr. Plunkett will do the History and Physical Reports; Discharge Summaries/Final Notes are signed by M. Brown, M.D., F.R.C.P.; Dr. Pelham completes Operative Records; Dr. W. Jarozenich completes Consultation Notes; and Dr. Emily Baret dictates the Delivery Report. All documents must be completed with all required information included.

ASSIGNMENT 11.6

The following assignment is to assist you in reading physicians' handwriting. Transcribe the physician's orders shown in Figures 11.36A and B line by line to a blank sheet of paper. Your instructor will provide you with the correct answers on completion.

TOPICS FOR DISCUSSION

1. The ward secretary is part of a multidisciplinary team. Who are be the other members of this team?

2. As a medical administrative assistant, the position of ward secretary is one that you would be qualified to apply for. What other positions within the hospital setting do you feel you would be qualified for?

CHAPTER 12

Hippocrates and Health Associations

CHAPTER OUTLINE

Hippocrates
Oath of Hippocrates
Codes of Ethics
Physicians Charter
Healthcare Associations

Associations of Importance to Medical
    Administrative Assistants
Topics for Discussion

LEARNING OBJECTIVES

After reading this chapter, you will possess a greater awareness of

- Who Hippocrates was and what medical symbols stand for
- The physician's Oath of Hippocrates
- The existence of codes of ethics
- Medical associations and organizations in Canada

- The College of Physicians and Surgeons
- The organizational structures of the previous associations

KEY TERMS

CMA: The initials *CMA* stand for the Canadian Medical Association.

Hippocrates: Hippocrates is known as the Father of Medicine.

Staff of Aesculapius: Aesculapius was the son of Apollo. He was known as the Greek god of medicine. The symbol depicts a serpent encircling a staff and signifies the art of healing.

HIPPOCRATES

FIGURE **12.1**   **Hippocrates is known as the Father of Medicine.**

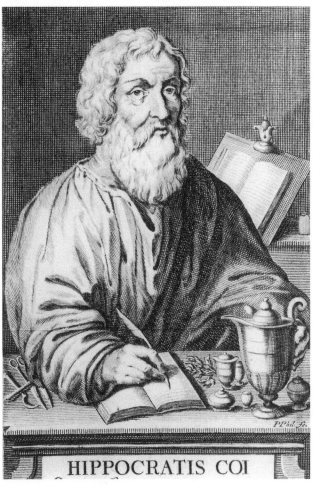

HIPPOCRATIS COI

SOURCE: Young, A.P. (2003). *Kinn's The Administrative Medical Assistant: An Applied Learning Approach*, 5th ed. (p. 17: Figure 2-2). St. Louis: Elsevier/Saunders.

Hippocrates is known as the Father of Medicine (see Figure 12.1). He was born in the island of Cos between 470 and 460 B.C., and belonged to the family that claimed descent from the mythical Aesculapius, son of Apollo. There was already a long medical tradition in Greece before his day, and thus he is supposed to have inherited chiefly through his predecessor, Herodicus; he enlarged his education by extensive travel. Though the evidence is unsatisfactory, he is said to have taken part in the efforts to halt the great plague that devastated Athens at the beginning of the Peloponnesian war. He died at Larissa between 380 and 360 B.C.

One of the works attributed to Hippocrates is the famous "Oath" (see Box 12.1).

Aesculapius, the son of Apollo, was referred to as the god of medicine. A common medical icon is the **staff of Aesculapius** (see Figure 12.2). It depicts

> ### 12.1   The Oath of Hippocrates
>
> I SWEAR by Apollo the physician, and Aesculapius, and Health, and All-heal, and all the gods and goddesses, that, according to my ability and judgment, I will keep this Oath and this stipulation—to reckon him who taught me this Art equally dear to me as my parents, to share my substance with him, and relieve his necessities if required; to look upon his offspring in the same footing as my own brothers, and to teach them this art, if they shall wish to learn it, without fee or stipulation; and that by precept, lecture and every other mode of instruction, I will impart a knowledge of the Art to my own sons, and those of my teachers, and to disciples bound by stipulation and oath according to the law of medicine, but to none others.
>
> I will follow that system of regimen which, according to my ability and judgment, I consider for the benefit of my patients, and abstain from whatever is deleterious and mischievous.
>
> I will give no deadly medicine to any one if asked, nor suggest any such counsel; and in like manner I will not give to a woman a pessary to produce abortion. With purity and with holiness I will pass my life and practice my Art.
>
> I will not cut persons laboring under the stone, but will leave this to be done by men who are practitioners of this work. Into whatever houses I enter, I will go into them for the benefit of the sick, and will abstain from every voluntary act of mischief and corruption; and, further, from the seduction of females or males, of freemen and slaves. Whatever, in connection with my professional service, or not in connection with it, I see or hear, in the life of men, which ought not to be spoken of abroad, I will not divulge, as reckoning that all such should be kept secret. While I continue to keep this Oath unviolated, may it be granted to me to enjoy life and the practice of the art, respected by all men, in all times. But should I trespass and violate this Oath, may the reverse be my lot.

a serpent encircling a staff and signifies the art of healing. The mythological staff belonging to Apollo, the caduceus, which is a staff encircled by two serpents, is often used as a symbol of the medical profession.

CODES OF ETHICS

Most health associations are guided by a code of ethics (see Figure 12.3). An example is the Canadian Medical Association's Code of Ethics. Each medical discipline has its own code of ethics.

> ### 12.2
>
> "The complete physician is not a man apart and cannot content himself with the practice of medicine alone, but should make his contribution, as does any other good citizen, towards the well-being and betterment of the community in which he lives."

SOURCE: The Canadian Medical Association *Code of Ethics* (April 1990).

FIGURE **12.2**   **Staff of Aesculapius and the Caduceus**

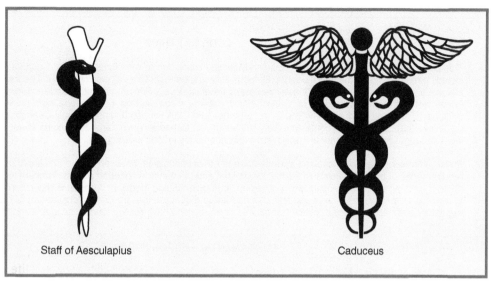

Staff of Aesculapius   Caduceus

SOURCE: Young, A.P. (2003). *Kinn's The Administrative Medical Assistant: An Applied Learning Approach*, 5th ed. (p. 17: Figure 2-1). St. Louis: Elsevier/Saunders.

PHYSICIANS CHARTER

The goal of Canadian physicians, in partnership with their patients, is to provide the best health care possible. The Physicians Charter expresses what Canadian physicians need to achieve this goal (see Figure 12.4). It complements **CMA** policies and the CMA Code of Ethics, which outlines the responsibilities of physicians to patients, society, the medical profession, and themselves.

HEALTHCARE ASSOCIATIONS

The range of health associations and organizations across Canada is extensive. There are associations relating to hospitals, physicians, medical secretaries, nurses, physiotherapists, nursing homes, health records administrators, diseases, and so on. It would be difficult to discuss in detail the purposes and bylaws of each association, so we will not do so here.

The organizational structures of health associations and organizations differ according to the specific group. However, many associations have national, provincial, and regional branches. For example, many physicians in Canada are members of the CMA. The CMA is a national organization with twelve provincial medical association branches. But these provincial branches also have municipal or regional medical association branches themselves. All physicians, healthcare associations, provincial

FIGURE **12.3** **Example of a Code of Ethics**

CODE OF ETHICS

This Code has been prepared by the Canadian Medical Association as an ethical guide for Canadian physicians, including residents, and medical students. Its focus is on the core activities of medicine—such as health promotion, advocacy, disease prevention, diagnosis, treatment, rehabilitation, palliation, education and research. It is based on the fundamental principles and values of medical ethics, especially compassion, beneficence, non-maleficence, respect for persons, justice and accountability. The Code, together with CMA policies on specific topics, constitutes a compilation of guidelines that can provide a common ethical framework for Canadian physicians. Physicians should be aware of the legal and regulatory requirements that govern medical practice in their jurisdictions.

Physicians may experience tension between different ethical principles, between ethical and legal or regulatory requirements, or between their own ethical convictions and the demands of other parties. Training in ethical analysis and decision-making during undergraduate, postgraduate and continuing medical education is recommended for physicians to develop their knowledge, skills and attitudes needed to deal with these conflicts. Consultation with colleagues, regulatory authorities, ethicists, ethics committees or others who have relevant expertise is also recommended.

FUNDAMENTAL RESPONSIBILITIES

1. Consider first the well-being of the patient.
2. Treat all patients with respect; do not exploit them for personal advantage.
3. Provide for appropriate care for your patient, including physical comfort and spiritual and psychosocial support, even when cure is no longer possible.
4. Practice the art and science of medicine competently and without impairment.
5. Engage in lifelong learning to maintain and improve your professional knowledge, skills and attitudes.
6. Recognize your limitations and the competence of others and, when indicated, recommend that additional opinions and services be sought.
7. Resist any influence or interference that could undermine your professional integrity.
8. Contribute to the development of the medical profession, whether through clinical practice, research, teaching, administration or advocating on behalf of the profession or the public.
9. Refuse to participate in or support practices that violate basic human rights.
10. Promote and maintain your own health and well-being.

RESPONSIBILITIES TO THE PATIENT

Patient–Physician Relationship

11. Recognize and disclose conflicts of interest that arise in the course of your professional duties and activities, and resolve them in the course of your professional duties and activities, and resolve them in the best interest of patients.
12. Inform your patient when your personal values would influence the recommendation or practice of any medical procedure that that patient needs or wants.
13. Do not exploit patients for personal advantage.
14. Take all reasonable steps to prevent harm to patients; should harm occur, disclose it to the patient.
15. Recognize your limitations and, when indicated, recommend or seek additional opinions and services.
16. In determining professional fees to patients for non-insured services, consider both the nature of the service provided and the ability of the patient to pay, and be prepared to discuss the fee with the patient.

GENERAL RESPONSIBILITIES

Initiating and Dissolving a Patient–Physician Relationship

17. In providing medical service, do not discriminate against any patient on such grounds as age, gender, marital status, medical condition, national or ethnic origin, physical or mental disability, political affiliation, race, religion, sexual orientation, or socioeconomic status. This does not abrogate the physician's right to refuse to accept a patient for legitimate reasons.
18. Provide whatever appropriate assistance you can to any person with an urgent need for medical care.
19. Having accepted professional responsibility for a patient, continue to provide services until they are no longer required or wanted; until another suitable physician has assumed responsibility for the patient; or until the patient has been given reasonable notice that you intend to terminate the relationship.
20. Limit treatment of yourself or members of your immediate family to minor or emergency services and only when another physician is not readily available; there should be no fee for such treatment.

SOURCE: *The Canadian Medical Association Code of Ethics* (Update 2004). Reprinted by permission of the Canadian Medical Association.

Communication, Decision Making and Consent

21. Provide your patients with the information they need to make informal decisions about their medical care, and answer their questions to the best of your ability.
22. Make every reasonable effort to communicate with your patients in such a way that information exchanged is understood.
23. Recommend only those diagnostic and therapeutic services that you consider to be beneficial to your patient or to others. If a service is recommended for the benefit of others, as for example in matters of public health, inform your patient of this fact and proceed only with explicit informed consent or where required by law.
24. Respect the right of a competent patient to accept or reject any medical care recommended.
25. Recognize the need to balance the developing competency of minors and the role of families in medical decision-making. Respect the autonomy of those minors who are authorized to consent to treatment.
26. Respect your patient's reasonable request for a second opinion from a physician of the patient's choice.
27. Ascertain wherever possible and recognize your patient's wishes about the initiation, continuation or cessation of life-sustaining treatment.
28. Respect the intentions of an incompetent patient as they were expressed (e.g., through a valid advance directive or proxy designation) before the patient became incompetent.
29. When the intentions of an incompetent patient are unknown and when no formal mechanism for making treatment decisions is in place, render such treatment as you believe to be in accordance with the patient's values or, if these are unknown, the patient's best interests.
30. Be considerate of the patient's family and significant others and cooperate with them in the patient's interest.

Privacy and Confidentiality

31. Protect the personal health information of your patients.
32. Provide information reasonable in the circumstances to patients about the reasons for the collection, use and disclosure of their personal health information.
33. Be aware of your patient's rights with respect to the collection, use, disclosure and access to their personal health information; ensure that such information is recorded accurately.
34. Avoid public discussions or comments about patients that could reasonably be seen as revealing confidential or identifying information.
35. Disclose your patients' personal health information to third parties only with their consent, or as provided for by law, such as when the maintenance of confidentiality would result in a significant risk of substantial harm to others or, in the case of incompetent patients, to the patients themselves. In such case take all reasonable steps to inform the patients that the usual requirements for confidentiality will be breached.
36. When acting on behalf of a third party, take reasonable steps to ensure that the patient understands the nature and extent of your responsibility to the third party.
37. Upon a patient's request, provide the patient or a third party with a copy of his or her medical record, unless there is a compelling reason to believe that information contained in the record will result in substantial harm to the patient or others.
38. Ensure that any research in which you participate is evaluated both scientifically and ethically and is approved by a research ethics board that meets current standards of practice.
39. Inform the potential research subject, or proxy, about the purpose of the study, its source of funding, the nature and relative probability of harms and benefits, and the nature of your participation including any compensation.
40. Before proceeding with the study, obtain the informed consent of the subject, or proxy, and advise prospective subjects that they have the right to decline or withdraw from the study at any time, without prejudice to their ongoing care.

RESPONSIBILITIES TO SOCIETY

41. Recognize that community, society and the environment are important factors in the health of individual patients.
42. Recognize the profession's responsibility to society in matters relating to public health, health education, environmental protection, legislation affecting the health or well-being of the community and the need for testimony at judicial proceedings.
43. Recognize the responsibility of physicians to promote equitable access to health care resources.
44. Use health care resources prudently.
45. Recognize a responsibility to give generally held opinions of the profession when interpreting scientific knowledge to the public; when presenting an opinion that is contrary to the generally held opinion of the profession, so indicate.

FIGURE **12.3**   **Example of a Code of Ethics, cont'd**   *continued*

RESPONSIBILITIES TO THE PROFESSION

46. Recognize that the self-regulation of the profession is a privilege and that each physician has a continuing responsibility to merit this privilege and to support its institutions.
47. Be willing to teach and learn from medical students, residents, other colleagues and other health professionals.
48. Avoid impugning the reputation of colleagues for personal motives; however, report to the appropriate authority any unprofessional conduct by colleagues.
49. Be willing to participate in peer review of other physicians and to undergo review by your peers. Enter into associations, contracts and agreements only if you can maintain your professional integrity and safeguard the interests of your patients.
50. Avoid promoting, as a member of the medical profession, any service (except your own) or product for personal gain.
51. Do not keep secret from colleagues the diagnostic or therapeutic agents and procedures that you employ.
52. Collaborate with other physicians and health professionals in the care of patients and the functioning and improvement of health services. Treat your colleagues with dignity and as persons worthy of respect.

RESPONSIBILITIES TO ONESELF

53. Seek help from colleagues and appropriately qualified professionals for personal problems that might adversely affect your service to patients, society or the profession.
54. Protect and enhance your own health and well-being by identifying those stress factors in your professional and personal lives that can be managed by developing and practicing appropriate coping strategies.

FIGURE **12.3   Example of a Code of Ethics, cont'd**

departments of health, Canadian healthcare associations, etc., can be found in the *Canadian Medical Directory*. Some Canadian associations are listed in Box 12.3.

12.3

Royal College of Physicians and Surgeons of Canada
774 Echo Drive Ottawa, Ontario K1S 5N8
Fax: 613-730-8250
Phone: 1-800-668-3740/613-730-6201
e-mail: publicaffairs@rcpsc.edu
Web site: http://rcpsc.medical.org

Canadian Medical Association
1867 Alta Vista Drive, Ottawa, Ontario K1G 3Y6
Phone: 1-800-267-9703/613-731-9331
Fax: 613-731-9013

College of Family Physicians of Canada
2630 Skymark Avenue, Mississauga, Ontario L4W 5A4
Fax: 905-629-0893 or 1-888-843-2372
Phone: 905-629-0900 Ext. 237
or
1-800-387-6197 Ext. 237
Web site: http://www.cfpc.ca

FIGURE **12.4**   **Physicians Charter from the Canadian Medical Association**

PHYSICIANS CHARTER

I.   Patient–Physician Relationship

Canadian physicians regard serving the health needs of their patients as paramount, and put this at the centre of the patient-physician relationship. A strong patient-physician relationship is one based on trust, honesty, confidentiality and mutual respect. In order to achieve the best patient-physician relationship, Canadian physicians need:

1. timely access to appropriate, quality health care for their patients
2. to be able to advocate for their patients' health care needs
3. patients to share appropriate information about their health so that they may receive the best quality care
4. to be able to hold information about patients in confidence, except when disclosure is consistent with the CMA's Code of Ethics
5. assurance that data generated by physicians in the context of clinical practice will not be compiled, sold or otherwise used in a manner that compromises the privacy of patients or physicians, except as authorized by law
6. to be able to refuse to accept a patient, or to discontinue a professional relationship, except in emergency situations and consistent with the provisions of the CMA's Code of Ethics

II.   Professional Integrity

Canadian physicians practise their profession in the service of their patients and society and collaborate with other health providers to this end. In order to discharge their professional responsibilities, Canadian physicians need:

7. to be able to practise medicine in accordance with professional and personal values, within the bounds of CMA's Code of Ethics
8. to be unhindered from complying with the CMA's Code of Ethics
9. to continue to be regulated by self-governing, professional medical bodies
10. to be free to practise medicine, subject to licensure
11. to be free to inform patients of all appropriate options relevant to their care and to have clinical autonomy in recommending care
12. to have adequate time and opportunity for career maintenance and professional development

III.   Fairness

Like all Canadians, Canadian physicians deserve fair treatment in matters concerning their individual and collective interests. Therefore, during training and in practice Canadian physicians need:

13. fair treatment with respect to access into, mobility and flexibility within, and exit from the health care training and delivery systems
14. procedural fairness with respect to policy, legal, contractual, administrative and disciplinary decision-making concerning themselves
15. assurance that appointment and reappointment procedures which include effective medical representation and appeal process, and that decisions will be based primarily on required professional credentials, competence and performance
16. to receive reasonable remuneration for the full spectrum of professional services, including administration, teaching, research and committee work
17. to receive reasonable consideration and compensation when facilities and programs are discontinued, reduced or transferred

IV.   Quality of Life

Canadian physicians strive to balance professional demands with their need for quality of life and personal health maintenance. Therefore, Canadian physicians need:

18. to be free from harassment, discrimination, intimidation or violence, both in training and in practising medicine
19. access to appropriate resources for dealing with personal or professional problems that affect their medical practice
20. to be free from reprisal when they report in good faith unsafe practices or conditions bearing on patient care
21. reasonable access to information needed to safeguard their personal health and safety, while respecting patient confidentiality
22. scheduling in the provision of medical services and physician training to be limited to reasonable hours, both to safeguard their ability to provide quality care and in consideration of their need to have time for a personal life and health
23. to be able to achieve adequate and affordable medical liability protection

SOURCE: Reprinted by permission of the Canadian Medical Association.

V.   Health System

Canadian physicians have a vital role in the health care system and can provide essential expertise about health system organization, funding and service delivery. In order to preserve and promote a quality health care system, Canadian physicians need:

24. to be consulted and involved meaningfully in health system reform and policy planning, and on issues related to service delivery, payment, funding, and terms and conditions of work, and to be assured that changes to the health care system will respect individual medical practitioners' liberty to choose among payment methods

25. valid methods of assessment, such as properly evaluated pilot projects to be applied to any proposed changes to the health care system

26. the health care system to respect the patient-physician relationship, continuity of care and the patient's freedom in the choice of a physician

27. date generated in the context of clinical practice and collected under legislative and administrative requirements to be interpreted with physician input and made readily accessible to physicians in a manner consistent with respect for the privacy of patients and physicians

28. to be free to associate for collective bargaining, and to be formally represented in negotiations on issues of health system reform, service delivery, payment, funding and terms and conditions of work

29. resources and funding for physician services to be negotiated by provincial/territorial medical associations or federations and allocated directly to physicians

30. sufficient resources to allow for the efficient, effective and professional delivery and management of medical care under reasonable and humane working conditions

FIGURE **12.4   Physicians Charter from the Canadian Medical Association, cont'd**

ASSOCIATIONS OF IMPORTANCE TO MEDICAL ADMINISTRATIVE ASSISTANTS

As a medical administrative assistant, you may be required at any time to write to or contact an organization or association relating to health care. At that time, you would use the information you have learned from this chapter as well as the reference sources available to you. There are, however, a few associations of direct significance to the medical administrative assistant.

National, Provincial, and Local Medical Associations

The Canadian Medical Association—As the governing body of the provincial associations, the CMA deals with the federal government and acts as the national voice of medicine. A portion of the fees paid by provincial members goes to the CMA.

Provincial Medical Associations—The provincial medical associations are voluntary associations of provincial doctors. The bylaws of the associations differ among the provinces, but these differences are minor. For example, in one province membership is voluntary, but in another a fee is mandatory.

We will use the Ontario Medical Association (OMA) as an example to outline some of the points relevant to the provincial bodies. Membership in the OMA is open to all doctors in the province as well as to medical graduates residing in Ontario and students enrolled in faculties of medicine at Ontario universities. Approximately 80 percent of practising physicians are members.

The objective of the OMA, broadly speaking, is to advance the practice and the science of medicine and public health by working for the improvement of medical education, hospital and other health services, and medical legislation, through study, investigation, and research.

The OMA represents the medical profession to the Ontario government, offering recommendations about legislation and regulations affecting medical practice and public health. The OMA produces a Schedule of Fees for medical services in Ontario and negotiates the Schedule of Benefits paid by the Ontario Ministry of Health. It publishes the *Ontario Medical Review*. The OMA also provides other services for its members, such as group insurance programs and support for continuing and postgraduate medical education.

The College of Physicians and Surgeons

Each province has its own College of Physicians and Surgeons. Established by provincial legislation, the College of Physicians and Surgeons is the official body that oversees the education, licensing, and discipline of doctors. In Ontario, as in other provinces, close liaison is maintained between the OMA and the College through a joint advisory committee of senior officers. These provincial colleges are completely separate and distinct from the provincial medical associations.

Hospital Associations

Many provinces have established hospital associations. Today, many of these provincial hospital associations have active memberships in other areas, such as mental health centres, district health councils, institutional associate members, nursing homes, senior citizen homes, private hospitals, and some educational institutions that provide healthcare student programs. All members pay annual dues, and usually only active members have voting privileges and representation on boards of directors.

The fundamental objective of hospital associations is to stimulate, encourage, and assist in the provision of the highest possible standard of hospital and other health services to the people of the province.

The Canadian Medical Protective Association

The Canadian Medical Protective Association is a mutual defence union of Canadian physicians. The association was founded in 1901 and had more than 66,000 members by December 2005. The purpose of the association is to provide its members with legal advice and counselling on any matters involving legal action. The association pays all legal costs incurred in the defence of such legal actions as well as any damages that the courts may award to the plaintiff. Members are also assisted with the defence of provincial governing body disciplinary actions, coroner inquests, and so on.

Medical Secretaries' Associations

There are medical secretaries' associations located in some provinces in Canada. In Ontario, the association is known as Ontario Medical Secretaries

Association-Health Care Associates or OMSA-HCA. Active membership is available to any person who is currently working in the healthcare environment or teaches in a medical administration program at a community or business college. Associate membership is available to any person who is not currently working in the healthcare environment but was previously employed in such for a two-year period. An international membership is available to any person currently working in the healthcare environment who is living outside of Ontario. Local chapters of the provincial associations generally meet on a monthly basis. Their purpose is to improve the status and knowledge of all medical administrative assistants. Students who attend their local chapter meetings are provided with excellent exposure to the profession. Speakers' topics are varied and provide valuable information, the majority of which concerns health-related issues.

The OMSA-HCA offers a Continuing Education Program. There are different ways that members can accumulate continuing education credits. Box 12.4 lists some examples.

12.4

- Attend a one-day seminar/workshop
- Enrol in a professional development course (e.g., CPR)
- Participate in the community (e.g., volunteer, blood donor)
- Attend a minimum of five branch meetings
- Hold an executive position in a local branch
- Enrol in a university or college credit course

The OMSA-HCA and MOAA (Medical Office Assistants Association) in British Columbia also offer a Certified Medical Secretary (CMS) program. This is designed for individuals who are interested in obtaining a professional designation through the association. Successful applicants are awarded the Certified Medical Secretary designation (e.g., Mary Smith, CMS).

Some medical facilities offer benefit packages to their office staff, but most private practitioners do not. Certain benefits are available through the OMSA-HCA and MOAA to members.

In 1990, the Ontario Medical Secretaries' Association Certification Program was affiliated with the Ontario Colleges of Applied Arts and Technology Office Administration—Medical Diploma Programs. Students who graduate with a 75 percent average mark from participating colleges can apply to the association for exemption from the certification examinations. For further information, contact the association's head office in Toronto, or visit its Web site at http://www.omsa-hca.org.

As previously mentioned, British Columbia has a provincial organization known as the Medical Office Assistants Association of British Columbia. The group is dedicated to the professional advancement of its members and also to providing networking that binds the groups together. Anyone who is employed in a medical office in an assisting capacity is eligible. Members include receptionists, secretaries, office managers, nurses, and technicians. The provinces of Ontario and British Columbia send out newsletters to their members with information about upcoming events and seminars and information from local chapters.

ASSIGNMENT **12.1**

Investigate the local medical secretaries' association in your area. If there is no active chapter in your location, write to the Ontario Medical Secretaries' Association, 525 University Avenue, Suite 300, Toronto, Ontario M5G 2K7 (or send an email message via the Web site) to obtain information. This address is for use by students who do not live in a province where there is an active association. For those who live in a province where there is an active association, use an appropriate reference source to obtain the proper address for your association's provincial head office.

Write a report on the organization, outlining the benefits to be derived from belonging to such a group. Prepare the report in proper form for submission.

This assignment should spark an interest in the association specifically related to your future profession. If there is no active chapter in your area, you may be interested in forming one after graduation. Ask your provincial head office for assistance. Office staff will be only too happy to provide you with guidance.

TOPICS FOR DISCUSSION

1. Read the Oath of Hippocrates and determine if it still applies to medicine in modern times.

2. If there is a Medical Secretaries Association in your area, do you think you would benefit from what it offers?

Doctors and the Law

CHAPTER OUTLINE

LEARNING OBJECTIVES

After reading this chapter, you will be able to describe

- Rules and regulations pertaining to the practice of medicine
- Proper names of various statutes that pertain to the medical environment
- Reporting procedures

- Various types of medico-legal problems
- Restrictions necessary to ensure patient confidentiality
- Minimum standards for medical records maintenance

KEY TERMS

Fraud: A deception deliberately practised in order to secure unfair on unlawful gain.

Mandatory: Required or commanded by authority.

Negligence: Failure to exercise the degree of care considered reasonable under the circumstances resulting in an unintended injury to another party.

Power of Attorney (POA): A specific individual chosen by you to act on your behalf should you become unable to do so.

Statutes: Established laws or rules; laws enacted by a legislature.

Because a medical administrative assistant acts on behalf of a doctor, the doctor may be held responsible for the consequences of the assistant's actions. Hence, an awareness of medico-legal problems is of great importance to the medical administrative assistant and is discussed in this chapter.

RESPONSIBILITIES OF THE DOCTOR

Rules and Regulations

Just as all other disciplines and human endeavours are subject to rules and regulations, so too is the practice of medicine. Doctors practise their profession under a well-defined and time-honoured ethical code. Even though doctors have the same general responsibilities as all citizens do, they have special additional responsibilities peculiar to their profession.

In order to practise medicine in Canada, a doctor must be licensed by the provincial College of Physicians and Surgeons or its equivalent, such as the Corporation Professionnelle des Médecins du Québec, the Provincial Medical Board of Nova Scotia, or the Newfoundland Medical Board. The profession and the college must operate under clearly defined rules as set out in the relevant provincial legislation and the regulations made under the medical acts. For example, each province has a *Physicians' Administrative Manual*, which discusses **statutes** relevant to the practice of medicine in that province. A *Physicians' Legal Manual* should also be available. All doctors and medical administrative assistants should obtain and read a copy of the legislation and regulations that apply to them. Copies of regulations and pertinent provincial statutes can be obtained by contacting the Queen's Printer for the province, or the province's government book store.

Healthcare facilities have facility bylaws, medical staff bylaws, and medical staff rules. Any physician with privileges to practise within that facility must abide by these bylaws and rules.

Other Statutes

Doctors should also be acquainted with other statutes that touch on or affect the practice of medicine in their province. Some of these statutes are listed in Box 13.1.

13.1
Child and Family Services Act
Coroners Act
Health Insurance Act
Health Protection and Promotion Act
Highway Traffic Act
Aeronautics Act
Nursing Home Act
Public Hospitals Act
Vital Statistics Act

Consideration should also be given to the fact that the practice of medicine may be controlled by certain federal statutes, most notably the *Food and Drug Act*, the *Narcotic Control Act*, and others.

Reporting

Practising physicians should be particularly aware that the statutes mentioned previously require **mandatory** reporting in certain circumstances. For example, reports may have to be submitted to the Children's Aid Society under the *Child and Family Services Act* (CFSA). Recent changes to the CFSA (March 2000) require that the physician make the report themselves. Reporting responsibilities can no longer be delegated. Reports may also need to be submitted to the Registrar of Motor Vehicles under most Highway Traffic acts or Motor Vehicle acts, to the Workplace and Safety Insurance Board under the *Workers Safety and Insurance Act*, and so on. If a doctor does not know how to go about reporting to these boards and agencies, a telephone call or letter to them will produce the desired procedures. A copy of *Determining Medical Fitness to Drive: A Guide for Physicians* (6th edition) can be obtained from the Canadian Medical Association, 1867 Alta Vista Drive, Ottawa, Ontario, K1G 0G8. Information about reporting communicable diseases can be obtained by contacting the local, regional, or provincial health department. Not reporting something that is required by law to be reported can result in the imposition of fines, or charges of professional misconduct, or both.

RESPONSIBILITIES OF THE MEDICAL ADMINISTRATIVE ASSISTANT

Medical administrative assistants and other medical aides who are employees of doctors are usually considered to be doctors' agents. Doctors are likely to be held responsible for the acts of their agents. Therefore, when a medical administrative assistant or other assistant acts on behalf of a doctor, the doctor may ultimately be responsible for the consequences of those actions. This puts a responsibility on the medical administrative assistant to be knowledgeable about the rules and regulations that govern the practice of medicine and the consequences that may occur if the rules are not followed. It should be noted that medical administrative assistants and other medical aides may also be held personally responsible for their own actions.

MEDICO-LEGAL PROBLEMS

Doctors may be faced with a number of legal situations, such as partnership agreements, contracts with employees, estate planning, leases, and so on. In addition, doctors can encounter problems of a medico-legal nature. Rarely will a doctor face a criminal charge related to the practice of medicine. However, **fraud**, violations of the *Narcotic Control Act*, and allegations of sexual assault are examples of possible instances in which a doctor could be charged. Most physicians will have a nurse or the medical administrative assistant present when a patient presents with a problem that requires a vaginal exam or is booked for an annual physical examination. A doctor is seldom charged with criminal **negligence** as a result of the professional care of a patient. (The term criminal negligence refers to reckless or wanton disregard for a patient's welfare.)

It is more common for physicians to face civil medico-legal problems. Medical malpractice actions can be brought against doctors in small claims or provincial courts or in courts of superior jurisdiction, such as the supreme courts or Court of Queen's Bench in each province. There may be one or several claims asserted for any one action.

A contract exists between a doctor and the patient. Although this does not take the form of a written document, a "contract" is implied when the patient requests examination and treatment from the doctor and the doctor makes a commitment, probably unspoken, to treat the patient. Either party could breach the contract: a claim by the doctor against the patient is likely to be related to the financial aspect of the relationship; the patient may feel that the doctor has not met the patient's expectations and may be tempted to start a legal action. The patient may claim that the contract was breached because the result of treatment was not what the patient thought was promised by the doctor.

More often, however, a medico-legal action is commenced against a physician from allegations of negligence. What is negligence? **Negligence** is a term used to describe the alleged failure of a person to exercise a reasonable and acceptable standard of care, thereby causing harm or injury to another.

Malpractice actions alleging negligence generally fall into one of two categories. The first category includes those cases in which a patient alleges that the treatment rendered by the doctor was negligent in a medical sense. For example, while the patient is undergoing surgery for removal of a gallbladder (cholecystectomy), his or her bowel is punctured by the surgeon. The second category, increasing in frequency, includes claims by the patient that the physician was negligent by failing to disclose sufficiently the risks of the treatment beforehand. Claims of this nature come under the expression "lack of informed consent" (see Box 13.2 for a definition of informed consent). The general rule is that, unless there is an emergency, before any medical treatment or medication can be undertaken, the patient must give his or her consent (verbal or written); without consent, there can be no treatment or medication (see Box 13.3 for the criteria for valid consent). The proposed treatment must be explained to the patient by the physician, never by the administrative assistant or the nurse. Consent can be witnessed by someone other than the physician after the proposed treatment has been explained to the patient.

13.2 Informed Consent

The patient must be aware of the nature and risks of the treatment, of not having the treatment, and of any alternative treatment.

13.3 Criteria for Valid Consent

The consent must be given voluntarily.
There must exist in the patient the mental capacity to provide the consent.
The patient must have the legal capacity to give the consent.
The patient's consent must be directed or related to a specific treatment or set of treatments.
The consent given by the patient must be an informed consent.
The patient must consent to the person who will be treating him or her.

If patients feel that they have received treatment for which consent was not given, they may allege assault and battery. Recent case law has established that for there to be a claim for assault and battery, the treatment carried out must be wholly unrelated to or different from that treatment discussed earlier with the patient.

Overriding the issue of consent is the "emergency rule," whereby in circumstances in which it is essential to treat someone in order to save the person's life or prevent serious permanent injury, and it is impossible to ask the person's consent, a health professional can treat that person. If the patient in an emergency situation refuses treatment, the health professional cannot act, assuming the patient is competent. For a definition of what constitutes competency, see Box 13.4.

13.4 Competent Adult

The person has the ability to understand the subject matter in respect of which considered requests are made and is able to appreciate the consequences of giving or withholding consent.

Other civil claims, in addition to medical negligence, lack of informed consent, or assault and battery, may be those that allege breach of medical confidentiality or defamation.

As well as, or perhaps instead of, suing a doctor, a patient may complain about the doctor's professional work. The complaint may be expressed directly to the doctor or to a member of the doctor's staff. It may be sub-mitted to officials of the hospital, to the local academy of medicine or medical society, or to the College of Physicians and Surgeons or its equivalent.

Complaints or claims against doctors sometimes arise out of certain aspects of the practice of medicine with which medical administrative assistants have considerable involvement. The competent medical adminis-trative assistant should pay heed to some of the following considerations.

CONFIDENTIALITY

Every patient has the right to expect that the information the doctor has obtained about him or her, on the basis of what the patient or others have told the doctor or what the doctor has discovered by examination and other means, will be kept confidential by the doctor. This duty applies also to the doctor's staff.

Information about a patient must never be revealed to anyone (except, of course, the patient) unless required by law or unless authorized by the patient or by the person legally responsible for the patient (in the case, for example, of a minor or developmentally handicapped patient). The physician can disclose patient information under the mandatory reporting requirements of certain statutes that require physicians to provide informa-tion that would otherwise be confidential. A physician who has questions about specific situations can contact the Physician Advisory Service or the Canadian Medical Protective Association (CMPA) through his or her provin-cial College of Physicians and Surgeons. (See Figure 13.1 for a list of Cana-dian Medical Licensing Authorities.) Unauthorized persons should not have access to appointment lists or other information, and certainly not to patients' records or to the information contained therein. Even the information that the patient was seen by the doctor should be considered confidential.

A doctor or medical administrative assistant should not release medical information to a third party unless properly authorized in writing to do so. An authorization should state clearly what is intended, and it should be dated. (The date should be reasonably current.) The authorization should be kept in the doctor's possession in case it is later alleged that a breach of medical confidentiality occurred.

If an inquirer, other than the patient, approaches a medical administrative assistant for information about a patient, it should be pointed out that the request for information should be put in writing and should be accompanied by an appropriate authorization, signed by the patient or the person respon-sible for the patient. Inquiries by the patient's lawyer, insurer, or employer must be in writing and must, like all other requests for medical information, be accompanied by the patient's signed authorization.

All patients have the right to know where and what their information is used for after being collected by your office. To protect these rights the federal government developed the *Personal Information Protection and Electronic Documents Act* (PIPEDA), which governs all "commercial activities"

FIGURE **13.1** **Canadian Medical Licensing Authorities**

ALBERTA
College of Physicians and Surgeons of Alberta
http://www.cpsa.ab.ca

#900 Manulife Place, 10180-101 Street Edmonton, Alberta T5J 4P8	Tel: (780) 423-4764 Toll-free: 1-800-561-3899 Fax: (780) 420-0651

BRITISH COLUMBIA
College of Physicians and Surgeons of British Columbia
http://www.cpsbc.bc.ca

400–858 Beatty Street Vancouver, British Columbia V6B 1C1	Tel: (604) 733-7758 Toll-free: 1-800-461-3008 Fax: (604) 733-3503

MANITOBA
College of Physicians and Surgeons of Manitoba
http://www.umanitoba.ca/colleges/cps

1000–1661 Portage Avenue Winnipeg, Manitoba R3J 3T7	Tel: (204) 774-4344 Fax: (204) 774-0750

NEW BRUNSWICK
College of Physicians and Surgeons of New Brunswick
http://www.cpsnb.org

One Hampton Road, Suite 300 Rothesay, New Brunswick E2E 5K8	Tel: (506) 849-5050 Toll-free: 1-800-667-4641

NEWFOUNDLAND
Newfoundland Medical Board
http://www.nmb.ca

139 Water Street, Suite 603 St. John's, Newfoundland and Labrador A1C 1B2	Tel: (709) 726-8546 Fax: (709) 726-4725

NORTHWEST TERRITORIES
Professional Licensing, NWT
http://www.behealthycanada.com/goto/62537

Department of Health and Social Services Centre Square Tower, 8th Floor Box 1320 Yellowknife, Northwest Territories X1A 2L9	Tel: (867) 920-8058 Fax: (867) 873-0484

NOVA SCOTIA
College of Physicians and Surgeons of Nova Scotia
http://www.cpsns.ns.ca

Sentry Place, Suite 200 1559 Brunswick Street Halifax, Nova Scotia B3J 2G1	Tel: (902) 422-5823 Fax: (902) 422-5035

NUNAVUT

Government of Nunavut
Department of Health & Social Services
Operations and Professional Practice
Nunavut Government Building, 2nd Floor
Box 390
Kugluktuk, Nunavut
X0B 0E0

Tel: (867) 982-7668
Fax: (867) 982-3256

ONTARIO
College of Physicians and Surgeons of Ontario
http://www.cpso.on.ca

80 College Street
Toronto, Ontario
M5G 2E2

Tel: (416) 967-2600
Toll-free: 1-800-961-3330
Fax: (416) 961-3330

PRINCE EDWARD ISLAND
College of Physicians and Surgeons of Prince Edward Island

199 Grafton Street
Charlottetown, Prince Edward Island
C1A 1L2

Tel: (902) 566-3861

QUEBEC
Collège des Médecins du Québec
http://www.cmq.org

2170 Boulevard René-Lévesque Ouest
Montréal, Québec
H3H 2T8

Tel: (514) 933-4441
Toll-free: 1-888-MÉDECIN
Fax: (514) 933-3112

SASKATCHEWAN
College of Physicians and Surgeons of Saskatchewan
http://quadrant.net./cpss

211 Fourth Avenue South
Saskatoon, Saskatchewan
S7K 1N1

Tel: (306) 244-7355
Toll-free: 1-800-667-1668
Fax: (306) 244-0900

YUKON
Yukon Medical Council

Registrar of Medical Practitioners
P.O. Box 2703 C-5
Whitehorse, Yukon
Y1A 2C6

Tel: (867) 667-5111
Fax: (867) 667-3609

FIGURE **13.1** **Canadian Medical Licensing Authorities, cont'd**

and came into force in January 2004. Hospitals are exempt from PIPEDA; however, physicians' offices are not. Federal law contains a provision stating that if a province can demonstrate to the federal government that it has legislation that is substantially similar in terms of the level of privacy protection it affords, the provincial law will prevail.

Ontario has introduced such a bill, called the *Personal Health Information Protection Act* (PHIPA), which was proclaimed as law in November 2004.

Medical offices in Ontario need to develop a privacy policy and the physician, or an employee delegate, must agree to take on the responsibility for compliance with PHIPA. Physicians in Ontario can access their medical association Web site for assistance with guidelines, forms, etc., if necessary. It is good practice to have your provincial Privacy Statement displayed where patients can easily read it (see Figure 13.2 for an example).

MEDICAL RECORDS

Proper medical records are considered an essential component of the physician–patient relationship. The main reason for making and keeping records is to assist the doctor in the continuing care of the patient. The importance of complete and comprehensive records from a medico-legal point of view cannot be overemphasized.

In some provinces, the regulations or bylaws of the College of Physicians and Surgeons or its equivalent specify minimum standards for maintaining, organizing, and retaining medical records by physicians. For example, a section of the regulations under the *Regulated Health Professions Act* requires that a member shall do the following:

(a) Keep a legible written or printed record with respect to each patient of the member containing the following information:
    (i)   the name, address, and date of birth of the patient
    (ii) if the patient has a health insurance, the health insurance number
    (iii) for a consultation, the name and address of the primary care physician and of any health professional who referred the patient
    (iv) every written report received respecting the patient from another member or health professional
    (v)   the date of each professional encounter with the patient
    (vi) a record of the assessment of the patient including
        a) the history obtained by the member
        b) the particulars of each medical examination by the member, and
        c) a note of any investigations ordered by the member and the results of the investigations
    (vii) a record of the disposition of the patient, including
        a) an indication of each treatment prescribed or administered by the member.
        b) a record of professional advice given by the member, and
        c) particulars of any referral made by the member
    (viii) a record of all fees charged which were not in respect of insured services under the *Health Insurance Act*, which may be kept separately from the clinical record
    (ix) Any additional records required by regulation

FIGURE **13.2** **Privacy Statement**

Privacy Statement

As your doctor, my staff and I are bound by law and ethics to safeguard your privacy and the confidentiality of your personal information.

This includes:

- collecting only the information that may be necessary for your care;
- keeping accurate and up-to-date records;
- safeguarding the medical records in my possession;
- sharing information with other healthcare providers and organizations on a "need to know" basis where required for your health care;
- disclosing information to third parties only with your express consent, or when necessary for legal reasons; and
- retaining/destroying records in accordance with the law.

Your request for care from me implies consent for our collection, use and disclosure of your personal information for purposes related to your care. As noted above, other purposes require your express consent.

You have the right to see your records. You may also obtain copies of your records – please see the receptionist for our fees for this service. Please speak to me if you have concerns about the accuracy of your records.

If you would like to discuss our privacy policy in more detail, or have specific questions or complaints about how your information is handled, please speak to me and I will try to resolve them.*

Oct 2004

*If your complaint is not resolved to your satisfaction by my office, you may wish to contact the Information and Privacy Commissioner of Ontario at (416) 326-3333 or 1(800) 387-0073.

SOURCE: The above Privacy Statement first appeared in the October 2004 issue of the *Ontario Medical Review*, and is reproduced here with the permission of the Ontario Medical Association.

(b)   Keep a day book, daily diary, or appointment record containing the name of each patient who is encountered professionally or treated or for whom a professional service is rendered by the member.

Generally speaking, entries in a patient's record should be dated and clearly written or typed. All significant information should be put into the record, including personal and family data, the past and present history obtained by the doctor, the doctor's findings, advice and recommendations concerning investigation and treatment, discussion of risks of treatment, alternative forms of therapy, and any other pertinent information about the patient's medical management. Events that may or may not involve the doctor should also be noted in the record—for example, vital signs taken by the nurse, changed or cancelled appointments, the issuance of printed instructions or pamphlets to the patient, referral arrangements, and so on.

If a patient is thought to be allergic to certain medications, the office record should contain a clearly discernible warning to that effect, so that this important information is readily available whenever a prescription is given to the patient. Likewise, patient charts should be "flagged" when follow-up appointments, review examinations, and so forth are necessary.

Some doctors use "Problem Lists" in their records. These are a type of flowsheet on which diagnoses and other important clinical information are recorded. Such information is thereby readily available to the doctor for review at the time of each encounter with the patient.

Many doctors find it useful to keep in the patient's record a copy of each prescription given to the patient. A notation should be made in the record whenever a prescription is given or renewed by telephone.

Retention of Records

The regulations under the *Regulated Health Professions Act* of Ontario require that a physician keep the records required by regulation for at least ten years after the date of the last entry in the record or until ten years after the day on which the patient reached, or would have reached, the age of 18 years, or until the member ceases to practise medicine, whichever occurs first. Other provinces have similar requirements. Apart from these statutory requirements, it is wise for doctors to keep their medical records for as long as there is an appreciable risk that the records may be required for the purpose of defence against a complaint or claim. Clinical records are often the most important single factor in the defence of a lawsuit arising out of a doctor's work. They are also often necessary when dealing with a complaint to the provincial licensing authority. A doctor should maintain control over records as long as possible; they should never be destroyed before ten years have elapsed following the last entry date. In some provinces, there is a small possibility that the doctor may be sued more than ten years after the last contact with the patient, even though that likelihood is remote.

When doctors leave practice because of retirement or for any other reason, or when they relocate their practices, they should ensure that their records are kept intact, that they are accessible, and that the information contained in them is available to their patients' new doctors. When a doctor dies, the estate should make appropriate arrangements for the safekeeping of records until there is no likelihood that a claim will be made against the estate. It is prudent for physicians to include in estate planning provisions for the care of their medical records. When a physician in family medicine and primary care ceases to practise medicine, the physician can either transfer records to a member with the same address and telephone number or notify each patient that the records will be destroyed two years after the notification. The patient may obtain the records or have the member transfer the records to another physician within the two years.

Production of Records

Occasionally, patients or relatives of patients will ask for their records for one reason or another. It is generally considered that the record is the property of the doctor or clinic and not that of the patient. However, patients are entitled to have access to and receive copies of their entire medical record, including all notes made by the attending physician and all consultation reports that are part of the attending physician's records, even where these are marked as confidential. This applies to information compiled in the context of the physician–patient relationship. Physicians may charge a reasonable fee for the preparation and copying of the records.

A physician may refuse to provide a patient with access to his or her records if the doctor believes that such access would result in a substantial risk to the physical, mental, or emotional health of the patient or harm to a third party. The physician must exercise this discretion reasonably and for very limited purposes. The patient may challenge the physician's decision in court. The onus is on the physician to justify the denial of access to records in such cases.

Medical administrative assistants should not give the doctor's office record (or a photocopy of it), or the information contained in the record (including consultants' reports, laboratory and X-ray reports, and so on), to a patient or a relative to read. Such records and reports frequently require interpretation for the patient, and the doctor's administrative assistant should arrange for the patient to have time with the doctor to discuss the information in the record.

Of course, if the doctor is presented with a court order to produce a patient's record, the doctor must comply, but steps should be taken to ensure that a duplicate copy of the record is kept by the doctor. The doctor should also retain a copy of the court order.

A second exception to releasing patients' records might arise when the doctor is served with a subpoena or a summons requiring submission of evidence in any legal action or other proceeding. The doctor may have to bring along a copy of the patient's office record. On occasion, a doctor may also be directed to forward a copy of a patient's record to the College of Physicians and Surgeons or its equivalent.

If a lawyer requests records, the physician can send only patient records that apply to the physician's direct patient care. Consultation notes, correspondence, and such from other physicians involved in the patient's care *must not* be released.

Transfer of Records

If a patient decides to transfer to another doctor's practice, the patient may ask the first doctor to forward the record to the second doctor, or the new doctor may ask for the record. A doctor should comply with such a request by sending a summary of the record or, if the first doctor prefers, a photocopy of pertinent portions of it. The first doctor should retain possession or control of the actual record. (On occasion, a doctor may have custody of another provider's record. Before transmitting such records or photocopies, the doctor might like to obtain medico-legal advice.) See Box 13.5 for a list of steps to follow when transferring patient records.

The doctor should obtain appropriate authorization from the patient (or the patient's legal guardian) even when transferring medical information or clinical record material to the patient's new doctor.

When a summary or photocopy of the record is sent to another doctor, a notation should be made in the record indicating when and to whom it was sent.

13.5   Transfer of Records

Obtain written authorization from the patient (Power Of Attorney or legal guardian).

Obtain a prepared summary or copy the pertinent information.

Send requested information, including a copy of the release of information.

Make a notation in the chart stating when and where the information was sent.

Retain the original chart for the first physician.

MEDICAL REPORTS

The Code of Ethics of the Canadian Medical Association adopted in most provinces states, "An ethical physician will, on the patient's request, assist him by supplying the information required to enable the patient to receive any benefits to which the patient may be entitled." This ethical duty is also affected in the province of Ontario by the regulations under the *Regulated Health Professions Act*, which requires the doctor to provide within a reasonable time "any report or certificate requested by a patient or his authorized agent in respect of an examination or treatment performed by the member." There is, therefore, a clear obligation, imposed ethically and by law, for a doctor to provide the patient or the patient's authorized agent with a report when requested to do so.

Unless reporting is required by legislation, as mentioned earlier, a doctor should obtain a signed authorization from the patient before releasing medical information. In other words, if a doctor is going to provide information about a patient to a third party, appropriate authorization must be obtained before doing so. When the information contained in the report is of a particularly sensitive nature, the patient should be alerted to the contents of the report. Whenever a doctor prepares a report, issues a certificate, or completes a form, a copy should be filed in the patient's chart. In some situations, the patient will not be entitled to receive a copy of the report from the physician and should be so advised.

A special kind of report is a medico-legal report, that is, one that is requested by a lawyer. The College of Physicians and Surgeons expects a doctor to provide a patient's lawyer with a report if requested to do so. The lawyer's request should be written, providing the doctor with an appropriate authorization, signed by the patient or, if the patient is deceased, by the executor or administrator of the patient's estate. This authorization should outline specifically what information is required. If a proper authorization (sometimes called a "direction" or "release") does not accompany the lawyer's request, the doctor should ask the lawyer for one before submitting a medical report. The doctor's report should be forwarded to the lawyer within a reasonable period of time. The doctor should keep a copy of the report.

If the doctor has reason to believe that the patient consulted a lawyer because of dissatisfaction with the doctor's care, the doctor may wish to seek the advice of a medical defence organization before responding to the lawyer.

MISCELLANEOUS

Problems that may have legal implications sometimes arise from the day-to-day events in doctors' offices and clinics.

Each medical administrative assistant should discuss with the doctor the type of advice he or she may give by telephone as well as the doctor's instructions about dealing with requests for appointments, referrals, reports, and so on.

Problems may be averted by an efficient system for handling incoming telephone calls and noting in patients' records the nature of the calls.

Medical administrative assistants who witness patients signing consent for treatment forms should assure themselves that the description of the proposed treatment on the form is correct. They should also satisfy themselves with the identity and competence of the patients who sign such forms. Should a patient have questions about the proposed procedure, the doctor should be specifically notified that the patient has unanswered questions and concerns.

FIGURE **13.3**   **Authorization for Release of Patient Information**

AUTHORIZATION FOR
RELEASE OF PATIENT INFORMATION

I hereby authorize _____
                           (Name of facility releasing the information)

to release the following information _____
                                          (Description of information to be disclosed)

_____

to _____
        (Name and address of person/agency requesting the information)

from the records of _____   _____
                           (Name of Patient)   *(Date of Birth dd/mm/yy)*

                     _____
                           (Address of Patient)

concerning treatment on _____
                              (Dates of contact/hospitalization)

I understand that this information is to be used by the recipient for the purpose of:_____

_____

_____

_____   _____
(Witness)   *(Signature of patient or person lawfully authorized)*

                                        _____
                                        (Relationship to patient)

                                        _____
                                        (Date dd/mm/yy)

NOTES: This authorization must contain the **original signature** of:
- the patient;
- where the record is of a former patient who is deceased, the personal representative of the patient;
- the parent or person who has lawful custody of an unmarried patient under sixteen years of age;
- a person lawfully authorized to make treatment decisions on behalf of an incapable person.

June 2000

FIGURE **13.4** **Consent to the Disclosure, Transmittal, or Examination of a Clinical Record.**

Form 14
Mental Health Act

Consent to the
Disclosure, Transmittal or Examination
of a Clinical Record
under Section 29 of the Act

Ontario

I, _____
(print full name of person)

of _____
(address)

hereby consent to the disclosure or transmittal to or the examination by _____
(print name)

of the clinical record compiled in _____
(name of psychiatric facility)

in respect of _____
(name of patient)   (date of birth, where available)

See
Notes
4 and 5.

_____   _____
(witness)   (signature)

_____
(if other than the patient,
state relationship to the patient)

Dated the _____ day of _____ , 20 ____ .

NOTES: 1. Consent to the disclosure, transmittal or examination of a clinical record may be given by the patient where
mentally competent or, where the patient is not mentally competent, by the person authorized under section
1*a* of the Act to consent on behalf of the patient. See subsection 29(3) of the Act.

2. Clause 29(1)(b) of the Act provides,
"(b) 'patient' includes former patient, out-patient, former out-patient and anyone who is or has been
detained in a psychiatric facility."

3. Clause 1(g) of the Act provides,
"(g) 'mentally competent' means having the ability to understand the subject-matter in respect of which
consent is requested and able to appreciate the consequences of giving or withholding consent."

4. Subsection 1*a*(1) of the Act provides,
"1*a*.--(1) A person may give or refuse consent on behalf of a patient who is not mentally competent if the
person has attained the age of sixteen years, is apparently mentally competent, is available and willing to
give or refuse consent and is described in one of the following paragraphs:
    1. The committee of the person appointed for the patient under the *Mental Incompetency Act.*
    2. The patient's representative appointed under section 1*b* or 1*c*.
    3. The person to whom the patient is married or the person of the opposite sex with whom the patient is
    living outside marriage in a conjugal relationship or was living outside marriage in a conjugal
    relationship immediately before being admitted to the psychiatric facility, if in the case of unmarried
    persons they,
        i. have cohabited for at least one year,
        ii. are together the parents of a child, or
        iii. have together entered into a cohabitation agreement under section 53 of the *Family Law Act, 1986.*
    4. A child of the patient.
    5. A parent of the patient or a person who has lawful custody of the patient.
    6. A brother or sister of the patient.
    7. Any other next of kin of the patient.
    8. The Official Guardian."
See sections 1*b* and 1*c* of the Act regarding patients' representatives.

5. Where the consent is signed by someone other than the patient, the relationship to the patient must be set out
below the signature.

SOURCE: © Queen's Printer for Ontario, 2005. Reproduced with permission.

The physician will assess whether or not the patient is competent. If there is any doubt, he will notify the patient's family, the legal guardian, or the person holding the **Power of Attorney (POA)** before obtaining consent.

A child of any age can give or refuse consent. The physician will asses the child's competency to understand the information presented in order to obtain informed consent. The child's consent must meet the criteria of the adult's consent.

Bookings for operative and investigative procedures should be exact and clear. Copies of booking slips should be retained. Notations should be made in patients' records about the arrangements that have been made.

Injuries sustained by a patient in a doctor's office can lead to a claim for damages. Those who work in medical offices should always be alert to situations that could put patients' safety in jeopardy.

Medical administrative assistants are important members of the healthcare team. A knowledgeable and caring medical administrative assistant can play a significant role in the interaction between patients and the providers of medical care.

Historically, the medical profession has been very aware of the confidentiality of patient information. The recent enactment of federal and provincial freedom of information legislation reinforces the importance of confidentiality. Before releasing any information concerning a patient, it is imperative that you secure in writing the permission of the patient. Figure 13.3 is a sample of a release of information form.

When working in a mental health setting, a Form 14 (Ontario) (see Figure 13.4) must be completed by the patient before information can be released.

ASSIGNMENT 13.1

The material for this test assignment will be provided by your instructor.

TOPICS FOR DISCUSSION

1. Euthanasia, or the aiding, abetting, or counselling of a suicide, is illegal in Canada. Discuss your feelings around this issue.

2. A patient has disclosed to you that the physician has done something inappropriate. The patient wants to report the doctor and is asking you for guidance on how to do this. How would you handle this situation?

3. Some statutes require mandatory reporting. What circumstances do you feel would require mandatory reporting under the *Aeronautics Act*, the *Coronor's Act*, and the *Child and Family Services Act*?

4. Medical administrative assistants and other medical aides act on behalf of the doctor. Discuss some scenarios in which the doctor may be held responsible for his or her staff's actions.

CHAPTER 14

Your Job Search

CHAPTER OUTLINE

Entry-Level Positions
Where to Find Job Leads
What to Consider

Your Letter of Application and Résumé
Interview Skills
Topics for Discussion

LEARNING OBJECTIVES

After reading this chapter, you will be able to

- Identify entry-level positions
- Identify considerations for your job search
- Recognize the importance of a letter of application and résumé

- Recognize appropriate formats to fit your résumé style
- Plan carefully for your interview

KEY TERMS

Networking: The term networking means a netlike combination or system of lines or channels (*Canadian Intermediate Dictionary*). Your personal network can exist of relatives, friends, or acquaintances who may have information or contacts to assist you.

Networking is information sharing; it is not one-sided.

Résumé: The term résumé simply means a summary. It is sometimes also referred to as a "curriculum vitae."

Your medical administrative assistant program has taken you through all the basic requirements for a position in a medical office or a medical environment. The next step is to find the "right" job. In today's society, education and experience are generally listed as requirements of the position in job advertisements. You have the education, but how do you gain the experience?

ENTRY-LEVEL POSITIONS

Most entry-level positions, such as file clerk and receptionist, do not require the same level of experience that would be required for, say, a medical administrative assistant in a physician's office or a ward secretary in a hospital emergency ward. It may be necessary for you to begin your career as a file clerk or a receptionist in order to gain the experience that will allow you to advance to a higher-level job.

Entry-level positions allow you to gain valuable knowledge and experience without having the responsibilities of a more senior job. Entry-level jobs also provide the opportunity to observe and learn the activities in your environment. You will receive ideas and constructive criticisms from your administrators and peers that will help you increase your knowledge of the requirements of your chosen career.

It is essential that you always practise the points covered in Chapter 1 concerning personal qualities and appearance, customer service, and skills.

WHERE TO FIND JOB LEADS

Several months before graduation, you should begin thinking about sources of information for your job search.

Most colleges have a placement office that publishes notices on a bulletin board or advises program instructors of employment opportunities. Some job opportunities are advertised in the classified section of the newspaper. Employment agencies servicing the medical profession will also be interested in your **résumé**.

Networking is often the best way to secure a job. Inform your primary care doctor that you will soon be graduating. He or she may hear of job opportunities through his or her medical network. It is unlikely that your primary care physician will hire you to work in his or her office if family members also attend the same physician, due to access to confidential information. Attend the local medical secretaries association (Health Care Associates) meetings if there is a chapter in your area. These meetings are an excellent opportunity to network, gain educational information, and keep updated on changes happening in your profession. The Ontario Medical Secretaries Association–Health Care Associates (OMSA-HCA) has a job bank that you can access if you are a member or a student member. Write to your local or provincial association for more information or access its Web site. The Ontario Web site is http://www.omsa-hca.org.

Job opportunities can also be found through the Internet, but do not make this the focus of your search. Visiting medical clinics or facilities is also important, as often positions at these locations are posted on a bulletin board. See Box 14.1 for a list of resources associated with job searching.

14.1 Job Search Resources

Networking
Newspapers
Employment agencies
Professional societies
Volunteering

WHAT TO CONSIDER

When beginning your job search, it is important to consider your expectations, needs, and abilities. For example, if you had difficulty with medical machine transcription, it would be unwise to seek a job as a transcriptionist. If you have a very pleasing personality, a pleasant smile, and enjoy meeting people, a job in the admitting office in your local hospital or as a receptionist in a complementary care setting might be of interest to you.

Another important point to consider is whether it may be necessary for you to relocate in order to get a job. Administrative skills are very portable. Can you think of any business that does not require some type of office skills? Providing there is no language barrier, your skills are required in all parts of the world. Of course, you may not have to move to the other side of the continent to get a job. However, if there is a shortage of jobs in your area, you may have to consider moving to another city or region. And if you are adventurous, you may find yourself in another country.

Investigate the salary level, skill requirements, location, benefits, and working hours of the position you want. Are the services provided by the organization in your area of interest? Is there room for advancement in the organization? Will the salary level allow you to reach a goal you have set, such as to buy a car or move into your own apartment? All of these things must be considered, because if you accept a position and you are not happy, you will not work to your fullest potential.

Because of today's job market, it may be necessary to accept a job that is not exactly what you want; however, work with the idea that you are gaining valuable experience and qualifications for when the right job comes along.

When you are invited for an interview, be prepared. You will be assessed based on your ability to communicate (i.e., maintain eye contact, use appropriate grammar, and provide descriptive answers to questions, rather than a simple "yes" or "no"), on your appearance (dress in appropriate business attire), and on your attitude (be courteous and positive). If you have any facial piercings, do not wear them to an interview.

14.2
Experience is an asset but not a prerequisite in acquiring the position.

Ask a peer to conduct a mock interview for practice. The person may point out mannerisms or nervous habits that are distracting, for example, finger tapping, voice inflections, or constant throat clearing. Be ready to sell yourself. Tell the interviewer about your achievements. Following the interview, send a thank-you letter.

YOUR LETTER OF APPLICATION AND RÉSUMÉ

Colleges often provide instruction in communication classes for writing letters of application and résumés.

When preparing your letter of application and résumé, talk to your peers and instructors and get their ideas. Research formats in textbooks, on-line, and in computer programs such as Windows. However, when you put all of the facts and ideas together, make certain that the finished product projects *you*. Do not copy from a textbook figure. The person reading the application wants to know about you, not a textbook character.

For students who have not had formal instruction on the preparation of a letter of application and résumé, we have provided a job advertisement (see Box 14.3), a letter of application responding to the advertisement (see Figure 14.1), and some examples of résumés. Figure 14.2 is an example of a contemporary résumé. Figure 14.3 is an example of a professional résumé. Both are formats available on many computer programs.

In developing your résumé, you should use a format that best reflects your skills and abilities and emphasizes the particular requirements of your job targets.

Figures 14.1 through 14.3 are examples of résumés responding to the ad listed in Box 14.3.

14.3
Medical Administrative Assistant required for busy family physician's office. Sound knowledge of terminology and anatomy, and office procedures (reception, appointment scheduling, billing, and records management) as applied to a medical office environment is required. Excellent communication and computer skills, medical machine transcription, time management, and problem-solving skills are essential. Apply to Dr. Jasbir Sandhu, 310 O'Connor Street, Ottawa, Ontario, J5Z 2X8.

Text continued on p. 317.

FIGURE **14.1** **Letter of Application**

1356 Gloucester Drive
Ottawa, ON
Z8X 1X9

October 21, 20__

Dr. Jasbir Sandhu
310 O'Connor Street
Ottawa, Ontario
J5Z 2X8

Dear Dr. Sandhu:

Subject: Application for a Medical Assistant Position

You can meet your requirement for a Medical Administrative Assistant as listed in the (paper) on (date) by positively considering my application. The enclosed résumé outlines my skills and experience that are most relevant in securing a clerical position in the medical environment.

Excellent administrative skills, a sound knowledge of medical terminology and anatomy, and demonstrated computer abilities will allow me to effectively meet the challenges of a busy family physician's office. Demonstrated time-management and problem-solving skills combined with my high energy level and positive, progressive attitude will provide you with a co-operative member of your healthcare team.

My education, background, and keen desire to succeed have prepared me to approach future challenges with enthusiasm and determination. A progressive and efficient family practice such as yours will enable me to work at my best while achieving your organizational goals.

I would appreciate a personal interview to allow a detailed discussion of my future contribution to your organization. I can be reached at (613) 555-0000.

Sincerely,

Daphne Smith

Attachment: Résumé

FIGURE **14.2**   **Résumé**

1356 Gloucester Drive,
Ottawa, Ontario
Z8X 1X9

613-742-9856

Daphne R. Smith

Objective

To work full-time in a Medical Office Environment

Experience

20__ to 20__   Dr. J.E. Plunkett   Ottawa
Office Assistant (Two-week consolidation)

- Performed reception and secretarial functions, medical machine transcription, filing medical documents, answering telephones and scheduling appointments.
- Prepared computerized billing and transmitted electronically to Ministry of Health using (insert name) system.
- Prepared consultation and medical correspondence.
- Effectively monitored patient flow and ensured records management.
- Assisted physician with medical tests.

20__ to 20___   Anytown Medical Centre   Anytown
Office Worker

- Handled high volume of bookings and all routine work for medical office including filing, reception, telephone.
- Input patient records, prepared and handled billing documentation for computer input.
- Accurately transcribed medical dictation.
- Organized and maintained a workable filing system of over 400 medical files respecting patient confidentiality.
- Assisted nurses with routine medical procedures.
- Handled high pressure situations and deadlines.

20__ to 20__   Anytown Hospital   Anytown
Teen Volunteer

- Assisted nurses with errand service.
- Transported newly admitted patients to rooms and patients for tests.

Education

20__ to 20__   Anytown College   Anytown

- Medical Office Administration Diploma.
- Recipient of Medical Secretarial Association Outstanding Student Award.

Interests

Squash, jogging, curling, skiing, singing, and crafts.

FIGURE **14.3** **Professional Résumé**

DAPHNE R. SMITH

OBJECTIVE

To work full-time in a Medical Office Environment

EXPERIENCE

20__ to 20__   Dr. J.E. Plunkett   Ottawa

Office Assistant (Two-week consolidation)

- Performed reception and secretarial functions, medical machine transcription, filing medical documents, answering telephones, and scheduling appointments.
- Prepared computerized billing and transmitted electronically to Ministry of Health using (insert name) system.
- Prepared consultation and medical correspondence.
- Effectively monitored patient flow and ensured records management.
- Assisted physician with medical tests.

20__ to 20___   Anytown Medical Centre   Anytown

Office Worker

- Handled high volume of bookings and all routine work for medical office including filing, reception, telephone.
- Input patient records, prepared and handled billing documentation for computer input.
- Accurately transcribed medical dictation.
- Organized and maintained a workable filing system of over 400 medical files respecting patient confidentiality.
- Assisted nurses with routine medical procedures.
- Handled high pressure situations and deadlines.

20__ to 20__   Anytown Hospital   Anytown

Teen Volunteer

- Assisted nurses with errand service.
- Transported newly admitted patients to rooms and patients for tests.

continued

EDUCATION

20__ to 20__   Anytown College   Anytown
- Medical Office Administration Diploma.
- Recipient of Medical Secretarial Association Outstanding Student Award.

INTERESTS

Squash, jogging, curling, skiing, singing, and crafts.

2

1356 GLOUCESTER DRIVE • OTTAWA, ONTARIO, Z8X 1X9 • PHONE (613) 742-9856

FIGURE **14.3   Professional Résumé, cont'd**

The functional/combination résumé in Figure 14.4 highlights the applicant's skills, strengths, and accomplishments that target specific job and work objectives. Work experience and abilities are listed by key functional areas in the order that best meets the requirements of the job. Those wanting to draw attention to a strong skill set required by a specific job and away from limited work experience, career change/redirection, or re-entry into the job market will benefit from this format.

INTERVIEW SKILLS

Plan carefully for your interview, and remember that the interview begins the moment you arrive in the office. The following factors will be evaluated by the interviewer:

- Punctuality
- Appearance
- Posture
- Mannerisms
- Courtesy
- Attitude

Arrive 10 to 15 minutes before your appointment. If you are going to be late due to transportation problems, call as soon as you can and explain the situation. If you are not sure where the exact location of the interview is, scout it out in advance.

Your appearance should be professional: for women a light scent, conservative makeup, minimal jewellery, and appropriate office attire; for men, a suit is preferable, and facial hair should be trimmed.

Colours should be subtle, as the focus should be on you and not on what you are wearing.

14.4   What Not to Do during an Interview

Do not chew gum or candy.
Avoid nervous gestures such as fidgeting, stroking your
    face, or tugging at your clothes.
Do not interrupt.
Do not argue, brag, or criticize.

14.5   What Does the Employer Want?

A person with the skills to do the job
A person who has a neat appearance and looks as if he or
    she fits the job
A person who is dependable and can prove that he or she is
    a reliable team member

FIGURE **14.4**   **Résumé (Functional/Combination)**

DAPHNE R. SMITH

1356 Gloucester Drive
Ottawa, Ontario
Z8X 1X9

SUMMARY OF JOB-RELATED SKILLS

- Work effectively in a busy medical office environment
- Knowledge of medical procedures, terminology and anatomy
- Familiar with computers
- Effective communication skills
- Ability to recognize and solve problems
- Effective time management

SKILLS AND ABILITIES

Medical Administrative Support

- Performed reception duties and secretarial functions: medical machine transcription, filing medical documents, answering telephones, and scheduling appointments
- Effectively monitored patient flow and ensured records management
- Knowledge of medical terminology, anatomy and physiology and paramedical studies
- Exceptional keyboarding and office skills
- Organized and maintained a workable filing system of over 400 medical files respecting patient confidentiality
- Assisted physician with medical tests and nurses with routine medical procedures and errand service
- Transported newly admitted patients to rooms and patients for tests

Computer Knowledge

- Computer software applications, Microsoft Word, Excel, and Power Point
- Prepared computerized billing and transmitted electronically to Ministry of Health using "xxs" system
- Entered all patient records and retrieved data from patient database
- Composed correspondence, prepared reports, completed hospital requisitions, merged letters with labels for mailing of 500

Time Management/Problem Solving

- As receptionist, answered and redirected heavy load of incoming calls and relayed messages to staff
- Handled high volume of patients while meeting appointment booking schedule
- Effectively handled high pressure situations and office procedures; met all billing deadlines
- Greeted patients and suppliers in a friendly and courteous manner

RELEVANT EXPERIENCE

Dr. J. E. Plunkett Medical Office   20__
Office Assistant (Two-week consolidation)

Anytown Medical Centre   20__ to 20__
Office Worker (Part-time)

Anytown Hospital   20__ to 20 __
Teen Volunteer

EDUCATION

Anytown Business College   20__ to 20__
Medical Office Administration Diploma

- Recipient of Medical Secretarial Association Outstanding Graduate Award for academic excellence

MEMBERSHIPS/CERTIFICATION

Medical Secretaries Association

- As student member, assisted with organizing 20__ Clinic Day.

Anytown Curling Club

- President – Junior Section
- Certified Curl Canada Instructor

RECREATIONAL ACTIVITIES

Squash, jogging, curling, skiing, singing, and crafts

REFERENCES

Available upon request

FIGURE **14.4** Résumé (Functional/Combination), cont'd

ASSIGNMENT **14.1**

If you have not been required to do so in another course, select an advertisement from the "Help Wanted" section of your local newspaper and prepare a letter of application and résumé.

Ask your instructor to assess the finished product and make suggestions for improvement, if necessary.

ASSIGNMENT **14.2**

Extract from your portfolio the rating sheet you completed in Assignment 1.3. Would your ratings in any of the categories change?

ASSIGNMENT **14.3**

Extract from your portfolio the skills and personal qualities inventory sheet completed in Assignment 1.4. Reassess your skill levels. Have you acquired any new skills? How would you rate those skills? Have any of your skills improved; how much?

Reassess your personal qualities. Would you rate any of your personal qualities as being stronger than in your original rating?

TOPICS FOR DISCUSSION

1. What are some examples of positive body language during an interview? What are some examples of negative body language?

2. Discuss appropriate attire to wear to an interview and inappropriate attire.

Common Abbreviations Used in the Healthcare Field

Following is a list of common abbreviations used in the medical profession for your reference.

abs. feb.	without fever
a.c.	before eating
ad	to; up to
adhib	to be administered
ad lib.	as desired
agit	shake, stir
alt. dieb.	every other day
alt. hor.	every other hour
alt. noc.	every other night
aq.	water
b.i.d.	twice daily
b.i.n.	twice a night
bis in 7d.	twice a week
BP	blood pressure
BUN	blood urea nitrogen
c or c̄	with
C	Celsius
ca.	about
Ca	cancer
cap.	capsule
CBC	complete blood count
cc.	cubic centimetre
c.m.	tomorrow morning
c.m.s.	to be taken tomorrow morning
c.n.	tomorrow night
CNS	central nervous system
comp.	compound
contra	against
CV	cardiovascular
d	day
/d	daily
D	dose
D&C	dilation and curettage
dr.	dram
dx	diagnosis
ECG	electrocardiogram
ECT	electroconvulsive therapy
EEG	electroencephalogram
EKG	electrocardiogram
EMG	electromyogram
e.m.p.	as directed
ESR	erythrocyte sedimentation rate
GI	gastrointestinal

gm	gram
gr.	grain
grad.	by degrees
Gtt., gtt.	drops
GTT	glucose tolerance test
h	hour
HEENT	head, eyes, ears, nose, throat
hgb	hemoglobin
h.n.	tonight
h.s.	at bedtime
hx	history
I.M.	intramuscular
IU	international unit
I.V.	intravenously
kg	kilogram
L	litre
liq.	liquid, fluid
mEq.	milliequivalent
mitt.	send
NYD	not yet diagnosed
os.	mouth
P	pulse
PBI	protein-bound iodine
p.c.	after meals
p.o.	by mouth
ppm	parts per million
p.r.	through the rectum
p.r.n.	as needed
q.h	every hour
q. 2h	every two hours
q. 3h	every three hours
q.i.d.	four times a day
q.l.	as much as wanted
q.s.	as much as needed
R	respiration
RBC	red blood count
Rx	prescription
s or š	without
s.cut., sc	subcutaneously
SGOT	serum glutamic oxaloacetic transaminase
SGPT	serum glutamic pyruvic transaminase
Sl	sublingual
stat.	immediately
suppos.	suppository
syr.	syrup
T	temperature

tab.	tablet
t.i.d.	three times daily
t.i.n.	three times a night
tinct.	tincture
TKVO	to keep vein open
ung.	ointment
ur	urine
top.	topically
UV	ultraviolet
WBC	white blood count
Wt.	weight
w/v.	weight by volume

Laboratory Medicine

Normal lab ranges will vary from laboratory to laboratory. Abnormal results will be flagged on the reports and the lab ranges will be identified.

BIOCHEMISTRY

Biochemistry—Analysis of routine, drug, and special testing on blood, urine, CSF (cerebrospinal fluid), and other fluids.

Following is a list of some laboratory tests and turnaround times for your reference.

Test	Routine	Urgent	Emergent
Acetaminophen	24 hr	3 hr	90 min
Alkaline phosphate	8 hr	na	na
Amylase	8 hr	2 hr	na
Barbiturates	8 hr	3 hr	90 min
Bilirubin total	8 hr	na	na
Calcium	8 hr	2 hr	60 min
Chloride	24 hr	na	na
CK (total)	8 hr	2 hr	na
CK-2 (MB)	24 hr	na	na
Creatinine	8 hr	90 min	na
CSF–protein	na	3 hr	60 min
CSF–glucose	3 hr	90 min	na
Digoxin	24 hr	na	na
Dilantin	24 hr	na	na
Drug screen	10	na	na
Electrophoresis	72 hr	na	na
Glucose	8 hr	2 hr	60 min
HDL–C	5	na	na
Iron	4	na	na
Lithium	2	na	na
Magnesium	8 hr	na	na
Occult blood	24 hr	na	na
Osmolality	8 hr	na	na
pH	1 hr	1 hr	20 min
Phosphates	8 hr	na	na
Potassium	8 hr	90 min	60 min
Pregnancy test	8 hr	2 hr	1 hr
Protein–CSF	na	3 hr	60 min
Protein–total	8 hr	na	na
SGOT (AST)	8 hr	na	na
Sodium	8 hr	2 hr	60 min
Triglycerides	8 hr	na	na
Urate	8 hr	na	na
Urea (BUN)	8 hr	2 hr	na
Urinalysis	8 hr	60 min	na

NOTE: Electrolytes = Sodium, Potassium, Chloride
Enzymes = SGOT, LDH, CK
BUN = Urea

The following information must be included when completing a bio-chemistry requisition:

Patient's name
Patient's birth date
Patient's medical record number (if an in-patient)
Attending physician
Ordering physician
Tests required
Date and time of collection
Diagnosis or relevant clinical information

See Figure B.1 for an example of a Biochemistry/Blood Testing Requisition.

CYTOLOGY

Cytology—Testing of gynecological cervical-vaginal specimens as well as a complete range of non-gynecological specimens.

Following is a list of laboratory tests and turnaround times (if applicable) for your reference.

Test	Routine	Urgent	Emergent
Bronchial washing			
Broncho-alveolar lavage			
CMV–screen			
CSF (for malignant cells)			
Fine needle aspirates			
Gynecological smears	5	na	na
Pericardial fluid (for malignant cells)			
Peritoneal fluid (for malignant cells)			
Pleural fluid (for malignant cells)			
Sputum (for malignant cells)			
Urine (for malignant cells)			

The following information must be included when completing a cytology requisition:

a. Gynecological Requisition
   Patient's name
   Patient's birth date
   Ordering physician
   Type of specimen

FIGURE **B.1** Combined Biochemistry/Blood Testing Requisition

PETERBOROUGH REGIONAL HEALTH CENTRE
LABORATORY MEDICINE - /BLOOD TESTING REQUISITION

□ PCH □ SJHC □ Haliburton □ Minden □ Other_____   □ **Emergent**

□ In-patient   □ Out-patient   □ Referred-In

Collection Date:m\d\yr_____Time:_____   □ **Urgent**

O.R. Date:_____   Time:_____

Relevant Clinical Information/Special Instructions: □ **Routine**

_____

Ordering Physician:._____   □ **Timed** ____

Nurse:_____

✓	HAEMATOLOGY		✓	CHEMISTRY		✓	CHEMISTRY		✓	SEROLOGY	
	CBC 2000	▐▐▐▐▐		CBG 3503	▐▐▐▐▐		GGTP 3190	▐▐▐▐▐		ANA 8200	▐▐▐▐▐
	DIFF 2010	▐▐▐▐▐		(NaKCl) LYTS 3052	▐▐▐▐▐		UREA 3020	▐▐▐▐▐		ANTI-DNA 8220	▐▐▐▐▐
	CELL MORPH. 2030	▐▐▐▐▐		GLUCOSE FASTING 3003	▐▐▐▐▐		TSH 3600	▐▐▐▐▐			
	RETIC 2040	▐▐▐▐▐		GLUCOSE RANDOM 3010	▐▐▐▐▐		FREE T4 3610	▐▐▐▐▐			
	MONO SCREEN 2060	▐▐▐▐▐		GLUCOSE AC 3003	▐▐▐▐▐		VITAMIN B12 3625	▐▐▐▐▐	✓	DRUGS / MISC	
	ESR 2050	▐▐▐▐▐		GLUCOSE PC 3014	▐▐▐▐▐		RBC FOLATE 3630	▐▐▐▐▐		ACETAMINO-PHEN 3380	▐▐▐▐▐
✓	COAGULATION			CREATININE 3030	▐▐▐▐▐		FERRITIN 3340	▐▐▐▐▐		BARBITURATE SCREEN 3390	▐▐▐▐▐
	INR 2500	▐▐▐▐▐		TOTAL BILIRUBIN 3220	▐▐▐▐▐		IRON 3310	▐▐▐▐▐		SALICYLATE 3470	▐▐▐▐▐
	A.P.T.T. 2510	▐▐▐▐▐		MICRO-BILIRUBIN 3120	▐▐▐▐▐		TIBC 3320	▐▐▐▐▐		ETHANOL 3430	▐▐▐▐▐
	BLEEDING TIME 2520	▐▐▐▐▐		CALCIUM 3100	▐▐▐▐▐		IRON 3315 SATURATION	▐▐▐▐▐		DIGOXIN 3410	▐▐▐▐▐
	D-DIMER 2540	▐▐▐▐▐		PHOSPHATE 3200	▐▐▐▐▐		CORTISOL AM 9350	▐▐▐▐▐		PHENYTOIN 3420	▐▐▐▐▐
	FIBRINOGEN SCREEN 2560	▐▐▐▐▐		MAGNESIUM 3110	▐▐▐▐▐		CORTISOL PM 9355	▐▐▐▐▐		PHENOBARB 3460	▐▐▐▐▐
				URATE 3210	▐▐▐▐▐		BLOOD GASES ART 3489	▐▐▐▐▐		CARBA- 3400 MAZEPINE	▐▐▐▐▐
				TOTAL PROTEIN 3240	▐▐▐▐▐		BLOOD GASES CAP 3519	▐▐▐▐▐		THEOPHYLLINE 3480	▐▐▐▐▐
				ALBUMIN 3250	▐▐▐▐▐		BLOOD GASES VEN 3504	▐▐▐▐▐		GENTAMICIN PRE 3440	▐▐▐▐▐
				AST 3160	▐▐▐▐▐		CHOLESTEROL 3270	▐▐▐▐▐		GENTAMICIN POST 3445	▐▐▐▐▐
				LDH 3170	▐▐▐▐▐		TRIGLYCERIDES 3280	▐▐▐▐▐		LITHIUM 3450	▐▐▐▐▐
				CK 3070	▐▐▐▐▐		HDL-C 3290	▐▐▐▐▐	✓	MISC	
				CK-2 3080	▐▐▐▐▐		LDL (CALC)			HAPTOGLOBIN 360	▐▐▐▐▐
				ALK 3180 PHOSPHATASE	▐▐▐▐▐		HbA1C GLYCATED PROTIEN 3350	▐▐▐▐▐			
				ACID 3260 PHOSPHATASE	▐▐▐▐▐		SPE 3580	▐▐▐▐▐			
				AMYLASE 3090	▐▐▐▐▐		IMMUNO- 3540 GLOBULINS	▐▐▐▐▐			
							C3 3545	▐▐▐▐▐			
							C4 3550	▐▐▐▐▐			

Form # JF 5048
July/98

SOURCE: Reproduced by permission of Peterborough Regional Health Centre.

        Date smear taken
        Date of last menstrual period (LMP)
        Relevant clinical information
  b. Non-gynecological Requisition
        Patient's name
        Patient's birth date
        Ordering physician
        Type of specimen
        Date and time specimen taken
        Relevant clinical information

See Figure B.2 for an example of a Non-Gynecological Cytology Requisition.
See Figure B.3 for an example of a Gynecological Cytology Requisition.

HEMATOLOGY

Hematology—Study of blood cells, bone marrow, and coagulation.
    Following is a list of some of the laboratory tests and turnaround times for your reference.

a. Hematology

Test	Routine	Urgent	Emergent
Leukocytes	4 hr	90 min	10 min
Hemoglobin	4 hr	90 min	10 min
Hematocrit	4 hr	90 min	10 min
MCV	4 hr	90 min	10 min
Platelets	4 hr	90 min	10 min
ESR	6 hr	na	na
Reticulocytes	6 hr	na	na
Mono screen	4 hr	90 min	na
CSF count	2 hr	90 min	60 min
CSF diff.	3 hr	2 hr	90 min
Malarial parasites	3 hr	90 min	60 min
Sickle screen	3 hr	90 min	60 min
Kleihauer stain	4 hr	na	na
Semen–fertility	36 hr	na	na
Semen–post vasectomy	6 hr	na	na
Bone marrow prep.	24 hr	2 hr	na

b. Hematology—Coagulation

Test	Routine	Urgent	Emergent
Prothrombin time	4 hr	90 min	30 min
Pro-time–anticoagulant	4 hr	90 min	na

FIGURE **B.2** Non-Gynecological Cytology Requisition

Patient's Surname   Given Name

Cytopathology Requisition
Non-Gynecologic Specimens   HEALTH   CENTRE

1 Hospital Drive
Peterborough, On
K9J 1C7
(705) 743-2121 Ext 3073

(FOR LABORATORY USE ONLY)
Cytology Lab No. C_____

Requesting Physician _____

____ ____ ____ ____ ____ ____ ____ ____   ____ / _____ / ____

Provincial Health No.(if not on addressograph)   Date of Birth dd/mm/yy   **Date and Time Taken** _____

Gender: ☐ Female   ☐ Male   (if not on addressograph)   (dd/mm/yy)

Specimen Type (one specimen per requisition)				
Respiratory	**Urinary**	**Serous Fluid**	**Fine Needle Aspiration Biopsy**	
☐ Sputum	☐ Voided	☐ Pleural	☐ Breast	☐ CSF
☐ Bronchial Wash	☐ Catheterized	☐ Peritoneal	☐ Thyroid	
☐ Bronchial Brush	☐ Bladder wash	☐ Pericardial	☐ Lung	
☐ Bronchial Lavage	☐ Ureter	☐ Peritoneal Wash	☐ Liver	☐ Other:
Site:	☐ Left	☐ Other:	☐ Other:	
_____	☐ Right	_____	_____	_____
Clinical Information and Diagnosis				

For Laboratory Use Only: # Slides Made: _____

Volume (mls): _____   Specimen description: ☐Cloudy ☐Mucoid ☐Clear ☐Bloody Other _____   ☐ Brush in Alcohol ☐ Prepared Slide(s) Received # ____ ☐ Received Unfixed

Cytotechnologist_____
FORM 5050 / rev Mar 2001

FIGURE B.3 **Gynecological Cytology Requisition**

Patient's Surname *Given Name*

Cytopathology Requisition
Gynecologic - Pap Smear

PETERBOROUGH REGIONAL HEALTH CENTRE

(705) 743-2121 Ext 3073

(FOR LABORATORY USE ONLY)

Cytology Lab No. C______________________

Provincial Health No. (if not on addressograph)

Date of Birth dd/mm/yy ____ / ______ / ____ (if not on addressograph)

Submitting Physician Dr.______________________

Collected By: ______________________

Date Smear Taken (dd/mm/yy) _____ / _______ / _____

L.M.P. (first day) : ____ / ______ / ____ dd/mm/yy

Specimen Type: (check all that apply)
- ☐ Cervix
- ☐ Endocervix (slide)
- ☐ Endocervix (brush in fixative)
- ☐ Vaginal
- ☐ Other____________________

Menstrual Status:
- ☐ Pre-menopausal
- ☐ Pregnant
- ☐ Post Partum
- ☐ Peri-menopausal
- ☐ Post-menopausal

Clinical Information: (check all that apply)
- ☐ Routine
- ☐ Previous Abnormal Cytology
- ☐ Repeat Smear Requested
- ☐ Oral Contraceptive
- ☐ I.U.D.
- ☐ Hormonal R_x________________
- ☐ Radiation R_x

Additional Information and Clinical Diagnosis:

For Laboratory Use Only:

FORM 5067 / rev Jan 2004

SOURCE: Reproduced by permission of Peterborough Regional Health Centre.

ACT PTT–heparin	4 hr	90 min	60 min
Bleeding time	4 hr	na	na
Thrombin time	4 hr	2 hr	60 min
Antithrombin III	3	na	na
Lupus anticoagulant	4 hr	na	na
Protein C	10	na	na
Protein S	10	na	na
Platelet antibodies	10	na	na
Platelet count	4 hr	90 min	10 min

NOTE: CBC = Hemogram

The following information must be included when completing a hematology requisition:

Patient's name
Patient's birth date
Ordering physician
Tests required
Date specimen to be taken
Relevant clinical information

HISTOLOGY

Histology—Routine surgical pathology reporting.
Following is a list of some specimens that are analyzed in the histological division of a laboratory and laboratory turnaround times for your reference.

Test	Turnaround Time
Intra-operative consultations	15-20 min variable
Prebooked elective	
Non-prebooked (elective or otherwise)	
Surgical pathology (without special stains, consultations, etc.)	24-36 hr
Fresh tissue for possible malignant lymphoma	24 hr
	48 hr (depending on time received by lab)
Estrogen receptors	2 wk
Renal biopsies	May be sent to another facility
Muscle biopsies	May be sent to another facility
Unstained slides	1-3 wk
Mammographically directed biopsies	24-48 hr
	48-72 hr (depending on time received by lab)

The following information must be included when completing a histology requisition:

Patient's full name
Patient's birth date
Sex
Type of specimen
Anatomic location
Pertinent history, including where and when previous diagnosis was made
Date of surgery
Preoperative diagnosis
Post-operative diagnosis
Submitting physician or surgeon

See Figure B.4 for an example of a Surgical Pathology Requisition.

MICROBIOLOGY

Microbiology — Testing and identification of bacteria, fungi, parasites, and viruses in patients' specimens.

Following is a list of some of the laboratory tests and turnaround times for your reference.

a. Microbiology (Routine)

Test	Turnaround Time
Abscess for C&S (culture & sensitivity)	48 hr
Acid fast bacilli	24 hr
Auger suction–C&S	48 hr
Bile–C&S	48 hr
Blood culture–C&S	72 hr
Blood culture–mycobacteria	8 hr
Bronchial washing–C&S	48 hr
Bronchial washing–fungus	4 wk
Bronchial washing–T.B.	8 wk
Catheter tip–C&S	48 hr
Chlamydia	3-6 d
Corneal scrapings	48 hr
CSF–C&S	72 hr
CSF–routine gram stain	24 hr
Fluid (body)–C&S	48 hr
Genital swab–C&S	48 hr
Genital swab–GC culture	72 hr
Genital swab–gonorrhea	72 hr
Gram stain–routine	24 hr
Lung washing–fungus	4 wk

FIGURE **B.4** **Surgical Pathology Requisition**

Patient's Surname

Given Name

Address

(if not on addressograph)

___ ___ ___ ___ ___ ___ ___ ___ ___ ___ ___   ____ / _____ / _____

Provincial Health No.   Date of Birth (dd/mm/yy)

Gender: ☐ Female   ☐ Male

Clinical Information and Diagnosis (print):
(e.g. relevant clinical, laboratory, or radiographic findings, surgery, hormonal or other therapy, etc - past and present)

☐ **INTRA OPERATIVE CONSULTATION REQUESTED**
     Purpose (print):

FORM 5089 / rev Nov 2001

Surgical Pathology Requisition

Lab No. _____

(705) 876-5014

Submitting Physician: Dr. _____

Copies to: Dr. _____

           Dr. _____

           Dr. _____

Date Specimen Taken: _____ / _____ / _____
                            (dd/mm/yy)

Specimen Sites (print):

1. _____
2. _____
3. _____
4. _____
5. _____
6. _____
7. _____
8. _____
9. _____
10. _____

Lab Use Only						
	A	B	C	D	E	F

SOURCE: Reproduced by permission of Peterborough Regional Health Centre.

Lung washing–G&S	48 hr
Lung washing–T.B.	8 wk
Mouth & gums	48 hr
Mycology (skin scraping/hair)	4 wk
Mycoplasma	10-14 d
Nails–fungus culture	4 wk
Nose–C&S	48 hr
Parasitology	7 d
Pinworm	1 d
Rectal culture	72 hr
Rectal culture–gonorrhea	72 hr
Skin–C&S	48 hr
Skin scrapings (fungus culture)	4 wk
Stool–C&S	72 hr
Stool–O&P	7 d
Stool–RSV	24 hr
Stool–*Clostridium difficile*	48 hr
Throat	48 hr

Throat washing– (virus)	7-10 d
Tissue	72 hr
Tuberculosis–respiratory	8 wk
Tuberculosis–urine	8 wk
Urine–culture & colony count	48 hr

b. Microbiology (Medical Emergency Requests)

Test	Turnaround Time
Blood Gram stain	<30 min
CSF and body fluid–Gram stain	<30 min
Lower respiratory Gram stain	<30 min
Wound Gram stain	<30 min

The following information must be included when completing a microbiology requisition:

Patient's name
Patient's birth date
Patient's medical record number (if an in-patient)
Attending physician
Ordering physician
Tests required
Date and time of collection
Diagnosis or relevant clinical information
Antibiotics currently being given or preferred by physician

See Figure B.5 for an example of a Microbiology Test Requisition.

BLOOD BANK

Blood Bank—Performs pre-transfusion compatibility testing before blood is issued. Serological testing is also performed to predict obstetrical sensitization and to aid in the diagnosis of certain immune disorders.

Following is a list of some laboratory tests and turnaround times for your reference.

Test	Routine	Urgent	Emergent
Blood Grouping–ABO	24 hr	10 min	10 min
–Rh	24 hr	10 min	10 min
–other phenotypes	24 hr	30 min	30 min
Antibody investigation–screen	24 hr	60 min	60 min
–identification	24 hr	60 min	60 min
Complex antibody identification	4 d	na	na
Blood group & antibody screen	24 hr	60 min	60 min
T&S (type & screen) (pre-op, prenatal, & poss. transfusion)			

FIGURE **B.5** **Microbiology Test Requisition**

Peterborough Regional Health Centre
Department Of Laboratory Medicine
Microbiology Test Requisition

Routine []   Urgent []

Ordering Physician _____

Collected By _____

Collection Date/Time _____

Clinical Information (Symptoms/Diagnosis): _____

Antibiotic(s) prescribed / Antibiotic Allergies: _____

*Specify Specimen Site/Type (tissue, aspirate, swab, other): _____

Test Request Menu:

Abscess Culture *	Dialysis Fluid Culture *	RSV Screen
Anaerobic Culture *	Drainage Culture *	Sputum Culture
Blood Culture	Ear Culture *	Stool Culture
Body Fluid Culture *	Eye Culture *	TB (Mycobacterium) Culture *
Bone Bank Culture	Fungus Culture *	Throat Culture
Bordetella pertussis (Culture/PCR)	Gonococcus Culture *	Tissue Culture *
Bronchial Brush Culture	Gram Smear *	Toxic Shock Screen
Bronchial Lavage Culture	Group B Streptococcus Culture	Urethra - Gonococcus Culture
Bronchial Washing Culture	Helicobacter pylori Urease Screen	Urine Culture
Cervix - Chlamydia trachomatis N.A.A	IV Catheter Tip Culture *	Vaginitis/Vaginosis Screen
Cervix - Gonococcus Culture	Legionella* (Culture/DFA)	Virus Culture *
Chlamydia pneumoniae PCR	Legionella (Urine Antigen)	VRE Screen
Chlamydia trachomatis Culture *	MRSA Screen*	Wound Culture* (aspirate or deep swab)
Clostridium difficile Toxin	Mycoplasma Culture *	Wound Culture* (superficial swab)
Corneal Scraping Culture	Oral Screen for Yeast (gram only)	Other (specify)
Cryptococcus Latex Screen	Parasitology Screen	
CSF Culture	Pinworm Screen	

Form # JF5048

Note: 1. All specimens must be labelled with patient name, patient number, collection date and specimen source.
2. Anaerobic Culture (which includes gram smear, aerobic and anaerobic culture) is only done on aspirate
(pus, body fluid) specimens, tissue, or deep wound swabs submitted in an anaerobic transport tube.

March. 2003   Over

Investigation of autoimmune hemolytic anemia	24 hr	2 hr	20 min
Direct antiglobulin test	24 hr	2 hr	20 min
Neonatal testing (D.A.T., ABO, & Rh)	24 hr	2 hr	60 min
Compatibility testing (ind. T&S)	24 hr	90 min	60 min
Investigation of transfusion reaction (non-hemolytic)	24 hr	na	na
Immediate spin crossmatch after type & screen	na	10 min	5 min
Issue uncrossmatched group O blood (trauma)	na	na	5 min
Group patient and issue uncrossmatched group compatible blood	na	na	10 min
Investigation of suspected hemolytic transfusion reaction	na	2 hr	20 min

The following information must be included when completing a blood bank requisition:

Patient's surname and given name (no abbreviation)
Medical record number for in-patients and birth date for out-patients
Location
Sex
Ordering physician
Priority of red cell transfusion
Clinical information or surgical procedure "type and screen"—check this
     area except when there is an order to transfuse the products, when the
     MSBOS (maximum surgical blood order schedule) calls for a
     crossmatch, or when it is an emergency situation.

See Figure B.6 for an example of Transfusion Medicine Services Requisition.

Computerized Reports

Many laboratory facilities now process their reports by computer. The requisitions have bar codes which can be scanned when ordering and processing. Figure B.1 is an example of a combined blood testing and biochemistry requisition. Figure B.7 is an example of a urinalysis and other body fluids requisition. The patient's name, date of birth, and ordering physician must appear in the top left corner of each report. The information would be handwritten or stamped with the addressograph card referred to in Chapter 11.

FIGURE **B.6** Transfusion Medicine Services Requisition

PETERBOROUGH REGIONAL HEALTH CENTRE
TRANSFUSION MEDICINE SERVICES
TEST / PRODUCT REQUEST

☐ PRH ☐ NHC ☐ CMH ☐ Minden ☐ Haliburton _____   ☐ Outpatient
☐ In-patient ☐ Out-patient ☐ Referred-in   ☐ **Urgent***(see below)
                                                                                                     ☐ Routine
Collection Date: dd/mm/yy _____   Time: _____   ☐ Pre-Op
O.R. Date: dd/mm/yy _____   Time: _____

Relevant Clinical Information Special Instructions/Surgery
_____
_____

Ordering Physician: _____
Nurse: _____

Armband checked, blood collected and tubes labelled by: _____

☐ TYPE AND SCREEN (RESERVE SERUM) blood   ☐ DIRECT ANTIGLOBULIN TEST   * **IN URGENT/EMERGENT**
  can be available within 10 minutes following a   (D.A.T.) ADULT
  negative antibody screen   **SITUATIONS CALL**

☐ CHECK FOR Rh IMMUNE GLOBULIN   ☐ COLD AGGLUTININS   **BLOOD BANK STATING**
  (Rh negative or Rh unkown)   (keep specimen at 37° C)
                                                                                                     DEGREE OF URGENCY
☐ CORD BLOOD

☐ FETAL MATERNAL HEMORRHAGE SCREEN   ☐ OTHER _____
                                                                            (specify)

PRODUCT REQUIRED	AMOUNT	DATE/TIME NEEDED	REASON FOR TRANSFUSION

☐ **RED BLOOD CELLS**
Special preparation e.g.:
☐ CMV neg   ☐ Irradiated
☐ Other_____
(specify)
 	
NB   dd/mm/yy   No Unkwn
Previous transfusions   ☐ _____ ☐ ☐
Previous pregnancies   ☐ _____ ☐ ☐
Previous transfusion reaction ☐ _____ ☐ ☐
	_____ units	_____ dd/mm/yy
		
		_____ hrs
			☐ Low haemoglobin with symptoms
			   (specify)_____
			☐ Radiation, chemotherapy
			☐ Trauma
			☐ Surgical
			☐ other
			   (specify)_____

☐ **PLATELET CONCENTRATE** ☐ CMV neg ☐ Irradiated	_____ units	_____ dd/mm/yy _____ hrs	☐ prophylactic-platelets < 15,000 ☐ platelets < 50,000 bleed or invasive procedure ☐ platelets < 70,000 trauma or major surgery ☐ other (specify)_____
☐ **FROZEN PLASMA**	_____ mls.	_____ dd/mm/yy _____ hrs	☐ coagluopathy ☐ factor deficiency ☐ massive transfusion ☐ other (specify)_____
☐ **ALBUMIN** ☐ 25% - 100 mL ☐ 5% - 50 mL	_____ units	_____ dd/mm/yy _____ hrs	☐ hypovolemia ☐ other (specify)_____

☐ RhIG   ☐ I.V. IMMUNE GLOBULIN _____ gm
Diagnosis (if other than gamma globulin deficiency)_____

☐ Other (see lab/nursing manual for availability and information required) specify_____

Consent for transfusion obtained   ☐ YES   ☐ UNKNOWN

FOR BLOOD BANK USE ONLY
Previous results Group_____ Screen_____ Antibodies_____ Comments_____   Hgb____ Plt. Ct (if applicable)_____

Current results Group_____ Screen_____ Antibodies_____ Comments_____   Stamp used on chart report

Time stamp ☐ Phoned re T&S only   by_____ to_____

Form 5088 – Sept. 2001

SOURCE: Reproduced by permission of Peterborough Regional Health Centre.

FIGURE **B.7** Urinalysis/Other Body Fluids Requisition

Peterborough Regional Health Centre **LABORATORY MEDICINE**

URINALYSIS/OTHER BODY FLUIDS

☐ PCH ☐ SJHC ☐ Haliburton ☐ Minden ☐ Other_____

☐ In-patient   ☐ Out-patient   ☐ Referred-In

Date Ordered:m\d\yr_____

Ordering Physician:._____

Nurse:_____

Specimen collected by:_____

Collection Date:m\d\yr_____Time:_____

☐ Random Urine   ☐ 24 Hour Urine

☐ **Emergent**   ☐ **Urgent**   ☐ **Routine**   ☐ **Timed**

O.R. Date: m\d\yr_____O.R.Time:_____

Clinical Information:_____

Special Instructions:_____

NOTE: USE MICROBIOLOGY TEST REQUISITION FOR ALL CULTURE REQUESTS

TESTS ON URINE	
ROUTINE URINALYSIS 3655	
MICROSCOPIC URINALYSIS 3660	
PROTEIN 3241	
SODIUM 3045	
POTASSIUM 3055	
AMYLASE 3092	
URATE 3215	
CALCIUM 3105	
OSMOLALITY 3142	
PREGNANCY TEST 3640	
CREATININE 3035	
CREATININE 3038 CLEARANCE (NOTE:SERUM CREATININE ALSO REQUIRED)	
PATIENT - HT.	
WT.	
OTHER	

TESTS ON URINE	
CHLORIDE 3065	
PO4 3205	
URINE 3595 ELEXTROPHORESIS	

OTHER TESTS	
SWEAT CHLORIDES 3670	

STOOL	
OCCULT BLOOD 3635	
OTHER	
OTHER	

STONES	
STONE ANALYSIS 9525	
OTHER	

BODY FLUID TESTING

☐ CSF   ☐ JOINT   ☐ PLEURAL

☐ OTHER _____

GLUCOSE 3013	
CSF PROTEIN 3243	
PROTEIN OTHER FLUIDS 3242	
CSF CELLS 2070	
CELLS OTHER FLUIDS 2090	
CRYSTALS (JOINT FLUID) 2105	
PHOSPHATE	
ELECTROPHORESIS CSF 3590	
LD 3172	
URATE 3212	
AMYLASE 3092	
ALK PHOS. 3182	
SPECIFIC GRAVITY (OTHER FLUIDS) 3662	
OTHER	

"FOR LAB USE ONLY: Specimen Volume:_____ mL   Surface Area:_____

☐ **PETERBOROUGH CIVIC HOSPITAL**
One Hospital Drive, Peterborough, Ont., K9J 7C6

☐ **ST. JOSEPH'S HEALTH CENTRE**
384 Rogers St., Peterborough, Ont., K9H 7B

Form # JF 5047

June/96

Pharmacology

Following is a list of the most commonly prescribed drugs by their generic names and brand names (where available) for your reference.

Antibacterials—Agents that have properties to destroy or suppress growth or reproduction of bacteria.

Generic Name	Trade Name
Amoxicillin/potassium clavulanate	Clavulin
Azithromycin	Zithromax
Bacampicillin	Penglobe
Cefaclor	Ceclor
Cefixime	Suprax
Cefuroxime axetil	Ceftin
Cephalexin	Keflex
Ciprofloxacin hydrochloride	Cipro
Clarithromycin	Biaxin
Doxycycline	Vibramycin
Erythromycin	Eryc, E-Mycin
Erythromycin estolate	Ilosone
Erythromycin ethylsuccinate	EES
Erythromycin ethylsuccinate	Pediazole/sulfisoxazole Acetyl
Metronidazole	Flagyl
Norfloxacin	Noroxin
Pivampicillin	Pondocillin
Phenoxymethyl penicillin	PenVee
Trimethoprim-sulfamethoxazole	Septra, Bactrim

Anticholinergics—Agents that block the passage of impulses through the parasympathetic nervous system.

Generic Name	Trade Name
Ipratropium chloride	Arovent (asthma)
Oxybutynin chloride (controls the bladder)	
Meclizine	Bonamine (motion sickness)

Anticoagulants—Agents that act to prevent clotting of blood.

Generic Name	Trade Name
Warfarin sodium	Coumadin
A.S.A.	Entrophen, Aspirin

Antihypertensives—Agents that control blood pressure.

Generic Name	Trade Name
Acebutolol	Sectral, Monitan
Amiloride	Midamor
Amlodipine besylate	Norvasc

Atenolol	Tenormin
Captopril	Capoten
Diltiazem	Cardizem, Tiazac
Enalapril maleate	Vasotec
Fosinopril sodium	Monopril
Furosemide	Lasix
Metoprolol tartrate	Lopressor, Betaloc
Nifedipine	Adalat
Sotalol	Sotacor
Spironolactone	Aldactone
Triamterene	Dyrenium
Verapamil	Isoptin

CARDIAC THERAPY

Generic Name	Trade Name
Digoxin	Lanoxin
Disopyramide	Rythmodan
Hydrochlorothiazide	HydroDIURIL
Isosorbide dinitrate	Isordil

LIPID-LOWERING AGENTS

(Lipid: heterogenous group of fats and fatlike substances)

Generic Name	Trade Name
Atorvastatin	Lipitor
Cholestyramine resin	Questran
Fluvastatin	Lescol
Lovastatin	Mevacor
Pravastatin	Pravachol
Rosuvastatin	Crestor
Simvastatin	Zocor

PERIPHERAL VASCULAR DISEASE THERAPY

Generic Name	Trade Name
Pentoxifylline	Trental

Analgesics—Agents that relieve pain.

Generic Name	Trade Name
Diclofenac sodium	Voltaren
Flunarizine	Sibelium
Hydrocodone bitartrate	Hycodan

Hydromorphone	Dilaudid
Ibuprofen	Motrin, Advil
Ketorolac tromethamine	Toradol
Ketoprofen	Orudis
Morphine	Doloral Morphitec, Statex, M.S. Contin
Naproxen	Naprosyn
Naproxen sodium	Anaprox
Oxycodone	Percodan/Percocet
Sumatriptan succinate	Imitrex

Anticonvulsants—Agents that control seizures.

Generic Name	Trade Name
Carbamazepine	Tegretol
Clobazam	Frisium
Clonazepam	Rivotril
Divalproex sodium	Epival
Gabapentin	Neurotin
Lorazepam	Ativan
Nitrazepam	Mogadon
Phenytoin	Dilantin
Valproic acid	Depakene
Vigabatrim	Sabril

Antidepressants—Agents that prevent or relieve depression.

Generic Name	Trade Name
Amoxapine	Ascendin
Fluvoxamine maleate	Luvox
Fluoxetine	Prozac
Doxepin	Sinequan
Moclobemide	Manerix
Paroxetine	Paxil
Sertraline	Zoloft
Trazodone	Desyrel
Trimipramine	Surmontil
Amitriptyline	Elavil
Citalopram	Celexa
Bupropian	Wellbutrin SR
Venlafaxine	Effexor

ANTIPARKINSONIAN AGENTS

Generic Name	Trade Name
Benztropine	Cogentin

Antipsychotics—Agents effective in the management of mood control.

Generic Name	Trade Name
Chlorpromazine	Largactil
Haloperidol	Haldol
Perphenazine	Trilaton
Prochlorperazine	Stemetil
Risperidone	Risperdal

Antipyretics—Agents that relieve fever.

Generic Name	Trade Name
Acetominophen	Tylenol
Ibuprophen	Advil/Motrin

Anxiolytics—Agents that relieve feelings of apprehension, uncertainty, and fear appearing without apparent stimulus.

Generic Name	Trade Name
Alprazolam	Xanax
Chlordiazepoxide	Librium
Diazepam	Valium
Lorazepam	Ativan
Oxazepam	Serax

HYPNOTICS AND SEDATIVES

Generic Name	Trade Name
Chloral hydrate	Novo-Chlorhydrate
Nitrazepam	Mogadon
Temazepam	Restoril
Triazolam	Halcion

Mania Therapy—Agents that control mood swings.

Generic Name	Trade Name
Lithium carbonate	Carbolith, Duralith

ASTHMA THERAPY

Generic Name	Trade Name
Beclomethasone dipropionate	QVAR
Budesonide	Pulmicort
Hydrocortisone sodium succinate	SoluCortef
Ipratropium bromide	Atrovent
Ketotifen fumarate	Zaditen

Methylprednisolone sodium succinate	Solu-Medrol
Oxtriphylline	Choledyl
Prednisone	Deltasone
Salbutamol sulfate	Ventolin, Airomir
Terbutaline sulfate	Bricanyl
Theophylline	TheoDur
Fluticasone propionate	Flovent
Tiotropium bromide	Spiriva
Salmeterol xinafoate	Serevent
Salmeterol xinafoate + Fluticasone Propionate	Advair
Ipratropium bromide + Salbutamol sulfate	Combivent

COUGH AND COLD PREPARATIONS

Antitussives—Cough suppressants

Generic Name	Trade Name
Dextromethorphan hydrobromide	DM
Guaifenesin	Robitussin
Naphazoline hydrochloride	Vasacon-A
Pseudoephedrine hydrochloride	Sudafed
Xylometazoline hydrochloride	Otrivin

APPENDIX D

Reference Sources

As a medical administrative assistant, you will need to be familiar with a wide range of reference material. You have already used some medical reference materials such as medical dictionaries, *The Medical Word Book*, and the *Compendium of Pharmaceuticals and Specialties* (CPS). There are, however, literally hundreds of more books of various types that you may use from time to time.

DICTIONARIES

You are, of course, now familiar with the standard medical dictionary. There are many such dictionaries available, from small pocket-size to large multi-volume editions. There are also many dictionaries available by specialty area. Some other types you should be familiar with are inverted dictionaries (in which the definition is given in alphabetical order, followed by the appropriate medical term) and dictionaries of abbreviations and acronyms, syndromes, diseases, hospital terminology, and so on.

DIRECTORIES

A directory is basically a list, and there are many lists available. The *Canadian Medical Directory*, published annually, lists most doctors practising in Canada. There are also international, national, and local directories of health organizations and institutions, hospitals, social agencies, and healthcare professionals. A directory can be anything from a large bound publication on a worldwide scale to a small pamphlet put out by your local association of pharmacists.

DRUG PUBLICATIONS

There are several varieties of publications dealing with drugs, but the one most widely used in Canada is the *Compendium of Pharmaceuticals and Specialties* (CPS). This book lists drugs by generic name (penicillin), trade name or monograph (Valium), manufacturer, type (antihistamines, oral), and so on. You will find a CPS in every practising physician's office and in all nursing units, Health Records departments, etc. The CPS is updated and published annually and is also available on-line. Individual drugs can also be looked up on specific available Web sites.

The CPS is divided into sections of different-colour pages as outlined in Box AD.1.

AD.1	CPS Divisions by Colour
Pink	Classification System Index
Green	Drug listing of brand and nonproprietary names
Glossy	White A picture guide to assist in the identification of products
Yellow	Manufacturers' Index
Mauve	Clinical information including the following: Poison control centres Selected resource agencies and literature Non-medicinal Ingredients Clinical monitoring
Blue	Patient information
White	An alphabetical list of each drug by name, including the chemical make-up of the drug; its use, indications, and contraindications; any precautions necessary when administering the drug; adverse effects; overdose symptoms and treatment; and appropriate dosages

MINISTRY OF HEALTH FEE SCHEDULES/DIAGNOSTIC CODES

Published by the provincial Ministry of Health, the *Fee Schedules and Diagnostic Code Listings* booklet can be obtained at the Ontario Government Book Store if needed. As mentioned in Chapter 6, diskettes or electronic transmission are sent to each practising physician's office to update his or her billing software.

HANDBOOKS FOR THE ADMINISTRATIVE ASSISTANT

Every medical administrative assistant should have at least one handbook close by for quick reference. There are several available in your school library, and you should take time to browse through them to familiarize yourself with the type of information that is at your disposal. If your office does not have at least one medical handbook available for your use, you should get one and use it frequently.

Whether you work in a one-doctor office or in a large hospital or clinic, you will be required from time to time to research certain information for your employer. The more familiar you are with the types of reference sources available to you, the more efficiently you will be able to find the information you need. Your school library has a large selection of medical reference material, and your reference librarian will be pleased to show you where this material can be found. Most medical journals and handbooks are available on-line. This will allow you to take specific information you require and develop and a handbook for your personal use.

A LIST OF SOME IMPORTANT REFERENCE SOURCES

Dorland's Medical Dictionary
Publisher: Elsevier Canada (http://www.elsevier.ca)
   1 Goldthorne Ave.
   Toronto, Ontario M8Z 5S7

Taber's Cyclopedic Medical Dictionary
Publisher: F.A. Davis and Company
Distributed by Login Brothers Canada (http://lb.ca)

Canadian Medical Directory
Publisher: Business Information Group
   12 Concorde Place, Suite 800
   Toronto, ON M3C 4J2
Online version available at: http://www.mdselect.com/

Sloane's Medical Word Book
Author: Ellen Drake
Publisher: Elsevier Canada
   1 Goldthorne Ave.
   Toronto, Ontario M8Z 5S7

The Surgical Word Book
Author: Claudia Tessier
Publisher: Elsevier Canada
   1 Goldthorne Ave.
   Toronto, Ontario M8Z 5S7

Health Information Management
Authors: Jennifer Cofer (editor) and Edna K. Huffman
Publisher: Physician's Record Company
     (http://www.physiciansrecord.com)
   3000 S. Ridgeland Ave.
   Berwyn, Illinois 60402

Medical Transcription Guide: Dos and Don'ts
Author: Marcy Diehl
Publisher: Elsevier Canada
   1 Goldthorne Ave.
   Toronto, Ontario M8Z 5S7

Dictionary of Medical Acronyms & Abbreviations
Publisher: Lippincott, Williams and Wilkins
Distributed by Login Brothers Canada (http://lb.ca)

Compendium of Pharmaceuticals and Specialties (CPS)
Publisher: Canadian Pharmacists Association (http://www.pharmacists.ca)
  1785 Alta Vista Drive
  Ottawa, Ontario K1G 3Y6

Index*

*b indicates boxes; f indicates figures; t indicates tables